Table of Contents

Book Dedications 1
Introduction - A Survivor's Tale 3
Childhood 4
Growing Up With the Lloyd family 12
First Stroke 23
Embrace Graffiti 30
Driving Life Into the Ground 33
Turning Martian 49
Change of Direction 58
Mission and the East Coast 67
The Big Beautiful O 89
Lake Superior 122
The NOT FLAT Prairies 155
Excited for the Mountains 178
Second Long for Life Fundraiser 184
The Hospital Stay 187
Post-stroke Shenanigans 212
Pain 215
Family and Friends 219
The Little Things 221
Post-stroke Effects 224
Things I Was Ungrateful For 231
The Power of the Mind 234
Learning to Walk, Bike, and Longboard 237
The Finish 244
Hard Work 287
Patience 289
Hidden Message 291

Book Dedications

This book is dedicated to the woman that gave her life to raise my two brothers (sisters, Ha!) and myself. To my incredible, strong, amazing, patient, and resilient mother, Karen Harrison. If it were not for you, I wouldn't have made it nearly as far as I have in this world. Thank you for everything you have done for all of us. There is no possible way I could ever repay you for what you have managed to accomplish. You were given the impossible task of raising three boys, by yourself. How you did it, I have no idea. But you have showed me what it really means to be a loving, caring, supportive, hardworking, and providing parent. I am incredibly blessed and honoured to have such a wonderful, dedicated, and strong mother as yourself. Your determination to make it through and push yourself through each day regardless of the physical or mental pain you are in, encourages me to do the same. You are my hero. I will always love you mostest!

This book is also dedicated to my crazy, strong, dexterous dad, Michael Floyd. Dad, you dropping everything and taking me on one incredible life-changing, mind-boggling, eye-opening trip, not only opened my eyes and mind in so many ways, but also unplugged me from the matrix of negativity I had buried myself in. Thank you for all your hard work, effort, time, blood, sweat, money, blood, and more sweat you put into helping me achieve my life's first ambition. It will never be forgotten, always thought about, honoured, and cherished. I love you man!

A tremendous dedication goes to the incredible woman that cut me open and meticulously operated on me for twelve and a half hours giving me another chance to live. Dr. Robin C. Eccles, if it wasn't for you, I'd just be a heartbreaking distant memory and another statistic in casualties caused by cancer. Instead, your years and years of schooling, hard work, resilience, patience, and more years of schooling have given me the blessing of not only having another chance at life, but to also be able to show others how to overcome the same crazy obstacles that have been thrown my way. Keep on being you, because you are amazing. Your dedication to help save kids' lives is honestly heroic; you too are my hero. I will always love and respect you more than you'll ever know.

Another tremendous dedication goes to my neurosurgeon, Dr. John Wong. Thank you for your countless hours reviewing my MRI, CT, CT Angio, and Gama-Knife radiation procedures. All the while making sure my operations are a smooth and easy process, as well as ending my risk of stroke. Thank you for your continued dedication to helping myself as well as other victims. You sir, are also a hero of mine.

To my (what seems like) two million PTs (physio therapists, OTs (occupational therapists), RTs (recreational therapists), STs (speech therapists), Nurses, doctors and all hospital staff that have helped me or just work in the industry, thank you for keeping the wheels of the machine oiled and making my recoveries go as productively as possible. I know you're over worked, underpaid, and very under-thanked, so on behalf of every patient you have seen or will see, THANK YOU SO MUCH. You guys are amazing!

This book is also dedicated to all the families that have taken me in over the years and treated me as their own. To the Wilkinson, Green, Lloyd, Bannack, Gaetz, Draper, Dennhardt and Tkachuk families. Thank you all for taking me in and having such a profound, positive impact on my life, while putting up with all my shenanigans and feeding me such good food; you guys are truly a blessing and a huge contribution to my life's story, success, and shaping the young man I am today. I love you all!

To all of my amazing aunties and uncles (blood or not) you guys are amazing. Thank you for being around and taking care of us, while providing a fun and loving environment to grow up in, as well for your continuous support in everything I do to this day. To all my friends who have stuck by my side through all the craziness that is my life, I love you guys. I wouldn't be the person I am today if it wasn't for you guys in my life sticking through my, crabby, fussy, annoying, and painful days. I honestly don't know how you guys put up with me some days. Just goes to show how patient and strong you all are. I appreciate and love you all till the end.

To all of my Martian family members out there, my heart and deepest condolences are with you, your families, and loved ones. Thank you guys for being here to talk me down when I get all riled up about these situations we are put into and forced to deal with. I love, respect, and appreciate you guys more than you'll ever know.

To the Phillips family, I thank you for giving me the opportunity and motivation to write this for the world. I feel very confident that this would not have happened if it wasn't for your unconditional love and belief to do so. I feel incredibly blessed an honoured to have met such a wonderful and strong family.

Introduction - A Survivor's Tale

My life started the same way the majority of yours did, with my mother and father having sexual intercourse (pretty picture isn't it) and my journey will inevitably end the same as yours, with death.

Over the past twenty-nine-years, I've had my fair share of near-death experiences and I am finally at a point where I am quite content with the fact that Death will come knocking at my door one day. But how many of you, like myself, are ready to answer the door with a smile and let him in. Not very many, I'd imagine. For years, like most individuals the thought of death or dying terrified me. It wouldn't be until shortly after my third near-death experience that the thought of death would turn from a tremendous fear, to one of the best life tools and one of the biggest, most incredible motivators in my life.

Think about this for a minute. Does the thought of you possibly dying now, today, or tomorrow make you want to take immediate action with your life now? Or does the paycheck at the end of the week motivate you to live your life to the fullest? If you died today, right now, would you be happy with the way your life went? Would you be content with the legacy you left behind? Would you be satisfied with what your memories here on the earth would be? These were the questions I started to ask myself when I was seventeen. At fifteen, I had to have the talk with my mom about whether to pull the plug if I ever ended up a vegetable on life support from another brain aneurism. It's absolutely terrifying to look back and think about how close I came to having that plug pulled. But for some reason I have the blessing of being here today to share my life and stories as a survivor.

However, before we start on this colossally fucked up expedition that is my life, I need to make something abundantly clear. My reckless past and my "I don't give a fuck" attitude, nor my past mischievous criminal behaviours DO NOT have any association with the companies, corporations, or individuals mentioned in this book. This book is solely the thoughts, feelings, expressions, and stories from one survivor to the world.

Childhood

Before I was even born, I was what you could consider "a problem child." I was causing all kinds of problems for my mom, as well as having some of my own. I started to grow sideways in my mother's womb. Day by day as I grew in my transverse position, I pushed harder and harder on my mother's spine and pelvis, eventually pushing them out of place causing an incredible amount of pain and discomfort for her. As I pushed on her vena cava, I would drop her blood pressure, and make her sweat and vomit. Meanwhile, unknown to everyone, my immature nerve cells known as Neuroblasts turned on me and instead of developing the nerves on my spine, they propagated bigger and bigger tumours as I developed.

My day of reckoning had come, and it was finally time to be taken out of my mother's womb. The day was Friday, September 10, 1993, in Calgary, Alberta. I was obviously upset at the doctor for disturbing my peace in my mom's womb because as soon as I was taken out—with my jet-black hair standing straight up—I started to urinate on the doctor as he held me. This was just the tip of the iceberg of problems, frustration, and anger I'd cause people in my life. My birth went as planned (aside from the doctor's shower) and a short time later I was able to go home.

About two and a half years later, my mom began an ordinary day by getting us both dressed and off to school. On her way to school, she dropped *me* off at daycare. Typically, I would go to daycare while mom was at school then she would pick me up and she, my older brother, and myself would go over to grandmas so mom could write her papers. One such day while at grandmas, I climbed under the desk and unplugged the computer. Of course, this was way before the days of autosave and Mom lost six or seven hours of work. Usually though, when I wasn't sabotaging Mom's efforts, Grandpa was helping my mom finish her schooling and grandma would review her work and help her with any edits that needed to be made. This went on for four years, with no summers off, until mom finished her schooling.

But that fateful day two and a half years after I christened the doctor at my birth, and an hour or two after my mom dropped me off at daycare, my grandma received a call from the daycare centre telling her to come pick me up as I wasn't doing well. My grandmother rushed over and picked me up before we went to her house and waited for my mom. When my mom got there, she saw me sitting on my grandma's lap in respiratory duress. She noticed I was having breathing problems. On top of that, I was being unusually quiet for me, I was oddly leaning forward, and she noted I had a tracheal tug. She then proceeded to investigate putting her nursing skills to practise. When she took off my shirt, she saw I also had 'in-drawing' on my sides when I inhaled. She packed a small bag and we headed to the Children's hospital on Richmond Road to get me looked at. There, I was treated with steroids and nebulizer for twenty-four hours because it was thought it was asthma. After that, a resident took a quick look at me and said, "He is fine," my mom started to argue the fact I still had in-drawing, a tracheal tug, and shortness of breath. After some arguing about how the resident needs to go back to school if he can't see I'm having troubles (and I'm sure a few motherly instinctive threats) she finally got his superior to give me a chest x-ray. He was reluctant because I was only two and a half years old, but he took me for an x-ray then sent us home.

We got home and went to bed but my mom got a call from the radiology department saying there was an abnormal shadow on my x-ray, and we needed to come back for more testing. By now, my mom had been up for nearly a day and a half so she asked if we could get a few hours of sleep and the doctor said it was okay. We had a quick nap before we headed back to the hospital where the triage nurse gave my mom sass about not coming back immediately and she got a mouthful from my mom like the resident. There, I was put in a CT scanner, had my blood taken, and had a few more tests done. Once I woke up, I was then put in a respiratory room that had other sick kids and their families. In the room, there were a few beds and about ten chairs in a big circle. At my side, my mom watched my in-drawing continue and couldn't help but anxiously worry.

Hours later, a doctor would come in and (in front of all the other families there) tell my mom that I had cancer, then left. My mom stood frozen in shock as the other families there came over and provided my mom with their undivided support. She then began to call friends and family to break the tragic news. After being scanned by a CT machine and having a variety of tests done over a few days, it was concluded that I needed even more advanced testing done so my mother and I were put in a taxi with a nurse and headed over to the Foothills Hospital for an MRI scan. It wouldn't be until after my scan, when the doctors realized the scope of the damage, and it was unbelievable.

The tumour was not so much doing damage as it was precarious in the way it was growing. The tumour itself was encapsulated with a malignant centre. It was the size of a soft ball and it was located between my heart and lungs. It had collateral vessels coming out of it. The biggest vessel was wrapped around my aortic arch and was squeezing it. The tumour had ganglioglioma that wrapped around my rib cage and onto my spine. All of this was making my heart and lungs work harder and put a lot of pressure on my organs. They scanned my spine from the base of my skull down to my tail bone and they found a Chiari's malformation, but that was something I could live with and didn't pose any threat. Little did we know if they just scanned a few inches higher, they would have found the biggest problem and threat to my life.

After my MRI, my mother and I were put in an ambulance and were taken back to the children's hospital where I had to have a bone scan and a bone marrow biopsy along with some other tests done. I had to have a full body bone scan to see if there were any other hotspots in my body for cancer. When the MRI results came back and the physicians realized how much more extensive my tumour was, they consulted a vascular surgeon in Edmonton and planned for him to fly in and assist Doctor Eccles in the operating room.

Due to the complexity of the operation, the odds of me surviving were roughly twenty-five percent, however without the operation, I was almost guaranteed to die. With my mom in the waiting room surrounded by other friends and family they all anxiously waited as I was operated on. They put me to sleep before they cut me open on my left side and debated if they needed to remove a rib to make more room for the operation, however it was not necessary. Once they got into my ribcage, they saw that my ribcage had cancer all over it as well. It was spread out "like a spider web" so they ended up removing the inner lining to my ribcage to get that cancer out. Hour after hour, my family waited. One hour turned into five, five hours into ten, and after twelve and a half gruelling day like hours they still waited, knowing at any time they could be coming back with the worst news any parent could ever hear. However, they removed the encapsulated tumour which was the easy part, then they had to use dental tools to get the cancer that cemented itself to my spine out of my body, they then put a tube in to drain fluids, they stapled me up with about twenty-three staples in my chest, and then stitched up the left side of my ribs with inline sutures. During the operation they took samples of the tissues surrounding the tumour and sent it to the lab for further testing.

From the operating room I was moved to the ICU (Intensive Care Unit) where I was supposed to be monitored for the next five to ten days. However, I was recovered and out of ICU within forty-eight hours. With my mom by my side, hour after hour she prayed for me to come through. From ICU I was going to be moved over to Q cluster (the cancer ward) in the children's hospital but after the slides came back from the lab negative, I was moved to N cluster (the surgical/cardiothoracic unit).

It was there the Calgary Flames would come visit some of the other sick kids and myself to give us hope. The enormous players came in and I looked at them and said "that's my mom" as I pointed to my mother. I didn't have anything else to say just "that's my mom." I remember the players looked like giants to me. They were huge, big, strong men and I hoped to be just like that one day.

The sick kid beside me had lost a lot of blood so they needed a blood transfusion to replace it. At one point, they brought in a bag of blood, put a spike in it, and then began to pump the blood into the kid. But after a short time, the spike came out of the bag of blood and blood started to spray all over my mom, the room full of equipment, people, and myself. It was quite the bloody chaotic mess for a bit.

It was unknown if I would need a secondary procedure like chemotherapy or radiation to make sure the cancer was all gone. Luckily for me, my body scan and lab results came back with good news, and I was a part of the select few that didn't need it. Chemotherapy and radiation can destroy even the healthiest of bodies and there was no way my mother was going to have me go through that unless it was absolutely one-hundred percent necessary; thankfully, it was not. However, I had to have a follow up every month for six months, then every six months for a few years, then only once a year for ten years.

It's hard for me to recall a lot of specific details about spending my early childhood in and out of the hospital. I'm not sure if it's because it was so traumatic, my brain blocked it out and suppressed it, or if it was because I was so young when I went through it all, I just can't remember. However, I do remember that I hated it. I hated it because it was a very confusing time in my life. I'd go to this strange place, where these strange people did all sorts of weird things to me. I remember always playing with wall toys and loving to watch the colourful fish swim in the fish tanks as we waited in the waiting areas of the children's hospital for endless hours. I would always find my favourite fish (usually the weirdest looking or most colourful one) and I'd watch it swim in circles for what seemed like hours on end. Sometimes I'd try to make sure no other fish would mess with mine. If any other fish dared to mess with my fish I'd bang or tap on the glass to try and get them to go away. Sometimes out of boredom, I'd tap the glass to watch them all scatter, then of course my mom would grill me about banging on the glass hurting all the fish.

I never understood why I couldn't eat or drink before I went to this strange place. I recall I'd feel like I'm starving or incredibly thirsty and, at most, I'd only be able to have a tiny sip from the water fountains leaving me frustrated that I was not allowed to eat. Once I was finally in for my appointment, they would take my mother and myself to a back room and I'd jump into a bed before they put a mask over my face and give me a number to count down from. "One-hundred, ninety-nine, ninety-eight…" next thing I know I would suddenly get incredibly sleepy and pass out even if I was wide awake and energized, and it always happened faster than I could understand what was happening. Sometimes I'd try and fight the sedation but I never could prevail; at most I was awake for an extra half second. But it was really freaky as a four- to ten-year-old child getting drugged to sleep on a constant basis. After that, I would wake up some time later in a complete state of confusion. I didn't know where I was, who these people were, or why I was even there to begin with. Luckily for me every time I woke up freaking out, worried, and confused, my mom would be there right by my side to assure me everything was okay and that I was fine. Then, she either took us out or home for a much-needed breakfast.

It would be some time following this routine before I learned that these strange nouns, and all these weird things they did to me were to make sure that I was okay and that the cancer I had didn't return. I couldn't eat eight hours prior to my appointment because of the procedures I had to have done. If there was a problem in my procedure and or I needed to be operated on, I had to have an empty belly. As time went on, going to the hospital for medical exams, checkups, x-rays, MRI scans, and needles got less and less freaky. The fear of the needle was still very much real but not nearly as bad as it once was. Although I never did get used to being drugged to sleep, it freaked me out every time. However, I was always intrigued how we as humans could turn off like a switch within a few seconds. Over time, this entire routine got less and less freaky and just became a standard part of life that everything else had to stop for.

It took me many years to understand what was happening to me, but many more years to finally understand the reason my mother wasn't at work and why I wasn't at school was because of the severity of my experience: A brush with death. Even my teachers never understood why I missed more class than the average student. I would tell them "I was at doctors' appointments" but not a single teacher could ask why, so teachers would know nothing until a one-on-one at parent teacher meetings when my mom had a chance to explain things in private. Which is partly why I think it was almost a secret I had cancer most of my life. I never talked about it, the teachers couldn't talk about it, and students don't just go around asking each other if they've had cancer. It was a subject on reality that was rarely brought up or talked about.

Once I was old enough, the doctors didn't have to drug me to sleep. I would walk with my mom to the MRI, CT, or x-ray department for imaging. However not being drugged to sleep came with its own problems. Mom and I would have to get up very early for my appointments and I'd show up ready for a nap. But they would put me in some sort of scanner like the MRI or CT scanner. I would be lying there, tired as ever, then the nurses and technicians would put a warm blanket on me before they put me in the scanner. With a warm blanket providing an extreme amount of comfort I'd quickly drift away to sleep. Then the machine would make a loud noise and wake me up. Waking up in a small, loud, white, confined space as a child was almost as freaky as being drugged to sleep. If I drifted to sleep in the machine and woke up flinching from the noise or freaking out by being in a tiny white tube, I'd ruin the images and they would have to do it all over again, keeping me in there for longer. It took me a long time to get comfortable enough to sleep through the whole process in the machines and even longer not to freak out whenever I woke up inside of them.

Once we got back home, I would either watch television, torment the crap out of my brothers, play with toys, or go play outside. I was mostly an outdoorsy kid my whole life. Always exploring and adventuring around the neighbourhood or biking and playing with friends. As a child, I was just fascinated by electronics and wanted to know how they worked so anything remotely electronic got savagely taken apart, dissected, examined, and then poorly put back together, if not just left in pieces. My mom would come home from work and I'd have her hair dryer taken apart; the motor would be glued to my Legos with a 9-volt battery to power it. "Look what I made mom!" I would say. She would roll her eyes and say something like, "oh my lord, not again," then I would get in big well-deserved trouble for obliterating all her belongings.

My mother had put herself back through school so she could provide for us three boys better. With mom always in school and our dads doing their thing, my papa and my uncle Tony spent a lot of their time watching my brothers and myself growing up. I always got super excited when Papa or Uncle Tony came by because Papa always brought my brothers, and I treats. I remember I would always get gum. My older brother always got smarties, I can't recall what my little brother got, but every time he came, he brought us something, so it was always exciting when Papa came by. Papa also rode a big red motorcycle that I was incredibly fascinated by. I wanted to take it apart and see how the bike worked but I knew that would be a grounding I'd never get ungrounded from. However, my brother and I always got to sit on it all the time when he came over.

When Tony came to watch us, it was always so much fun. He would help us build forts out of blankets, pillows, and couch cushions, or we would wrestle, go to the park to play for hours, and he would throw me in the air and catch me or flip me over as I tried to take him down. I remember one day I piled all the couch cushions and pillows I could find and put them in the middle of the room. I then climbed on the couch, and I would jump off to body slam into the pile of softness. I decided the couch was not high enough, so I started jumping off the kitchen table. For some reason, I had a thing for climbing on tables. When we were living by the Heritage train station on Haddon Road, I was on the table pretending to be superman or something as I watched this guy cut the grass in the courtyard. I ended up falling off the table and smashing my face off the edge so hard I sliced the frenulum open in my mouth (the thin skin flaps in your inner lips), as well as killed my tooth. Mom had to take me to the ER. This is when we found out that all the radiation I had with my cancer testing affected the development of my adult teeth. I was missing my adult canine teeth.

When the kitchen table wasn't high enough for my satisfaction, I tried to put a chair on top of the table. Tony came around the corner and saw me trying to climb onto the table with the chair on it and immediately stopped that from happening and I started to complain. He told me I had to be safe and that this was not being safe. I asked if he could help me. "You can't tell Mom," he says as he helps me onto the kitchen table. He then holds the legs of the chair so I can climb on the chair. I get to the top and realize its way scarier than I was expecting but I leaped anyway. BAMB. I hit the big pile of cushions and lost all my breath. Now I am out of breath from being winded for the first time of my life, literally thinking I'm dying. Tony stood by my side assuring me I'll be okay and shortly after I caught my breath, I asked him "Can we do it again?" He was reluctant but just made sure I kept my mouth shut so my mom didn't kick his butt later. Back to the top I went and again I jumped. This time I made sure to land on my butt, and on the big couch cushions so I didn't get winded again.

Then there were the times Uncle Tony would bring his daughter, my cousin Brittney over. No matter what brother or cousin I was with I would always torment the heck out of them, as I was always a little brat and troublemaker. You could easily go as far as calling me a little shit disturber. I remember one day Brittney was over and I was bugging her like crazy until she said, "If you don't stop, I'm going to punch you." But did I listen? Nope. I kept bugging her and bugging her until she got so fed up, she punched me right in the face. My nose exploded with blood, so I freaked out and started crying and the blood everywhere made Brittney start crying as well. Mom comes in and gives Brittney crap, cleans me up, and ten minutes later I was back to pestering her, I was probably about five years old at the time.

It wasn't all fighting with Brittney though. One day she came over and while my mom was cooking, Brittney took me into my mom's room, got her makeup out, and started to doll me up to her liking. My mom's cooking then she thinks to herself, "Gosh it's quiet, too quiet." Her motherly instincts quickly kicked in and she went on a children hunt. She walked into her room and there I was in full makeup. Blush, eye liner, mascara, I think I had it all. Even in a pair of my mom's shoes. Mom took one look at me and hysterically laughed her head off. Then of course took a picture of me, cleaned me up and we sat down to eat.

When I was just five months old Uncle Tony was out for his birthday on February 4th. At some point the night turned and he was attacked by a much bigger guy, high on cocaine and drunk. After Tony defended himself and kicked the guy's ass, he tried to walk away. The coked-out drunk tackled him to the ground, sat on him, pulled out a nine-millimetre handgun, and then shot Tony in the side of the head, right outside a family restaurant and bar in downtown Calgary. Tony's friend immediately called the police and began CPR hoping to save his life. Miraculously he did and Tony survived. Even after being shot in the head at point-blank range Tony was the only person to survive a shooting during the big gang crime wave that year. He instantly became my hero after I was old enough and able to comprehend the reality of that situation. How one takes a nine-millimetre slug to the side of the head and lives to tell the tale, I'll never understand. Maybe it was luck, maybe it was his strength, or his determination to live for his face-punching little girl. Perhaps it was a fluke or a combination of the above. All I know is that he showed me anything was possible at a very young age. His strength, determination, and will to be able to walk out of the hospital on his own two feet will always inspire me and remind me how resilient, strong, and determined humans can be.

Even when I began school, I was trouble and causing fights all while being a klutz. One day at recess, I ran up to this one guy I didn't even know then kicked his foot as he walked (the same way I watched him do it to his buddy) and then I ran away. Then I came back to do it again, and again. Each time he would tell me to bugger off or he was going to do something about it. Did I listen? Of course not. I ran up to him and kicked the bottom of his foot mid-stride one more time, and he lost it. I didn't even get a step away when he grabbed me and picked me up, holding me over his head in the air against the dark brown wall of the school. It looked like game over for me.

As I'm up there being held against the wall five feet in the air, a teacher walked around the corner and I started screaming for help like I was being attacked. The teacher then gave that guy so much shit as I ran away free to go play with my friends. Months later, I was running around with some people playing tag when I tripped on my untied shoelace and ran face first into this poor kid so hard that I ended up breaking his collar bone with my forehead. I thought he was just being a big cry baby as I didn't think I ran into him very hard. He even screamed out, "AHHHHH I think you broke something!" I didn't believe him until the next day when I was in the principal's office with him in a sling after the poor kid went to the hospital to find out I very much did break his collar bone with my head. I felt so terrible, even though it was an accident. With such a mix of kids, that school got out of line at times. On the days the older students cleaned out their lockers, someone almost always lit a garbage can full of paper on fire and the school would be evacuated while the fire department came in to deal with it. It was like clockwork every year. "Garbage day" then became "fire day" and all the students and probably the staff expected to be evacuated on those days.

I was always being a disturbance in class, so I was constantly getting kicked out of the room and sent to the hallway. One day after being kicked out of the classroom, I decided to climb into the boot rack where I lay singing, "I'm all alone and there's no one here beside meeeee!" just continuing to be a disturbance.

After the playground was rebuilt, some kid was lying under the new bridge that bounced. He had put his legs up against it as he laid on the ground underneath. Right when he put his legs up someone jumped on the bridge and snapped the poor kid's leg like a twig. At that same school, I'd stick my tongue to the frozen pole of the baseball fence. Yup, you only do that once, when I think about it, I can still see the white stringy pieces of what must have been my taste buds on the pole. I then ran inside with my tongue profusely bleeding because it was missing a huge piece.

After school, I would usually come home and either go play with friends or go see my aunt Schniedy who was living just next door to us. With Schniedy being a hairdresser, we got her to cut, dye, and style our hair for "funky hair day" at school. Only when my brother and I showed up to school with our funky hair the next day, it wasn't funky hair day and we walked around looking like weirdos all day. After grade two, we all moved to the small town of Chestermere just east of Calgary.

Growing Up With the Lloyd family

This chapter is dedicated to the late Lisa Lloyd: The beautiful angel on God's shoulder.

When my family moved to Chestermere, Alberta in the early 2000s, I had the blessing of moving in next to the Lloyd family. We lived right on Chestermere Lake with just one house in between ours. At the time, Chestermere was a very small town with a ring of houses and cabins surrounding the small manmade lake. Only a few parts of land were developed at the time. The land right behind our houses was still dirt and we would spend hour after hour riding dirt bikes and quads on the empty land. When it was really hot out, we would blow up the tubes and go ride tubes being pulled by a Sea-Doo or boat on the lake.

That, at times, got a little extreme when we would make it a mission to toss the other person off the tube or even off the back of the Sea-Doo. You would know you were about to go flying when whoever was driving started doing circles to make waves. With every circle the waves bounced off each other creating bigger and bigger waves. After a few circles they would get you going and turn you into the monstrous waves. Once you hit them, it was game over; you'd go flying fifteen to twenty-five feet in the air. Most of the time, the impact from hitting the wave would be enough to make you let go of the tube and if you did, goodbye. You were going for a flight and hoping for a soft landing. When the town started to develop the land behind our houses the dirt bike riding was moved into the big back yard on the lake where we would continue to ride for hours making little jumps and stuff everywhere. With us just learning to ride I'm pretty sure the back yard was torn to shreds from the back tires spinning when we popped the clutch and drifted around the trampoline or fireplace.

When we weren't ripping dirt bikes, quads, or Sea-Doo's we would be hanging out in the little tree house or the fort beside their house. They even had built a little half pipe in their backyard for us to ride skateboards on. However, I was okay going one way but coming down backwards always freaked me out so I was pretty bad at it. I'd launch myself off the side and off the ramp and do mid-air tricks and try to land them on the grass. Sometimes I would climb on top of the dog house and ride off of it in the front walkway.

The Lloyds, to this day had the only dog I've ever seen (in person) that loved to ride a skateboard. When Jake and I started to learn how to ride, their dog, Bailey, did as well. He actually got pretty upset with you when you didn't give him his turn on the board. The dog would jump on the board with his front two legs and run with his back two legs and then hop up on the board with all four once he got some speed. It was comical and super cute.

When winter came along, the town of Chestermere would drain the manmade lake about five or six feet for the winter before it froze over. Once the lake was frozen solid, I'd throw on some skates and go for a skate on the swept path that went around the entire lake. If the ice was solid enough, we would get the quad down onto the ice and go rip it across the frozen ice for hours until we couldn't take the cold faces, feet, and hands any longer. I remember one Christmas I got a sled and the next day we tied a rope to the back of the quad and pulled each other around on the sled. It was kind of like knee boarding only it hurt a lot more when you fell and skipped off the rock-hard ice instead of water. I think that sled lasted maybe two days of that before it was destroyed. Chestermere was very small only a few thousand people lived there at the time so you could bike, walk, roller blade, or skateboard pretty much everywhere. I'd get on my bike and go to the canal and bike the paved pathway till it ran out and turned into gravel about halfway to Calgary; then I'd turn around and head back or bike around the lake adventuring for hours. Sometimes, when I was bored, I would just ride around the lake to the camp and back.

We were living there when I woke up all happy and stoked one day because it was my birthday the day before. Then my mom came home from work, ran right to the TV and turned it on, which wasn't like her to do. There, we watched the second plane crash into the World Trade Centre, then saw the two buildings crumble to the ground like a controlled demolition. My mother and I were in a complete state of shock, along with the rest of the world. However, I was too young to really know the gravity of what happened. My mom had to explain how New York was being attacked. Scared and worried, I finished getting ready and went to the bus stop. At school all morning, we didn't really do anything but sit in silence from the state of shock and as a respect to the 2,000 people who lost their lives on that horrendous day.

Another day, a while later, I got up and ready for school. While waiting for the bus, I was standing on what I thought was solid ice. The drain ditch with the pipe that ran under the road appeared to be frozen, so I was stepping on and sliding on it bored while I waited for the bus. Next thing I know, my right leg fell through the ice into the frigid water. My breath was taken from me in a nanosecond. It was only about thigh high but as I tried to get out my left leg fell through as well.

Now I was really struggling to catch my breath. However, with both legs now in the ice water I was able to touch the bottom and jump up to get myself out of the hole. I then started walking back home in my soaking-wet clothes in the minus thirty-degree weather. With each step I could feel my jeans solidifying and turning into a solid piece of ice. I got home and called out for my mother. She came to the door to find me freezing cold, soaking wet, and literally half frozen. When I took off my pants, they were frozen in one solid piece with the legs and waist open like I was still in them which I found funny. Mom went and got some towels and a change of clothes and warmed me up. I don't think I went to school that day because I spent that day, and the next three, sick and freezing cold even when I was under five blankets.

Getting ready for school one morning, I was on the chair in the living room when I stood up and took off toward my room to get my Scholastic book order that was due that day. I made it about halfway down the hall to my room when I blacked out, fell into the bathroom, and hit the counter in the bathroom with my face. I woke up with my nose pouring blood. Apparently, I stood up too fast in excitement to get my book order in and passed out for a second. Because of it, I had to stay home and be monitored by Nurse Karen for the day and…missed out on my order.

One day, my older brother and one of his friends were hanging out over at our place and I was being me, bugging them relentlessly, being a little shit. They would catch me, hog tie me, and give me a beat down but I would always come back to bug them for revenge. They finally had enough of me so my older brother put me up on a stepping stool next to the support beam in the basement and, with his friends' help, they taped me to the pole with Tuck tape. After that, they kicked out the stool so I was just hanging there taped to the pole, suspended a foot in the air. As they stood there laughing at me, I started screaming and cussing at them to get me down but that only made them leave the house. It would be an hour later when my mom came home from work to find me taped to the pole in the basement screaming for help. I told her what happened (minus me being a brat, of course) and she cut me down. Then I relaxed while we waited for my brother to come home so I could watch him get in trouble.

When the Lloyds moved from Chestermere to Langdon, just east of Chestermere, they got a nice piece of land with a big beautiful home and had to renovate the entire basement. So, the basement was in shambles for a bit. But the big, open basement had lots of room for us to play. They had some electric scooters; we would rip in circles around the big basement. It got a little competitive at times when we would kick, crash, or try to push each other off the scooters to win the races.

Then the BB gun wars came. We would lock and load as many BB guns as we could then we would have wars running around the basement like crazy kids shooting each other and hiding, having full on wars for hours at a time. Not even thinking about what we were doing to the walls when we missed each other. For years after (and probably to this day) you could see little dents in the walls everywhere. I was never a big fan of BB guns or guns in general because of Tony being shot and when they lived in Chestermere, I accidently shot Jake with one point blank by mistake just handling one. I felt horrible and terrified of guns at the same time. I didn't know how it went off so I was never a fan of guns. But there we were running and screaming from excitement and pain as we ran around shooting each other. Then we mixed the scooter races and the BB gun wars and that was good fun, chaotic, but fun. It was probably starting to look like they were going to have to renovate the basement, again.

When we weren't inside causing a chaotic mess destroying the place, we were outside riding the quads, dirt bikes, doom buggies, or golf carts all over the property again tearing up the land, creating a mess. At one point, they had made a little dirt bike track behind the barn for us to go shred for hours on end. I remember I was on a little dirt bike and I was trying to do a wheelie after we were already riding for hours. I hit the throttle and pulled the front end up and got going for maybe ten feet when I fell off the bike. The extremely hot, overworked motor of the bike somehow fell on the inside of my upper arm and gave me a huge burn on an incredibly soft, tender spot. I spent a few weeks draining the white clear pus from the burn, it was terrible. About a year or two later, we were riding that same dirt bike for hours and I was an idiot not thinking, wearing shorts on the hot summer day. At one point, the left inside part of my leg touched the motor and it gave me a nice big burn, again. This time, however, you could see the "S" of the Suzuki that was now branded into my leg, I thought that was kind of funny, but was going to be really mad if I had it forever embedded on my leg, but luckily it healed nicely.

Jake was doing doughnuts on the big 250cc quad they had and he was on gravel, but once the gravel was all spit away, the tires caught onto the hard ground and the quad suddenly went to flip. The tires caught and the quad went straight up on its side balancing on the left two side wheels. Jake looks at me in the golf cart looking at him with a "holy shit" look in his eyes and he just leans his body to the right and the quad fell back on all four tires. We just looked at each other for a second, Jake with a butthole puckered up look and me with a "holy crap you almost squished yourself" look. Then we went back to ripping around the property. I remember Jake's older brother Cody was riding his dirt bike and he did the same thing I did with trying a wheelie, only on a bike that was five times bigger and ten times more powerful going probably fifty times faster than I was. He hit a bump in the land and flipped the bike. Only he didn't just have the bike fall on his arm. All that was left of the bike when he fell was the bent frame. Everything from the handlebars, seat, exhaust, clutch, gas tank, and the break lever all broke off as it rolled over the land. The beautiful blue bike was completely unrecognizable and he was left with a gnarly concussion and a bad back injury. I'm actually surprised he didn't have more damage after seeing the bike reduced to nothing but the bent and mangled frame.

Shortly after the Lloyds moved from Chestermere to Langdon, my family moved from Chestermere to Cranston in Calgary with my mom. It was now about a forty-five-minute drive away but Cal or Lisa would always find or make the time to come get me and bring me over. I got into an argument with my mom one day and I ran out of the house and tried to find somewhere to go so I called Jake and he said they could come get me. I snuck back into the house, grabbed some clothes, wrote a note to my mother saying where I'd be, and left.

My mother never did see or get that note and assumed I ran away. Of course, this was right before she went on a medical mission to Africa. Unknown to me, she had filed a missing person's report with the police. I was out on their acreage and Cal put us boys to work for a while before we went into town to take a break and grab a few drinks from the local convenience store. We were driving down the highway and we sped past an RCMP officer who quickly turned around and pulled us over. The officer asked the guy driving if he had smoked any marijuana and as a joke he replied, "Not yet, officer." The officer took all our names then ran them. Both Jake and the driver were good, but I of course had a missing person's report, so the officer threw me in the back of the car and held me there until a family member picked me up. I tried to explain how the people I was with were like my family. I tried to explain how Jake's father and mother were a father and mother to me for years of my life, but he couldn't release me into their custody because of my age. When Jake and Jay got back, Cal asked where I was and they told him, "In the back of the cop car on the highway." Cal was like what the... and immediately came to get me but even with the both of us saying I was fine the officer wasn't able to release me into his custody, so I had to call my grandmother in Chestermere to come and get me. Needless to say, my mother and grandmother where not impressed with me for almost causing my mom to cancel her medical mission to Africa.

When I started longboarding for fun, I had nothing to do one weekend so I called Jake to see if I could come over. I thought he said that I could, but his dad couldn't come get me. It was a nice sunny day out so I thought I would longboard over. I packed a bag and got the longboard that I was borrowing from Jake because someone stole mine. I got on the highway and started to push east. However, the thirty-plus-kilometre trip was much further than I thought and after hours I had only gotten to the spot to turn left going north through the small town of Langdon then continued on down that highway to their acreage. While I was heading north on the road, Jake and his dad drove right past me in the oncoming lane. Jake's dad probably wondering if he was tripping out or if that was actually me says, "Was that Brandon!?" They went into town to get some things and I got to their beautiful home before they got back. I put Jake's longboard down out front, went inside, and drank about five huge cups of water, none of them satisfying my thirst. I ran out of water outside Langdon and didn't even think to go to Cal's restaurant to fill up.

Once they got back, Jake told me I actually wasn't allowed to come over as they were busy that weekend but after longboarding over thirty kilometres there, they weren't going to make me longboard thirty-plus kilometres back. I can only guess the amount of stress and grey hairs I caused Cal and Lisa over the years with being the lazy, klutzy, accident-prone kid I was. But their patience and kind hearts kept them from strangling me and they continued to love and treat me like one of their own.

After refusing to listen to my mom's rules and always doing whatever I wanted, I moved into my dad's when I was fourteen and one night when I was about to sit down for dinner, I got a call from Jake on the house phone. I answered and said, "Hello," and Jake's only words to me were, "Do you want to go to the Dominican?" Just as he asks me this, my dad's girlfriend told me to get off the phone and sit down for dinner, but I wasn't exactly going to hang up after hearing that. I replied, "Do I what?" He repeated, "Do you want to go to the Dominican?" I walked over to my dad at the table and asked him "Umm, can I go to the Dominican with Jake?"

My dad says something like, "That is something we are going to have to discuss but sit down were having dinner." I told Jake I'd call him right back after dinner and he shouts out, "My dad is going to pay for you!" I replied, "What no way!" He reassured me he would and I said, "Okay, I'll call you back after dinner." I put the phone back before I went and sat down at the table and started to talk to my dad about going on an all-expense paid trip to the Dominican Republic.

I didn't have a passport so I went through that whole process to get one, then got all the documentation I needed to be able to leave the country with another family. I believe we went around the end of December 2006 or early January in 2007. Cal came and picked me up from my dad's house on the other side of Calgary before we went over to their house for the night as we were leaving bright and early around three or four the next morning. Jake and I were both filled with excitement and decided to just stay up all night until we had to go. Hour after hour we played Nazi zombies on Call of Duty on the projected screen that went from floor to ceiling in the basement. Once it was time for us to get going, we threw our mountain of gear into the limo and the driver took us to the airport.

We arrived at the airport a while later and began the joys of airport security. Once through, we boarded our plane. I was really nervous as it was only my second time flying in my life. I had not need to worry, though, because we had a smooth flight there. As soon as I got off the plane, I was punched in the face with humidity that I've never felt before. I was also overtaken by the strong smell of marijuana. I had a laugh about the whole country seeming to smell like marijuana as we walked through the airport in the Dominican.

As we walked through the airport, I noticed the difference in their security. The only security I saw were people with dogs and soldiers with big machine guns walking around and I couldn't help but think 'damn, they're ready to fight.' From the airport, the six of us caught a cab and drove over to the resort where we were greeted by more guys with big guns guarding the gate. Jake and I got our own room so we stopped there and dropped off our things. After we all knew where we were staying, we made a secret knock to let each other know it was us, and got settled in for the night.

The next day, I woke up clueless to where I was until I looked outside and was incredibly ecstatic to remember I was in the Dominican with my buddy. We got up and went over to Cal and Lisa's room to check in. We said good morning and Cal gave us some money to have some fun down at the beach but told us to make sure we check in later when we get back. Wristbands on, cash in our pockets, we visited all the small, touristy places and bought overpriced, unnecessary goods all afternoon before returning to the resort. It was around this time that I was told about these drinks at the resort called a "special" which was an amazing ice-cold slushy type of drink with a shot of rum in it. I tried one and it went down like water so I had another and another. That's when Jake told me they had rum in them so I waited a bit before I had another. They were so good I couldn't even tell they had alcohol in them. After checking in with Cal and Lisa, we hung around the pool as I snuck specials on and off until bed. The next morning, we checked in with Cal and Lisa before we went off to buy more touristy things down the beach.

At every resort they had a swim up bar and a normal bar so we stopped at a few of them and I had a drink and chatted with the bartenders for a few minutes. As I was talking to one of them, I discovered that everyone in Canada is either from Toronto or lives in igloos. This one bartender Francesca asked me those two questions: "Are you from Toronto?" and, "You guys live in igloos, right?" I don't think I've ever felt more disconnected from my home in my entire life.

After returning to our room with a bag full of mementoes, we went over to check in with Lisa and Cal. But first I grabbed a special on the way that was finished before we even got around the corner. We got into their room and Jake and I went upstairs to check out the hot tub they had in their suite. As Jake and I walked up the spiral metal staircase that led to the big tub, Jake's foot slipped on the wet metal stairs and he jammed his toes into the metal bars so hard he tore open the webbing between two of his toes. Blood started to gush out everywhere and we came right back down the stairs. He went right to the bathroom to try and clean it up leaving a blood trail from the stairs to his parents' bathroom. Even on the dark, wet staircase you could see the thick, bright-red puddles of blood that came down. Then all across the white tile floor was a gnarly, bloody footprint every few strides. It almost looked like a scene from a horror movie.

Once Jake got his foot in the bathtub, they poured alcohol on it to disinfect it and I couldn't even imagine the sting that must have caused Jake. Just looking at the open wound gushing blood and watching the alcohol run over it made me cringe. After the disinfecting, they tried to stop the bleeding, but nothing seemed to work and after a while it was decided he had to go to the hospital to get his foot stitched up.

Jake, Cal, Lisa, and I got in a cab after walking over the blood all over the floor of the suite and drove over to the local hospital that seemed to be forever away. As soon as we walked into the hospital, I noticed the smell of marijuana only intensify. It smelled like we just walked into an indoor grow operation, not a hospital. Stepping off the plane smelled like a bag of mediocre doubles whereas walking into the hospital smelled like a bag of Snoop Doggs' quadruple A private stash. Jake was taken for stitches as Cal, Lisa, and I patiently waited. After he was given some pain meds and stitches we left and headed back to the resort.

With the fresh open tear between his toes, Jake was given direct orders from the doctor to not go onto the sandy beach, into the ocean, or even into the pools for at least two days to let it heal. It was one of our first days there, so the timing was brutally unfortunate. After the hospital trip Cal took us all out for a delicious dinner at one of the nearby restaurants and we all hung out and relaxed for the evening.

The next day we went walking back and forth down the beach and I tried a special from every one of the bars on the way between the little shops they had at the resorts. I felt really bad Jake couldn't go do anything in water or on the beach, or drink with his new meds so we just walked around buying useless stuff for us and our friends and family back home, eating lots of food along the way.

It was my first time being somewhere you can literally drink everywhere so Jake and I checked in with Cal and Lisa before I convinced Jake to take me to the resort bar and ignoring everything Cal and Lisa asked of us I took shot after shot to the point even the bartender asked if I was going to need an ambulance. Little did we all know I could have dropped dead on the spot. After I had my fair share of shots for Jake and myself, we walked around the resort for a while and just as I was starting to feel the effects of the rum we stumbled upon an unattended wheelchair in the middle of nowhere and of course, like a drunk asshole, I ran up and got in it not even thinking Jake could use it with his torn foot, or thinking of the person it was originally intended for.

Once I was in the abandoned chair, I took a quick feel in my pockets for electronics and I had none so I rode the wheelchair as fast as I could down the path, around the right corner, and jumped it into the deep end of the nearest pool. Jake comes walking around the corner to see me in the wheel chair in our hotel pool and just laughs while he shakes his head and walks over to me. I told him to jump in but he reminded me of his foot so that was a bust. In the pool, I got on the back two wheels of the wheelchair and was balancing on them when a guard with an AK47 around his shoulders came ripping over to us on a dirt bike. Jake and I showed him our wristbands and I fell backwards out of the chair in the water in the process. The guard then asked me, "What are you doing, man?" I just said, "I'm hanging out not doing much, just enjoying the night." He then rode off down the beach as I pushed the chair over to the shallow end and pulled it out.

With the wheelchair and myself dripping wet, we went back over to the bar I just had shots of rum at. This time the bartender sees me in the wheelchair still dripping wet and, like Jake, just shook his head in an obvious state of thinking, 'What the fuck?' The bartender then asks, "Why are **you** in a chair now, man?" I told him, "Because you gave me too many shots, man, I can't walk." Then I jokingly asked for another shot as I laughed thinking I wasn't going to get one. That was until he started filling the shot glasses. He poured Jake one as well but he told the bartender he couldn't drink because of the medications he was on. So, I did a shot with the bartender as I wasn't going to be able to take two back-to-back after already losing count. After the stop at the bar, we made our way back to our hotel room and I dropped off the wheelchair where I found it before we passed out for the night.

As I tried to sleep, I got the worst spins I've ever had in my life. Even with me and my friends getting plastered from my mom's liquor all the time I had never been really drunk like that before and I wasn't very impressed with myself as I struggled to fall asleep while feeling like I was on the spinning rides at the Calgary stampede. If I thought I was unimpressed with myself trying to fall asleep, I was very upset and angry at myself the second I woke up the next morning. The first thing I did was run to the bathroom and spew into the toilet for about fifteen minutes. I felt like absolute garbage, so full of resentment of going irresponsibly hard the night before. I wondered why people got really drunk to begin with. It was my first time having a real hangover and between the spins, lack of sleep, puking, and the headache, with gut rot. I was at a loss to why people did this to themselves. "I'm never going to drink again," I told myself as I sat beside the toilet trying to recover in between dry heaves.

After I pulled myself together, we checked in with Lisa and Cal before doing our usual pondering around the resorts. We got a few resorts down when the weather drastically changed and Jake and I got caught in a nasty storm. The raindrops felt like water balloons with the amount of water in every drop that hit us. We hid out where we could and made our way back down to our resort. We got back just as the storm stopped and the sun came out. Right when we got back to our resort, one of the shop owners who had seen us around for the past few days came up to us and asked if we could take his jug and go ask the bartender to fill it with orange juice for him. I thought nothing of it so I grabbed it and walked around the corner to get it filled then brought it back to the guy. Just as I handed the guy his big coffee mug, we ran into Cal who was out and about trying to find us so we could go to dinner.

With my hangover I think I only had maybe one or two specials that day. 'So much for never drinking again,' I thought to myself as I drank the delicious ice-cold drink. I'm pretty sure I was probably still drunk from the night before as well, so I just relaxed and ate all the tasty food I could fit in my angry stomach before completely dying on the bed that night. Jake wanted to go out but I was so hungover, unable to drink or function. So we just stayed in that night and put on the television. We couldn't find anything worthy besides the Spanish rap channel. Even though we couldn't understand what they were saying, it still sounded alright so we left that on as we rummaged through our new belongings. I was super stoked about my new necklace I got until Jake told me he got the same one the last time he was here, and he got it for half the price. I had bought it without trying to negotiate a deal, like I did with everything and suddenly got super chapped at myself.

The next afternoon Jake's foot was healed enough that we could wrap his foot and sneak him onto the beach and into the ocean. Jake, his brother, his brother's girlfriend, and I went on a banana tube ride in the ocean. We rode around through the waves for a bit then the driver of the boat took us right into a big wave and Cody's girlfriend went flying but Jake quickly caught her by one of her arms and got her back on the tube. Later we laughed how he should have left her to be a goner in the big ocean or caught her by the arm, looked her in the eyes, then let her go just for the laughs.

After our tube ride, we all went over to one of the restaurants for another delicious meal then we went out and watched a performance on stage before going over to the pool again where I had more of my new favourite drink in the world. You guessed it, another special. The ones at most of the resorts were good, but the specials they made at our resort were on a dangerous level of delicious.

Jake, Cody, and Cody's girlfriend and I hung out in the pool where Cody and his girlfriend played with the underwater camera as they swam around, and Jake and I just hung out at the swim-up bar and relaxed in the pool all afternoon. At some point, Cody noticed the scars on my left side from when I had cancer and asked how I got them. I told him I had cancer as a child and he was shocked as he said, "Crazy, I didn't know you had cancer." That's when I first realized that I never talked about my cancer story. Here was a family that I had known for the better part of a decade and not a single one knew I had cancer, because I never talked about it. I went back to our hotel room and called my mom to check in with her again before we all went out to dinner. After another great dinner we walked around for a bit before jumping in the hot tub and relaxing by the pool for the evening. The next afternoon we were up and back off to the airport to head home.

That morning, I got up and was sad that our week stay there had come to an end so fast. It felt like we just got there and I didn't want to go back home. I definitely didn't want to go back to Canada mid-winter. I thought and joked about how they should just leave me behind and say that they lost me and I'll stay until I get kicked out but that wasn't going to happen. I packed my bag and my now way overfull suitcase with hundreds of dollars in funky necklaces, candle holders, chains, t-shirts, and bag upon bag of touristy bought artifacts. I literally had to sit on my suitcase and get Jake to zip it closed, it was so full. We all piled into a van after one last meal at the resort and drove back to the airport. As usual, my flying nervousness got the best of me as we arrived. We all walked through the maze of dogs and armed guards in the open concept airport. I loved how everything there was an open concept. Nothing was enclosed off like back home. They had no need for four walls and a roof, they just had roofs. On the hot blistering days, the wind would come through the buildings and give you a nice much needed cool down.

We got through security and onto our plane for our eight-hour flight. I somehow managed to calm my nerves, **just** as the plane started to take off. About that same moment, the exit sign that hung from the top of the fuselage above me fell off from the vibrations and landed by my feet. 'Oh great,' I thought, 'We're not even in the sky and the plane is falling apart…But maybe I can bring this exit sign home!' By now the *Final Destination* movie was going through my mind and I wanted to puke from the nervousness. Thinking of that really made my nerves unsettle. I tried to casually kick the exit sign under my seat so I could steal it and bring it home as a souvenir, but one of the flight crew saw me trying to casually and discreetly kick it under my seat. She looked at me, smiled, then came and picked it up ruining my hopes and dreams of bringing airplane pieces home. Once we got to our maximum cruising altitude, we hit some turbulence and the plane started to violently shake. Between the sign falling down and now the whole plane shaking in my first turbulence experience I was incredibly uncomfortable with being on the plane and wanted to be on the ground then and there. With nothing else to do and still feeling like hot garbage from all my excessive drinking I tried to sleep the whole way home.

Once we finally arrived back in Calgary, before we even got off the plane, we could feel the dry, ice-cold, fresh air ripping through the fuselage as soon as they opened the plane door. It was super weird and very uncomfortable going from somewhere so hot and humid to coming home to a place that's incredibly dry and cold. After we got off the plane we went through customs and a lady looked at me and said, "Your bag needs to be searched." But after the lady saw the five others with me, she changed her mind and let us go instead of searching all our bags. Outside, we waited for their limo driver to pick us up and they dropped me back at my dads in Calgary before taking the long trip back to Langdon themselves. The next day it was back to school and getting slapped with a pile of work I had missed over the last week but continued with my day-to-day life missing the Dominican Republic and ready for my next trip out of the country.

First Stroke

I was fifteen years old and living at my dad's house in the southwest Calgary area. Being a rebellious, angry child who refused to listen and refused therapy, or any help at all, my parents thought it would be better if I was with him so he could watch me more as my mom worked twelve-hour shifts at night all the time. So, with Mom, I'd be grounded with nobody home and I could just hop and skip out the door and sneak out whenever I wanted. But there, with Dad, nothing changed. I was now angrier than ever and instead of walking out the front door I'd just sneak out the basement window. I don't think they or most people realize that when you're a modern-day slave at work for sixty plus hours a week, you're going to let kids do whatever they want anyway. So, I moved there and nothing really changed except for my anger being amplified because now I was hours away from all of my current friends.

Once I made some new friends, I was up to the same-old, no-good things. I had made a two-foot bong one day and one of my friends told me to sneak out and come get her. So, I snuck out and walked over to her place with this bong hidden under my coat. I got to her house at the agreed time. She said she was home alone so I could knock on the door or ring the bell which I did. Only unknown to me, her older brother unexpectedly came home early and she forgot to tell me. So, I showed up to her house at two or three in the morning with a huge bong in my coat and was greeted by her older brother. Needless to say, he was not impressed and started to scream at me and tear me a new butthole. My friend came upstairs to see me at the door getting cursed out by her brother. He slammed the door in my face and told me to "fuck off" so I roamed around the neighbourhood until her and her friend where able to sneak out an hour or so later.

At school, some other friends and I made a plan to sneak out and go to the "shed" to hang out one night. I told them I'd be there at around 2:30 a.m. Around 2 a.m., I crawled out of my window with my longboard. Once I got down the street, I got on my board and pushed over to the school the shed was at. Upon arriving to the school parking lot, I could hear my friends having a good time. I could smell the marijuana and could tell they were all drunk by how loud they were. Me being me, I decided to mess with them. I got off my board, picked it up, then quietly walked over into the shelter and I listened to them talking for a few seconds as I stood outside the door of the shed. Then I gave three or four obnoxiously loud bangs on the door before I went into a really deep voice saying, "Calgary Police, open the door now and put your hands in the air where I can see them." As soon as I said that they all went from drunk and rowdy to being so quiet you could have heard a pin drop. I turned on the flashlight on my phone, then ripped the door open really fast and shined the light into their faces so they couldn't see who I was. All five or six of my friends sat there with their eyes wide open and jaws to the ground with the infamous "We are so fucked" look on all of their faces. I couldn't help it, the look on their faces had me burst out laughing so hard and I said, "What's up guys?" I had a good laugh but they definitely didn't as they all thought they were getting in huge trouble for a second. They were upset with me, until I told them how far away I could hear them, so unless they really wanted the actual police to arrive, we had to be quieter.

Then one chilly December morning, I got up and grabbed some clean clothes before I headed for the shower. I was in the middle of my shower when I got this really weird head rush and blacked out. This head rush wasn't my average stand up too fast and blackout head rush. This head rush was different in the sense that I literally felt the center my brain vibrate when the light-headedness came. A few seconds or minutes later (I don't really know) I woke up. I immediately noticed that the bottom half of my peripheral vision was missing. I only saw blackness where there was once light. First, I thought perhaps I had gotten something in my eyes, so I started to flush them out with the running water. After a few minutes of this nothing had changed, I was still missing a large portion of my vision. I got out of the shower and also noticed I had a massive, intense headache. It felt like someone had stuck a knife in my brain and was cutting through my brain matter. I grabbed the bottle of Tylenol out of the medicine cabinet, took a few, and after getting dressed I started walking to the bus stop to go to school. My vision was still partially gone but it wasn't enough that my stubborn ass was overly worried, I just continued on as it were any other day like an idiot. I took a few more pills on the bus to help with my headache that seemed to not be subsiding. I remember being really confused on why my vision was missing as I sat in the middle of the bench on the back of the city bus. I got to school and took another few doses of Tylenol as my headache was still incredibly painful and debilitating.

It was after English class, I noticed I had taken about half the bottle of Tylenol. I looked on the back and read, "Adults take 1-2 tablets every 4-6 hours as needed." I was probably six to eight pills deep by that point. I immediately started to freak out a little bit thinking I might have just killed myself. This caused one of my friends to notice something was going on with me and he asked me what was going on. I told him about my headache, bottle of swallowed pills, and my vision loss. He then took me out the back doors of the school and as we walked it was decided I was going to skip the rest of the day. He pulled out a joint and lit it as we walked through the parking lot of Westbrook mall. He asked if I wanted a puff and I said, "Sure." I grabbed it figuring it couldn't possibly ruin my day more than it has already been. I took a long, slow puff, then I inhaled. Instantly before I could even exhale my blistering, knife-like headache was gone. I looked at him and I said, "What the fuck, my headache is now gone." But so was the bottom of my vision. We went to his house and played video games for a bit until he went back to class.

I walked with him back to the school and found some friends out front playing hacky-sac while they were on a spare. I quickly joined in the game but was such a terrible player that day. Every time it came to me it would go into my new blind spot and I'd lose it and miss my kick or just not kick it at all. I think I spent more time that game picking it up and serving it to people than kicking it. After school, some friends and I waited around the school until the rush was over, then I got on the bus and headed home. When I got there, I told my dad's girlfriend what happened to me earlier that morning. When I told her, she shrugged it off in disbelief which left me feeling absolutely hopeless, pissed off, and about to steal her car to drive myself to the doctor. I then called my mother who was working at Rocky View General Hospital. She informed me to come to the hospital immediately. So, I asked my dad's girlfriend if she could drive me to the hospital; that was around 5:30 p.m. She said she couldn't because her youngest had a piano recital at 8 p.m. that night. So, I called my dad who was at work and also in denial of my symptoms. My mom lost it when I told her this so she left work and came to pick me up right then and there.

At the Rocky View General Hospital, they were unsure what to do with me because of my young age of fifteen and being a huge, chubby, adult-sized kid. After my mom gave them my medical history, they decided I needed an MRI scan to see what was going on in my brain. Only problem was I had braces on my teeth. An MRI machine uses something like 300,000 times the force of gravity that will pull on and remove any metal objects that go into the massive, magnetic machine. Therefore, the braces needed to go. So, bracket by bracket they grabbed, wiggled, pulled, pushed, and tore every cemented bracket off my teeth. The one bracket on my right K9 tooth was really cemented onto the tooth and instead of breaking off the bracket, they ripped out the entire tooth. After that, the nurse held my tooth in her two fingers and used the fingers on her other hand to pull the bracket off my tooth that was now ripped out of my face. Knowing that was my only K9 tooth I was so mad and wanted to start swearing and cursing but my mother was there, and I would have gotten a "momma bear beat down" or a "knuckle sandwich" so I stayed quiet. After the MRI scan, we sat and waited for the results. A short time later, the doctor came in and told me I had a brain aneurism that caused a massive stroke which was the cause of my sudden blindness. I then spent weeks in the hospital being monitored.

I was in utter disbelief. What in the hell was a brain aneurysm? And all I knew at the time was strokes are what happened to older people, or people that are close to death—I was fifteen. After a short talk, they decided to transfer me to the children's hospital. So I flopped off the bed and onto a stretcher. As I lay on the hard stretcher, I couldn't help but think how messed up this whole situation was. I wondered what was going on with my life, now more confused than I've ever been. They put me in the back of an ambulance and we were off. Lights and sirens blaring we sped over to the new Children's hospital. It was my first time in an ambulance with lights and sirens and I loved how we didn't ever have to stop. I'm not sure if the suspension of the ambulance was broken or not but I recall it was a very hard and uncomfortable ride the whole way. After a day of monitoring me and giving me advice on how to not cause a stroke by doing everyday things they released me and I moved right back into my mom's house in the southeast Calgary area.

I was in a state of shock and pure disbelief for some time. I was in disbelief that a stroke could happen to a fifteen-year-old. This was when the mental tormenting began. Every single morning, I now began to wonder "Is today the day I'm going to die?" I had to deal with every day, every situation, and every moment possibly being my last. The amount of anger, rage, depression, and anxiety that put me in, was unfathomable. Day by day I hated the world more and more. I saw it as unfair and wanted the world to burn as I watched. I couldn't help but wonder 'why me? Why now? Is today the last day I'll get to see? Is this life even worth living?' The more I wondered the more angry I got and the more I both hated the world, life, and started to not care about anything including myself, friends, family, and loved ones. This was only amplified by slowly figuring out I was lied to by society my whole life. Things such as 9-11, the black Jews out of Egypt, the reason our names are in all capital letters on every piece of government issued ID, and the way a "Pagan religion is carefully hidden, woven into the holidays of a Christian" (*Internally Bleeding*, Immortal Technique) As well as how we live in a system that's inevitably set for failure all started to come to light. But out of everything, nothing pissed me off more than the realization that I solely exist to be monetized by the government. My anger, frustration, depression, and hate for the world only kept growing immensely. Now on top of the daily questioning of my existence, I was questioning why I survived these things to begin with. Did I really survive cancer and a massive hemorrhagic stroke only to spend the rest of my life being used for nothing but profit? I'm sure you already know the answer; yes. That was the worst life realization ever, which caused the anger and rage to reach its "I don't give a damn" boiling point. I couldn't comprehend caring for a world that doesn't give a damn about any of us.

Now I had to deal with every day possibly being my last, on top of that I was going to have to spend those possible last days as a modern-day slave. 'Fuck that, I'd rather die young' I clearly recall telling myself upon this realization as I stood in my light-green bedroom looking at the rocky mountains out of my west-facing window. If I was going to die today, I was going to spend that day doing whatever I wanted to do and if someone didn't like what that was, well tough tits, they had a tomorrow and just like that, the government mentality of only caring for myself and nobody else was imbedded into my mind body and soul.

Then came the fights with everyone. With my mom, my brothers, even some of my friends. I quickly started to rebel harder and harder not caring about anything or anyone, especially myself and life. It was around this time I started to abuse and experiment with drugs. It all started with my free, prescribed opiates and alcohol which provided a great escape from my reality, but really it was just exacerbating the problem. The doctors thought giving the fifteen-year-old me a bunch of opiates to help manage my headaches would be a good idea. Only problem was, when I took a pill or two and my headache didn't go away I'd take another one or two and if my head still hurt, I'd eat some more. Doing the same thing I did with the bottle of Tylenol the day I had my stroke, I just ate pills trying to relieve my pain. Only unlike Tylenol, when you take more opiates than recommended, you end up getting higher than a space shuttle, and I didn't know that until I was melting on the couch in the living room feeling really damn good. Being in that high was where I realized drugs took me—out of the reality I was in. It was there in that state I realized I wasn't worried or stressed or in an endless mind loop of "Am I going to die today?"

Three weeks (two weeks of monitoring and a week of tests) after my stroke I was back in school. I honestly can't even remember how the few first days went. I was in an utter state of shock and fear all the time. It was almost like being in love. When you're in love you wake up and the first thought of your day is your significant other, you then spend all day thinking about her or him and as you fall asleep your thoughts are still completely enveloped with them, and the love you have for them. Only for me, my significant other was death, and I was not at all in love with him, he absolutely terrified me. I've never been abused (except by life) in my twenty-nine years on the planet but I can only assume it was what being in an abusive relationship would feel like. Sure, you're in a relationship but when that other person comes around you don't feel safe, you don't feel secure, nor do you feel protected. When they come around, you're petrified in fear, you're scared, you're more uncertain than ever, all the while riddled with the worst anxiety you've ever felt. Only this wasn't a person or a thing that I could take an alternate route home to avoid. This abusive, fearful, life-destroying individual was nobody but myself inside my own head. It wasn't a person in physical form that I was fearful of, it was my own thoughts. Thoughts that had me suddenly frozen in life like a Woolly Mammoth frozen in a glacier. I was unable to move, think, or process my new unexpected reality.

I realized that while I was in my science class now struggling with reading and writing with my blindness and debilitating headaches. I had my textbook and binder out like I was prepared for class but I wasn't ready at all, I was simply there going through the motions. The teacher was writing notes on the white board while I was just sitting there staring off into space in a complete daze of confusion, misery, anger, frustration and more hate than any individual should ever have. He was writing but I was not taking any notes. To me it was like there was no white board and I was staring beyond the wall that suspended it in the air. My teacher would speak to explain the significance of what he was writing and not a single word was registering with me as I was too busy thinking if my next fight, gym class, sneeze, cough, fall, or bowel movement would kill me. When this happened, I was only able to live in the now, and in the moment of impulsive self-satisfaction. I suddenly stopped caring about everything in my life, especially my future. Why would you focus on a future when you didn't even have one? That to me sounded like a waste of time and the dumbest thing ever, all I cared about was having fun and living in the moment because to me that's all there was. When you're in a constant fear of death I think it would be hard for any individual to think clearly about, well, anything. Especially where they want to go or what they want to do in life, let alone a fifteen-year-old kid.

Once I got into that negative routine of impulsive self-satisfaction living day by day, I really started to run my life into the ground and at a much faster rate than ever before. I found my escape from reality by using drugs and alcohol, as well as being a little, mischievous neighbourhood brat running around causing all kinds of havoc for the adrenaline rush. From playing 'ding dong ditch' to throwing snowballs at passing cars trying to get a chase out of someone. My friends and I would hide in specific spots on the bus route and we would hit the bus with snowballs as it came into the community then after the bus did the lap around the community, we would hit it on the way out. We would do this for hours till random people got off the bus and gave chase trying to catch us. It was purely an adrenaline rush and I loved it because it was the only time besides being asleep or high that I wasn't in that constant state of fear about dying because of this ticking time bomb with no timer in my head.

There were some close calls though. I remember some friends and I were in between two houses throwing snowballs at cars, like idiots. One guy pulled over, got out, and started chasing us. We ran behind the houses and down the alley with the mad stranger right on my slow chubby tail. I made a left turn in the alley and there was a jeep there so I stopped and quickly rolled underneath the vehicle. The stranger turned the corner to see I had disappeared. He makes an "hmm" noise out of confusion and continues on after my friends that went further down the alley while I laid there frozen from not only the cold, but the fear of the fact that there is a very mad person around looking for me after we all pelted his car with a few snowballs. If we did get caught by an angry stranger, we would just tell him it was a kid named Denis. We had a friend named Denis, but he was never with us so anytime we got caught we would just tell them, "Denis did it and he ran that way," and point off into a random direction in a desperate attempt to get the heat off us.

One time a big, buff guy ran out of his apartment and caught us only a block from his home. One of my stupid friends had picked something up and threw it at his patio door then just took off running without saying a word to the other three of us. Once he caught him, he was on a mission to get us in trouble and made my buddy walk us to his house to talk to his parents. Once there, we told them "Denis did it and then took off somewhere." His mom made us call Denis multiple times to try and find out where he was. To this day, I'm still glad he didn't pick up the phone because we would have been busted right there. But it was her stupid kid that caused the situation to begin with, so my two friends and I were able to go home without trouble.

After the mischievous faze of aggravating people till they gave chase, came the mischievous graffiti stage. Graffiti was a lot of fun and it involved some of my favourite activities like longboarding, adventuring, and painting. Not to mention once you found the spot you wanted to hit and started painting, it became therapeutic and there was almost nothing else on your mind and it caused that adrenaline rush I desperately craved. The only problems I had with graffiti was I lacked the artistic mind so I wasn't any good. I also couldn't afford the paint as drugs, booze, and longboards was where my money went. I also caused a lot of trouble with other graffiti writers because of the 'street rules' I didn't know of or give a damn about. Life was still all about me and my daily escape whether it be drugs, alcohol, graffiti, or causing mischief in the neighbourhood. Nothing else mattered to me. It was my way of escaping from reality. They were the only things that kept me somewhat sane and going from day-to- day without jumping off a bridge or in front of traffic.

Not being able to afford paint, meant I was stealing all the change and money out of my mom's purse that I could. When I couldn't do that I, like most graffiti writers, would do what's called "racking" this is just a street term for stealing paint. My friends, or just myself, would go into a store with a backpack and big baggy clothes on, walk into the paint isle, and just start filling our pockets and bags with as much paint as possible, then walk out, maybe grabbing a job application before walking out to try and avoid suspicion.

I had found myself becoming a little too comfortable with going into stores and racking paint. I would go maraud the same stores two or three times a week. It really became an addiction and mental escape of its own. From the rush of going into the store and racking paint, then the rush of painting itself. There is also an incredible adrenaline rush when you are climbing up the sides of buildings or bridges trying to get to "heaven spots." A heaven spot is pretty self-explanatory. It's a spot you climb to on top of a building or bridge to paint that is incredibly dangerous and will take your life if you slip. I am so terrified of heights that I was never one to go out of my way to hit a 'heaven spot' the highest I would go is about two or three stories. If I went higher than that the fear of falling would overtake the joy for painting and I would mess up my painting and do a very poor job at it, even worse than I already was. So as much as I enjoyed painting, that wasn't really for me.

I was surprised to see even the risk of death won't stop some of these kids because of how much they love writing. If anything, it makes them want to do it more. The rush of it all is so intense and provided a profound way to escape from reality, which was my selling point and I'm sure it is for many others. Yet the city spends countless dollars trying to fight it. When the reality is, like the war on drugs, it's a war that will never be won.

Embrace Graffiti

Years ago, the city of Calgary had a great idea. They decided to drop something like ten-thousand spray paint cans at the Millennium Skate Park downtown Calgary so the graffiti writers could go nuts and paint all they wanted at the skatepark. So, they drop a stupid amount of spray paint cans there and left it all up to the public. It was a good idea in theory I suppose, but what ended up happening was all the immature kids grabbed cans and drew pictures of male reproductive organs with sayings like "fuck the police" and all sorts of really stupid, ugly things and destroyed the entire park. So basically, the city sponsored and paid for the most vandalism they ever saw in one place. The project was a huge failure and a disgrace to the City of Calgary's management, and it demonstrated their lack of basic knowledge of the world of graffiti. But if they understood the graffiti world, I believe it could have and would have been a tremendous success.

You can't just drop thousands of spray paint cans at a skate park in the heart of downtown with little kids and immature teenagers and zero supervision then expect things to go the way you want. It would have worked and been a great success with lots of amazing art if they did it right. I think they needed to have volunteers there and maybe a police presence to keep an eye on any of the immature people drawing penises, vulgar language, and what not. They should have had a volunteer tent where you had to go up with your rough sketch on what you wanted to paint and registered it with the volunteers.

This way they could see what will be painted, who will be painting it, and where it will be painted. It would have been a really simple way to weed out the immature kids and get some nice artwork up for the public to see and admire. Also, they needed to run it for more than one weekend. If there was more time the actual good graffiti writers would have been able to put up some nice pieces of art. Then over time, the bad graffiti would get covered up with good graffiti and it would weed things down to nice clean art with positive, non-vulgar language. Anyone breaking these rules could be subject to the same $1000 and $5000 fines as if it were illegal. This would be a huge deterrent for anyone fighting the urge to draw a six-foot penis on the cement walls.

If there were lots of good artwork up, the people that aren't good (like me) wouldn't go up there and attempt to paint over it. In the graffiti world you need to cover a "piece" with a "piece" (a piece is a complex intricate piece of art that usually takes hours or more to paint). Then you are supposed to cover a "throw up" with a throw up (a throw up is something you can throw up in 30 seconds to a couple minutes and get going, then you have your "hand styles" (a hand style is like a graffiti writer's signature). It's just a quick scribble of their name. That's the way it is supposed to work, but not everyone follows the rules. Someone will spend five or six hours working on a big beautiful "piece" then someone will come along and put a "throw up" on top of it and ruin their piece they spent hours on in less than a minute and destroy it. This causes lots of drama and tension in the world of graffiti and it's a quick way to start fights or drama on the street.

If you did put a throw up over a piece, the graffiti world would tear you apart and cuss you out and you will lose your street credibility as a writer if you didn't get jumped and beaten for it. So over time, the "throwups" would be covered with nice "pieces" and fade out the terrible unappealing art. For example, if you go to Vancouver, there is amazing graffiti everywhere. You'll still find your little "hand style" scribbles everywhere. However, people need to understand it takes that little scribble to slowly get to that big beautiful complex piece of art. You can't just expect a new writer to put out amazing pieces without slowly getting to that creativity, opening their artistic mind, and finding their writing style. I'm sure Leonardo Da Vinci didn't paint the Mona Lisa without first scribbling on something that wasn't a canvas once or twice.

I think Calgary should lose the "goodbye graffiti" organization that goes around "buffing" (removing or painting over) all the graffiti. Like the war on drugs, it will never be won. For as long as people want to do drugs, they will find a way to get them and do it. It is the same in the graffiti world. For as long as these people want to paint, get back at society, destroy things, or escape, they will. They can buff all the graffiti they want but that will never change the attitude or mind of the graffiti writer. It just pisses them off and gets them to come back the next night. In my opinion, they will never be able to stop and say "goodbye" to graffiti. As long as this world is disgusting and as long as we keep selling out generation after generation to a government that doesn't care about the health or wellbeing of its people, there will always be plenty of people to lash out, rebel, and get back at the government through things like graffiti.

The best any city or government could do is accept that fact, and try to at least manage it. I think they could do this by setting up designated painting areas, they could have designated painting areas that are monitored by the city and police coming by. They can have an organization (like goodbye graffiti) have these writers come to them saying I want to paint this here. Have them register their name, graffiti name, and what they want to paint, then let them go paint it in peace. They're going to go paint whether the city likes it or not. So why fight a never-ending battle. Why waist endless tax dollars trying to stop something they can't stop? Why not spend that money giving people a way to peacefully express themselves in an artistic manner?

The "golf dome" off the red LRT line is a great example of them being able to control it. I heard they were doing an "anti-graffiti" thing there as it is a highly painted spot for graffiti writers. So, what they did was get a bunch of decent graffiti writers to paint their artwork all over it. There's some nice clean artwork on it and it hasn't been touched by other writers for years because it's good and no one wants to start a bunch of drama on the streets by bombing (painting) over it. So, month after month, year after year the art stays there for the public to see. I'm sure some people don't like it, but I'm sure some people (like me) do like to see some art on the massive white and green eyesore of a dome. Thankfully over the years, Millennium Skate Park was improved and now holds some nice art in places as well.

I think it would be incredibly beneficial to both the writers and the city if they had more designated spots like that all over Calgary. I could see the risk of two graffiti crews meeting in a spot and causing a problem, but if they were given a place and time to be there or had one police officer around or even a volunteer from the city overseeing it all (only stopping any violence), I don't think it would be an issue. If there was video surveillance, they could see who is at fault for what as well as catch any writers bombing there illegally. They could use this to see who writes what, who they write with, and what part of town they bomb in. As well they could enter in the names of the graffiti writers into a data base and when there is an unregistered piece of graffiti, or graffiti where it shouldn't be they can look them up and issue them a ticket. It would be much easier and cheaper instead of sending out six police units with dogs to find them and write them a ticket they can't afford, wasting lots of tax dollars and valuable police time. I think graffiti is like illegal marijuana; it's not even worth the time of the police or tax payers' dollars. The police should be going after the heroin, crack, fentanyl, and Carfentanil dealers who are killing people and not waste their valuable time chasing lost fifteen-year-old kids like myself through neighbourhoods with police dogs, just to issue a ticket and arrest them for something like graffiti.

Driving Life Into the Ground

When I moved to Cranston there wasn't very much to do because it was still all farmland being developed. Some friends and I would just walk around exploring and sometimes sneak into some of the empty construction houses. We would climb up into the rafters or try and get onto the roofs and just hang out while we smoke a joint or something. A friend and I were in the basement of a construction house when a worker came walking in upstairs. We both instantly panicked and started booking it for the nearest basement window to make our escape. We both jumped for the tiny window at the same time, only my friend gave me a little push mid-air to the side.

SPLAT. I ended up hitting the concrete wall of the basement while he climbed out of the window safe from any trouble. By now the worker upstairs hears the commotion in the basement and comes downstairs to investigate. I went and hid in the boiler room behind the furnace. My knee was sore from meeting the concrete wall so I now couldn't jump out. The worker walked around each room clearing them out one by one. He then comes in the furnace room. My heart is now beating like crazy because I'm stoned and now know I'm about to be busted and get in so much trouble. The man comes into the room and walks around the furnace counterclockwise. As he does this, I am slowly and as quietly as possible walking around it counterclockwise. He then goes clockwise so I change directions and start going clockwise around the furnace. He does two laps around the room then I hear him go "hmmm" obviously confused and then walks back upstairs and left. To this day, I'm still so glad there wasn't an opening in the furnace where he could see through because I would have been caught.

I met up with my friend a block or two away and told him the story. He bursts out laughing because he was the reason I almost got caught. I slugged him one in the arm and told him he was an ass while he argued his mid-air push wasn't intentional but just a natural reaction to the situation and we continued our random adventure through the neighbourhood and developing farmland.

Later, I was catching a bus home with a friend when a group of graffiti writers spotted us. My friend informed me that they were the ones that jumped him and sucker punched him a while back. So I got off the bus with a mini bat up my sleeve and they were all in a group fingering us and cussing us out. Pissed off at the world, I ran up to them all and started to scream my head off trying to provoke a fight with all four or five of them. Hoping they give me a reason to unleash all my anger and inner demons. However, very-angry me is not something anyone wants to voluntarily go after so they all just backed up towards the fence. I slid the mini bat out of my sleeve and they all started calling me names saying I was a pussy for having a weapon. By now, my friend gets off the bus and I'm there screaming at these kids and once they called me out for having a weapon, I just threw it away. It hit the fence and landed right by them so my friend casually walks over and grabs it off the sidewalk while I'm unleashing years of anger and frustration at these kids trying to fight them. None of them individually, nor all of them collectively, wanted to come near me. As I'm losing my shit on the side of the road trying to fight these kids that are about my age, a lady pulls her car over and she says she's calling the cops, so we got back on the bus and went home without incident.

On a March morning, I got up and like any other day, I had nothing to do but look for my next form of mental escape or form of numbness, so I called a friend to see if he wanted to hang out. He said he was interested to paint in his back yard or garage. I had no paint, but I told him, "I'll go rack a few cans again and head over." I jumped on the bus, headed to the store, walked into the paint isle and took a quick peek around. I didn't see anyone, so I opened my backpack and started filling it with paint. After putting five or six cans in my bag I turned around to see a woman just standing there watching me. I kept my head down, closed my bag and headed for the door as fast as I could. They kept on calling a code over the intercom and I was hoping it wasn't for me. The lady didn't appear to work there, she just looked like a shopper so I thought if I could get out fast enough, I'd be okay. I was not okay.

I got to the door, walked outside thinking I'm home free. Then out of nowhere this massive guy grabs me by the arm without saying a word. Not knowing who he was or what he wanted, I hit his arm as hard as I could to get him to let me go and I started running. I got about five steps when he dove for me like a football player and tackled me to the ground. He held me down with his 250-pound body rubbing my face into the concrete as we waited for the police. Once the police arrived and took me into custody, a lady who saw the first guy tossing me around came up and told them to relax and stop being so rough on me. From there, we went right to the district eight police station only a few blocks away. I had to call my mom to see if she would pick me up. After rightfully getting yelled at by my mom (to the point that I had the phone two feet away from my ear as both the cop and myself heard the screams coming from the phone) I hung up and called my dad who I expected to be out of town. However, he wasn't.

My father picked me up and drove me back to my mom's. When I got there, my suitcase was outside with some of my things. I knocked on the door and my mom told me I wasn't coming in. I asked to just get a few things from my room, so my older brother watched as I grabbed some clothes and other personal belongings. I then called my buddy and told him what had happened before I asked if I could crash at his place. He told me to come crash there so my dad drove me over to his place. My dad's wasn't an option because he was always back and forth between Alberta and Ontario at the time.

The first night as I tried to sleep on my buddy's couch, I remember thinking 'I can't believe my mom just kicked me out.' I then started reminiscing over the last few years of my life and how I was literally just driving it into the ground. Then I suddenly found myself wondering 'why did it take her so long to do so?' For years, I had given her more than enough reason to do so, but it wasn't until now that she did. I realized that night as I tried to sleep, what a coward, a loser, and horrible son I was over the years. That she finally kicked me out was truly a blessing in disguise. I know it must have been hard for her to do, but to this day, I'm glad and grateful she did it.

Still a homeless burden on my friends family from summer into the winter, I was sitting on a computer chair in my friend's room. We were watching the Boston playoff series on his TV like typical Canadians. While I was sitting there, out of nowhere, I got a sudden massive, intense, sharp headache. Right after that, I felt the need to vomit so I ran to the washroom and puked for a good five or ten minutes. When I returned to my buddy's room, he took one look at me and says, "You don't look so good man." I told him, "Yeah, I don't feel so good, I just spent the last five minutes puking in the toilet." I gave my emergency nurse mother a quick text of what happened and my symptoms. She was concerned. She wanted me to come in, so she paid for me to cab over to the Rockyview Hospital. After a brain scan, the conclusion was I had some trouble walking, left-sided weakness, and a massive headache caused by another, even bigger stroke. Once they saw I had a stroke, I was shipped to the Foothills Hospital.

Days later, while I was there, I got a call from my disgrace-of-a-legal-aid lawyer who asked, "Why were you not at court today?" I told him, "I'm at the Foothills Hospital recovering from a stroke," to which he replied with something like, "Oh okay." I then thought 'Oh great, so now I have a warrant out for my arrest.' As if having a second massive stroke at seventeen wasn't enough. My second stroke just reassured me that my time on this earth was very limited and I honestly thought I wasn't going to see my twentieth birthday now. It was a terrifying place to be. All my second stroke did was make the anger, frustration, depression, hatred, and pain in me rise to an unfathomable level. My lifestyle of living day-to-day solely looking for an escape from this just intensified the problem and anger I already had inside of me. But the escape was all I had. I had no idea what else to do, where to go, or how someone just becomes okay with dying in the beginning of their life. If I thought I was in a mental prison before my second stroke, the second stroke took me from a minimum, to a maximum-security mental prison and I felt, knew, and truly believed my death was going to be soon. I was in the hospital for about eight days with a wobbly walk and issues with my left hand.

I was still at my friend's house that spring when he got a call from his girlfriend's (abusive) ex-boyfriend saying that he and his friends were outside his girlfriend's house and they were going to start smashing windows if he didn't go fight him. So two of my friends, I, and his girlfriend at the time got into his green jeep to drive over to her house to see what's going on. We got there and there was nothing out of the ordinary so we slowly drove down the street looking to see if they were even out.

All of a sudden, my friend's girlfriend jumps out of the jeep yelling and screaming. I look in the back of his jeep and saw a small sports store. There was a bag of golf clubs, a baseball bat, and he's probably the only person you'll find driving around in the summer with ice skates, a hockey stick, and a hockey puck. I moved the football over and grab the bat before I jumped out. As a friend and I jumped out we saw my friend's girlfriend running down the dark alley towards a dark figure. Once she got close, this dark figure took a hail maker of a swing right for her head. I asked my friend if he just saw what I did, and he confirmed it. Fighting my friends and getting your ass kicked was one thing but hitting and attacking a woman because you can't get to or won't come to us, was another thing completely.

My buddy and I both took off running after her. Once the ex-boyfriend saw me coming, he took off running down the alley. Still with a bat in my left hand, I kept running after him down the alley, across the street, and into the adjacent parking lot where he went inside a 7-Eleven to try and hide from me. He had a hand on each door and his feet up against the doors leaning and pulling back as hard as he could trying to hold them shut to keep me out.

I walked up, smiled at him, then grabbed one of the doors with my right arm and ripped the door wide open. When I pulled the door open, it pulled him outwards towards me so he immediately backed up and went over to the counter. I walked up to him at the counter, and he then pulled a small pocketknife out on me. I thought about swinging the bat for a second till I realized I was in a store full of cameras and a witness so decided against it. But if the knife came near me, I'd be breaking an arm for sure. Knowing I can't beat his ass right there, I grabbed him and threw him into the counter as hard as I could before I told him, "If you ever hit a girl again, I'll find you and you won't be able to walk away once I'm done." He then slid to the floor with awe written all over his face.

I then see my friend pull up in his jeep and all sorts of commotion going on outside. I see the lady at the 7-Eleven is now on the phone with, who I'm assuming is, the police and I noticed her trying to make out the licence plate of my friend's jeep. I ran outside through a cloud of excess mace someone had sprayed and popped the hatch back on my friend's jeep so his licence plate was now up, and no one could see it. I then jumped in through the open hatch and told him to peel out. We ripped out of the parking lot and made a right onto the street where my friend, who was driving, saw one of the friends of the woman beater and swerved at him to scare him. I was still in the back trying to close the hatch of the jeep properly and when he swerved, I bounced off the right side of the jeep, then bounced off the left side of the jeep, lost my balance as I tripped over the small sports store in the back, and fell.

I fell into the hatch of the jeep and it flew wide open. As I fell out of the back of his moving jeep into the middle of an intersection. I heard "BOB!!" My friend's girlfriend screamed bloody murder as I'm falling out of the moving vehicle with some golf balls. I hit the pavement hard then rolled once or twice before I stopped. It was no worse than a fall off a longboard, which I was plenty use to by then. I quickly stood up to see the friend of the guy I just chased down into the store. Now all bloody with road rash and torn clothes I asked, "What's up? You want to go, mother fucker?" He just says, "I'm good," and kept on casually walking over to his friends at the store. I got back into the back seat of the jeep and we drove off but just as we got to my friend's girlfriend's house again, we got pulled over by the police. The cops took us all out, took our names, and then left. I was really confused on why we didn't get taken or interviewed harder. It would be some time later while I'm at work that I'd find out why.

At this point, all the legal issues I was currently dealing with were only going to get worse. On September tenth it was my eighteenth birthday and shortly after the 7-Eleven brawl I got up and got ready for work at a restaurant where I was working dish pit to make a little bit of money, but mostly to keep my goldfish probation officer from sending me to jail as my stunt at 7-Eleven got me an extra twelve months of probation with conditions such as maintaining full time employment, no contact orders, community service, and weapon restrictions. I spent all afternoon working and one of the girls heard it was my eighteenth birthday and offered to buy me a drink after my shift, so I stayed behind for an extra ten or fifteen minutes. Little did I know that one drink would spark more shitty events in my life.

After my rum and coke, I said thanks and goodbye to my co-worker before I skated over to the train station, got on the train, and sat down. The train made it two stops when I saw a buddy of mine get on the train. He was going to my friend's place where I was staying at the time, so I was stoked I now didn't have to walk by myself. We got off the train together and shortly after we started walking down Haddon Road, our buddy came ripping by us in is green jeep. He saw us and decided to pull a quick U-turn to pick us up. Only as soon as he pulled a U-turn, a cop turned the corner.

The officer saw him pull a U-turn and then pull over beside us. Before any of the three of us could speak, Woop Woop! the red and blue lights start flashing and a quick siren came on as the officer pulled up behind my buddy's car. The officer got out and asked for everyone's IDs. Dubious of the situation I pulled out my wallet and gave him my ID as he walked by to collect my other two friends' drivers licences before going back to his car. After running our names, he came back out, pushed me against the side of my friend's jeep, patted me down, and arrested me for breaching my probation conditions. One of my conditions was not to be anywhere near the buddy I was living with (unless in the presence of law), nor was I allowed to be carrying a knife. I got thrown into the back of the cop car and my two buddies got into the jeep and drove away. Despite the situation I was in, there was a good Gorillas song playing on the radio and I just sat there bobbing my head and quietly singing along as we drove downtown.

Once downtown they threw me in the drunk tank for holding until I was processed. Meanwhile, one of the officers started laughing at me and mocking me because it was my eighteenth birthday and I had been arrested. Knowing full well if it wasn't my eighteenth I'd be let go, but instead, I get to go to jail. The officer's teasing me, in return provoked me to tell all the jokes about me and the other officers banging his wife. I stood there at the counter going back and forth with this officer in an acrimonious discussion. Once I finally lost my temper, another officer had to come out and pull me away from the counter and put me back in the holding cell.

A few hours later, they took my mug shot and my extensive medical history before taking my fingerprints and putting me back in the holding cells. As I waited to see the JP (justice of the peace), an officer came by with a juice box and cheese sandwich for all the detainees to eat. I ended up falling asleep sitting on the floor with my arms crossed and head on the wooden bench. I was woken up in the middle of the night and put in the back of a van with another inmate. From there we headed out of town to the Remand Centre. Once we got to the Calgary Remand Centre, we were stripped nude, searched, and processed in again. After some time waiting in a separate room, an officer brought me to my first cell. It was about two or three in the morning at this point, and I was put in a two-man cell with two other people. I put my bed on the ground and I fell asleep right away. I was woken up again very early in the morning and was transferred to another cell. I was again placed on the ground for the day due to overcrowding.

The next morning, I was woken up and brought out to go to the courthouse downtown. I had my crappy coffee and orange and waited with the other inmates going to the courthouse as well. On the way I mentioned to another inmate that I was pissed about my $3,000 bail, and he laughed then mentioned his $30,000 bail for armed robbery. About a half hour later, we arrived and were taken into the basement of the courthouse where the holding cells were. As I sat in the cold, dark basement, I could hear the Calgary transit trains passing above every few minutes which let me know I was on the south side of the building underground near seventh avenue.

An officer came and got me a while later and took me into this small room that had a little television in it. He said someone would be there shortly to speak with me. A few minutes later a lady appeared on the television and started asking me questions. After making sure I was the right person, she then asked me why I had breached my probation conditions. So, I told her how I had probation conditions that stated I wasn't supposed to be around the person I was living with. She found it as silly as I did and didn't have anything to say after that.

After my short CCTV conversation with this lady, I was then put back in a cell for a few hours till my ride took me back to Remand. Once I was back there, I was back in another cell with my two cell mates. There, I watched as inmate after inmate would bring my one cellmate bread, jam, and peanut butter. I think he must have been a high-ranking gang member as I was thrown into a gang unit because I had my pocketknife on me when I was arrested. Which apparently automatically means I'm a gang member to the illiterate courts. I wasn't a gang member nor did I want or inspire to be one, I just wanted to live life before I died. But knowing I was in a gang unit had me stay quiet and just keep to myself.

The next day, I thought I should try and give my girlfriend a call to tell her what's going on if she didn't already know. As soon as the one hour of rec time came and the cell doors opened, I ran down the flight of stairs to the phones. I picked it up and tried to dial her number only jail phones you can't just pick up and dial there is a process to it. There's that and you can't just be going and grabbing first dibs on phones in a gang unit. As I was trying to figure out how to make a call, I hear a guy start screaming at me, "You better get off the phone, mother fucker." He was pissed off and coming straight for me. "Really man, you're going to fight me over a phone and be in jail longer because of it?" I asked. I wasn't interested in fighting a random inmate and starting shit in a gang unit, nor was I interested in extending my stay, so I hung up the phone and walked away. He started calling me a "bitch" and all sorts of names as I walked up the stairs back to my cell. I had no idea how long I was going to be in there and no one could or would tell me either. With an important yearly anniversary with my girlfriend now only a few days away I needed to get out of there sooner rather than later and a fight with a random in jail was not the way to go about it.

That night and the night after I couldn't sleep for the life of me. I was just staring at the walls. All I could think about was my upcoming anniversary, as well as wishing I was outside somewhere quiet and peaceful on my longboard. My entire life I was told I would be headed here and I always said that I didn't care, or so I thought. Now that I was here, reality set in, and I honestly didn't feel like living again. I realized I'd rather die outside in the vast open space of the wilderness than in a cell. With nothing to do but think, my mind went a bit stir crazy with anxiety.

I honestly couldn't imagine how a person facing life in prison must feel. I lay there for a few days telling myself 'I'll be out in time for my anniversary' and that 'I can make a change for the better before I died' I couldn't help but think back to every person that ever said I was going to end up a lowlife scumbag in jail. There I was, lowlife scumbag now complete. The piece of garbage that would never amount to shit in life was in full swing. Pondering the purpose of existing, life, and the world. I was wondering 'Why I was the one that survived. Why couldn't I have just died? How come my strokes or cancer couldn't have just taken my life?' That way I wouldn't have been here to deal with anything. If I died, I wouldn't be here suffering from my own poor choices and negative decisions. But I was very much alive and in the deepest darkest hole I ever dug for myself. Once again, I had found myself contemplating suicide for the rest of the night.

Next thing I noticed it was morning time and I was still super tired from my sleepless, mind wondering nights. I literally spent the morning lying on the ground. I didn't eat, I didn't read, I didn't go to the bathroom, I didn't do anything but lay there in my depressed-like state thinking how I'm in both a physical and mental prison at the same time. I realized I could drop dead right then and there and I'm confined to this brick room. I wasn't happy, I was not at peace with my life or myself, and I was unquestionably not at peace with my mind, body, or soul. What was the point of going through life if you were unhappy and miserable, especially when you had the risk of dying without warning at any given second? I realized I could have another stroke and die right then and there. I then thought about dying within the walls of the jail. I wondered if I'd even get the medical attention I needed or if they would just shrug it off like my dad and his two-faced girlfriend and wait till they found my unresponsive body. That led me to then think about what I would have left behind. I found it would have been nothing but pain, frustration, more pain, sprinkled with a dump truck load of stress, and more frustration, nothing else. I had no education, no life, no purpose, no direction, and no way out of the mental or physical entrapment I was currently in at the time.

I couldn't let my life end like this. **No matter what** I did, I had to change, or die trying. But how does one change? How does one shed eighteen years of insurmountable anger, pain, depression, and frustration without doing drugs, beating the shit out of people, and ending up here? I just did my best to **remember to** tell myself 'I can and will change my life for the better.'

As I'm thinking about all of this, the intercom in the room went off and asked for me. I replied and the voice told me to come down to the den where all the officers were caged in behind the protective glass. I walked up to the protective octagon and asked what they wanted. They told me I was being processed for release and to go gather my things, drop off the mat I was sleeping on, and wait until they call me. I got all excited thinking I was going to be able to go home. But I had no home, I torched that bridge six months ago. I anxiously waited and waited and waited with my things ready to go, but I never left. I sat by the door waiting all night ready, excited, and believing I'm about to go. However, I was there another sleepless night because of "administrative things". I could see the rain outside the tiny slit of a window at the top of the west cell wall and couldn't help but think 'well at least I'm inside and not being released into the pouring rain.' Giving up on waiting to be released, I called the officers to bring me my mat back so I could try to go to bed, but they had none for me.

The next day, I went down and checked out some books killing time, trying to be patient with the officers but ended up going over to the den and complaining how I was told I was going to be released the day before, then slept without a bed on the concrete and I was still there. The officer said, "Oh okay. I'll look into it for you." Again, I was just staring through the concrete block walls expecting to be released soon. I told my roommate I should have been released last night and he said I would be that morning; then he asked if he could have my breakfast tray saying, "You can go get some real food once you're out." I couldn't argue about that. I still hadn't eaten anything but a couple oranges, a terrible breakfast tray, a terrible supper tray, a crappy coffee, and zero actual cups of water within the last week. I had absolutely no appetite. After waiting all morning and into the afternoon I began to regret giving my roommate with the massive Scarface scar my breakfast and lunch trays, by mid-afternoon my hunger caught up to me and my stomach started screaming gurgling noises at me.

Finally, they called my name, so I brought my things down ready to throw a fit if they slow rolled me on my release again. They verified who I was, gave me my belongings and a bus ticket, then told me to walk down the road back to the city and take the bus home. After getting all my things, I walked out of the building, jumped on my longboard and headed for the city; but where was I to go?

With nowhere else to go, I went back to my buddy's house (where I still had the conditions that I couldn't be around him as nothing got resolved from my honesty with the judge on the CCTV) after eating some food and taking a huge hoot of cannabis oil that was there waiting for me. I got a hold of my girlfriend and took off to see her at our friend's house for the night. We hung out and I had some hoots with our other friend while I told them all about my awesome eighteenth birthday, the long work week trip to jail, and how stupid the whole situation was. Then it was back to the whole endless circle of drugs fighting and frustration. Only after going to jail, I had more anger and frustration pent up ready for the next person.

I went to pick up my girlfriend from her school sometime later. After I walked and skated over to the school, I met with her. At some point we were walking down the hallway in her school when the brother (of the woman beater) turned the corner and saw me. He looks right in my eyes and said, "What's up, Brandon," in a stupid voice as he walked with a friend giving me a stupid shit grin. I snapped back with, "What's up, you fucking bitch." I was overly sick of him, and his brother and I didn't try to hide that fact at all. He then came up to me raising his hands ready to fight so right then and there we just started to throw down in the middle of the hall of a school I didn't even go to. My girlfriend just broke down crying and ran away from the random, chaotic scene as I was swinging away.

We continued to fight for a bit when he tried to put me in a head lock or something while simultaneously trying to punch me in the back of the head. It felt like my mom lightly rubbing her knuckles into my head giving me a noogie as a child. I grabbed his arm and twisted it enough that I got out of his hold. I fed him a few shots, then grabbed him, and threw him face first into the lockers (like I did to his brother at 7-Eleven into the counter). When he connected with the lockers, it made a really loud face-on-hollow-metal-box BANG. It was like someone just booted it with steel-toed boots. He got up noticeably wobbly for a second and tried to give me a jab in the face but missed the first try as I backed up. I walked back up to him again and he finally got a little hit on me, square in the face. That pissed me off a bit, so I threw him around the empty hall some more and gave him a few more blows. While we were fighting, a teacher came running out of his room into the hall and broke it up. The brother not wanting to get in trouble immediately ran the other way. The teacher then grabs me trying to hold me back. Filled with adrenaline from the unexpected fight, I took a serious look at him and said, "Look man one of your students just assaulted me, so I defended myself. You have absolutely no right to touch me, so unless you want to start fighting me next you better let me go." He knew I was right and got noticeably flustered so he let me go and I took off to find a bathroom for my now bleeding nose and to find my girlfriend.

These brothers seemed to be really persistent in trying to get us in trouble. Not long after that, they called me and my friend a few times telling us to come fight them. We would show up to their house or wherever they said to go, and then they would just call the cops. We would have no choice but to leave so I didn't get arrested again, but we always came in case they decided to man up one day.

My roommate got that call from them a while later. We were more than fed up with them and ready to fight at a moment's notice so as soon as he got off the phone we got in the jeep and drove off. We were driving down Canyon Meadows when a Nissan Skyline flew by us and cut us off. I turned to my buddy and said, "What a dick, this guy," as I pointed to the car. That's when my buddy noticed it was one of our other friends by the decals on the back. This friend is always down to brawl and fight as he's a very rowdy, rambunctious person just like his older brother. They're not the type of people I would want to upset that's for sure.

So, I called him up, he answers on speaker as I asked, "Are you driving down Canyon Meadows and just cut off a jeep?" He laughed and said, "Yeah, how do you know that?" sounding confused. I told him we were the ones in the jeep, and we were on the way to fight the brothers, then asked if he wanted to come. He's heard all the stories about the brothers and doesn't even hesitate to tag along with us. We got to the parking lot of the same 7-Eleven (that I also have conditions I'm not allowed to be around) and the brothers were actually there. I got out and started walking towards them. As I'm walking up to them across the parking lot our other buddy, rips through the parking lot in his Skyline, rips his e-break, puts it sideways, gets out, and starts screaming his head off at them. One of the brothers told the other to call the cops as usual. I didn't even give him the chance and I just started swinging. He put the phone to the right side of his head; so, in an attempt to break him and the phone I punched the phone into his head and they both went flying. I was so fed up with them constantly instigating and provoking a fight, then calling the cops, I kept swinging. Next thing I know, my other buddy was swinging at him too so after his fair share of a beat down I stopped. The brothers quickly backed off and as they tried to run away, I saw my one friend punch one of the brothers so hard in the back I felt it in my chest, I felt the punch a good twenty feet away. I shouted at the brothers one last time before we got in our cars and went home like nothing happened.

At first, I felt kind of bad at how badly the one brother and his phone got it. But then I started to think about it, and when you call someone to fight two on two then get your ass beat two on two, what do you really expect. Plus, when you're threatening to beat and attack women in the process, to me you more than deserve a good ass beating. It could have been three on two and we could have done some considerable "send them to the ER" damage, but the third person wasn't even necessary.

A few months later, a few friends and I were at another friend's having a few drinks when I went inside to pour myself another. I realized I had left the chase (pop) in my friend's car so I ran out to grab it. I go outside, down the steps, and over to the car parked on the street. That's when a group of four or five people (the same graffiti ones from the bus stop incident months prior) spotted me and instantly start calling me out. I quickly ran inside and screamed that there was some beef going on outside so come out front. As I ran back outside, I grabbed a broom stick I saw on the ground along the way and brought it with. The group of guys were still there screaming and hollering at me out front on the street. I ran at them and screamed, "Let's go, mother fuckers!" But they just scattered everywhere so I ran after some. I was now in the adjacent alleyway with a few of them that were still threatening me and calling me names. One of them was grabbing rocks from the alley and throwing them in my direction trying to hit me with no success. I stood my ground in the dark alley at one or two in the morning and backed them up back into the street where I can see one of my friends using a spray paint can and a lighter as a flame thrower to defend himself from the people that sucker punched him before and were now again threatening him. Another one of my friends came ripping beside me in his big truck swerving at the group of people making some distance between them and myself so I could get away.

As I ran over to my friend with the flaming spray can, I heard something to my left, so I looked and there is an older gentleman standing on his stoop in his robe talking on the phone looking directly at me. I shouted out, "K, it's time to go, guys." I had the option to jump into my friend's car who I was living with but still had probation conditions so I couldn't be around him. Because of that, I chose to go with my other friend in his car. He got in the driver's, a friend got in the front, and I jumped in the back seat behind the driver before we took off.

We made it about two blocks away when a cop car flew by us before immediately slamming on the breaks and turning around. As soon as we saw them turn around, we all knew we were about to get pulled over and we were right. The lights and siren went on, so we pulled over. As multiple police cars group around and behind us an officer got on the intercom and tells my friend to turn off the car, then to step out with his hands up, and proceed to walk backwards towards his voice with his hands in the air. He did the same for our friend in the front who I'm sure was scared and confused on what was going on. She knew that our friend was sucker punched a while ago but probably didn't know it was by one of those guys I just unexpectedly ran into.

Then the police got me to come out. I stepped out and raised my hands, I placed them on the back of my head with my fingers interlaced like the officer said and started to walk backwards towards what seemed to be the entire district-8 police force. As I was walking backwards, I took a peek over my left shoulder to see where I was going and if there was anything in the way. I didn't see anything in the way but I saw five or six squad cars, a few police-issued, twelve-gauge shot guns, and several hand guns pointed at me everywhere. They ran my friends' names and they were let go when they came up clean. I, on the other hand, had a warrant out for a ticket I didn't **remember to** pay, so I was put in the back of the cop car, again. As I sat in the backseat handcuffed, I looked at the officer's computer screen and saw the neighbour's call into the police. It said there was "reports of people fighting in the streets with sticks and flamethrowers." Then a description of me and only me. Not a single other of the ten people, just me. It wasn't till later I'd find out if I went with my other friend (who I had probation conditions not to be with) I would have been fine, but I avoided it because of the legalities with it. 'So much for trying to do the right thing for once' I said to myself when I found that out.

After sorting out that legal issue, I was at work for the day. My boss asked me to go do inventory in the walk-in freezer and fridge. I grabbed the clip board and went into the freezer. As I'm checking off how much of what is there, I hear a loud bang on the door. The door opens slowly and I looked up to see a fully uniformed police officer. I had no idea why he was there. He looks at me and asks, "Are you Brandon Harrison?" I replied hesitantly and slowly say, "Umm yeah." Right then and there in the freezer, I was thrown in cuffs and arrested. My boss came up and asked the cop if he could take me out the back door and not walk me through the lobby in cuffs in front of all the customers. The jerk said, "Nope. Car is out front." Then dragged me through the lobby and out the doors to the cop car. I was then taken to the 8th precinct again to be officially charged with assault from the 7-Eleven incident a few weeks before. No idea why it took a few weeks. I thought if I would have been charged, it would have been when the cops pulled us over right after the incident, that night. Turns out the one brother (who was punched in the back by my friend) lied and told the police it was me that attacked him with a bat and tried to play the poor innocent victim like always.

I guess the brothers decided they couldn't win face to face, so they would screw me over one last time and filed a false report against me, even though they provoked and started nearly every altercation we ever had (besides the fight in the school). I was released on a "promise to appear" in court and let go. I then ran back to work to get my stuff only to find my girlfriend came by and picked it up for me but forgot to tell me, so I went back and had a chat with the boss about what just happened. I told him about chasing the cowardly woman beater down and throwing him into the counter of a 7-Eleven after watching him punch my friend's girl. I told him I didn't regret it and if I had to, I'd do it all over again. He appreciated my honesty, but after missing a week of work because of getting arrested on my eighteenth birthday and now being arrested in work and missing more, I rightfully lost all the respect and work ethic I put in over the months and I was fired. I then began the second walk of shame through the lobby that day. Now expecting to go to jail as soon as my P.O found out I no longer had a job. I was again majorly pissed off at everything all the while looking for more work.

After I talked to the JP and judge when I was in jail and told them I had conditions I could not be around the person I was living with I made the terrible assumption of thinking they would remove that condition for some stupid reason. This would prove to be a terrible assumption. It was probably around 1 or 2 a.m. one December morning when my buddy and I went to go grab a late-night bite to eat at McDonald's. We got in the jeep and took off. We got there, placed our orders, got our food, and then proceeded to head back to his house. We turned right out of the drive-through and headed south on McLeod Trail and immediately a police car pulled out of the night club parking lot that was directly beside the McDonald's and came out behind us. I thought 'Oh great. Here we go again.' The cop followed us down the road and turned right onto Southland Drive, continuing to follow us for an unusual length of time. At this point, I knew we were going to be pulled over. "Woop woop" The red and blue lights start flashing just as my buddy turned right onto Haddon Road and pulled over. Now we were in the exact same spot we were in when I got arrested on my eighteenth birthday, not even twenty feet from that very same spot.

My buddy told me to pretend I'm his brother and try to get off that way, but I knew if I was caught in a lie, I'd probably have some sort of charge added onto the probation breach and worsen my situation. The officer comes up and asks us for identification. I reluctantly give him my ID and he goes off to run our names. He quickly comes back and says, "Hey Brandon, I'm going to need you to step out of the car for me." 'Fuck sakes,' I thought as I comply and get out of the car. He says, "You're under arrest," and reads me my rights. He says he pulled us over because of a busted taillight, but it was working just fine when I looked at it on the way to the cop car. They followed us for so long looking for any reason to pull us over and when they didn't have one, they just made one up.

'You slimy pieces of shit, I'm getting really sick of these cops, lawyers, and shitty court system' I couldn't help but think as I went back downtown to jail for processing. We got there, I had my picture and prints taken, went through my extensive medical history, and after being in the cell all night I was released on another promise to appear for court. I was confused on why I only kept getting arrested and not my friend as well, so I asked the cop. The cop says, "you have conditions you can't be around him unless in the presence of law, but he doesn't have conditions, so he can be around you." I said, "That's the most illogical thing I've ever heard of. So, he can just roll up to me in his car without me knowing (like he did on my eighteenth) and that's enough to send me to jail? Seriously, who makes up this crap?" I asked. He said something like "it is what it is man" as he gave me a bus ticket and sent me on my way to get my belongings and go home.

At the same time that I was starting to believe I wasn't going to see twenty years old, I had to go to court every other week. On top of the garbage of court, I had to go see this probation officer that had the people skills of a goldfish. A goldfish that was left for a month, went belly up, then was flushed. She seemed to get a raging hard-on for threatening me with jail time if I breached my conditions. Every meeting it was the same: Belittle me for being a low-life piece of shit, then kick me out the door to have to come back the next week and repeat the cycle. When she didn't believe I had a second stroke and that's why I missed court, my mom showed up to her office and explained everything. My P.O then decided to take this confidential conversation with my mom to my dad and started a bunch of crap between them. After that, my dad called my mom about what she told him, so my mom called my P.O and went at her with "both barrels". After my mom put her right in her place, my P.O stopped trying to pry in their business and went right back to mine.

It started to feel like I literally had the weight of the world on my chest. The hate, anger, frustration, depression, and rage in me just continued to compound which made me look for an escape from reality more than ever. I used this compiling anger and frustration to fuel the rages behind my fights with cowards, thieves, graffiti writers, and anyone that wanted to go against me. With believing I wasn't going to be alive for much longer anyway, I started to mentally long for a way out. I desperately needed to find a way to change my life's course and get on the right path, the path I have never seen in my life. But switching onto the right path wasn't enough. I needed a purpose, I needed to find myself, I needed direction, and more than anything else, I needed to find my inner peace and happiness.

Every day, I had this "I don't give a damn" kind of attitude because I honestly didn't expect to live very long and that had me not caring about anything, especially life itself. I didn't care about life, death, morals, kindness, or anything at all. I only wanted and looked for my next escape and day by day, week by week, and month by month I became more of an ungrateful and unscrupulous asshole. How was one supposed to respect life when it was horrible, disgusting, unfair, and painful? I became incredibly ungrateful for the things I had because my anger, rage, bitterness, depression, and hate blinded me. Then once the drugs came in, it blinded me even more, but that is exactly what I wanted. I wanted out of the reality I was in. Drugs helped provide me with that escape. But when you came down from your high, you realized your life is still the same pile of shit as it was before, so you went back on a mission to find another escape. I found myself getting caught in the endless cycle of the drug life. I found the addiction isn't the hardest problem to quit. It's not only breaking the habit of addiction that is hard. The habits of quickly stealing cash, emptying your bank to go score, the going to get your drug of choice, then the choice to go use it when and wherever you can, all had to be broken. Then there's the debating to go use it when you're stressed, which for me was an everyday occurrence from morning to night. Then there are the people that came with the drug life that all had to go.

For example, I gave my so-called friend money to go get me some drugs when he went to meet his guy. It was a couple days later when I called him to bring my stuff or my money back. He told me to go screw myself, so of course we started arguing. He then told me I was a bitch and told me to come fight him at the windmill in our neighbourhood. I told him I would be right there. I hung up the phone and started to look for some sort of weapon because I knew it was going to be an unfair fight. I knew I would probably need one for self-defence purposes so I'm looking around the garage, basement, and my closet for something. I then suddenly realized I had my pocketknife on me. I only ever used it as a handy tool so the thought of it being used as a weapon never crossed my mind until then. I grabbed my longboard and started to skate to the windmill. As I'm coming down the main drag I'm pushing as hard as I can, just flying down the street. I then saw him standing there with four others. He was apparently still chirping saying, "He's not coming, he's a pussy," till he saw me ripping down the street doing close to the speed limit. When I saw the group of people at the windmill, I began to push even harder and flew right through the T-intersection of the road and went right for him. With the speed and momentum of me flying down the street, I rode into him and pushed him. He went airborne for a bit before he hit the grass and rolled two or three times and I told him to give me my money. Instead, he got up and punched me in the face. So, I started to throw some back and after two or three swings I connected to the left side of his face and he dropped to the ground like a sack of potatoes. While he was on the ground, I went to give him another pop but his brother came at me, so I started to swing and fight him too.

While I'm fighting his brother, one of their friends reached into a backpack and threw a baton at the brother that stole my money. He whipped out the metal baton and took a sturdy swing. The hard baton cracked across the back of my head hard and confirmed to me that this was going to be an unfair fight as I'm now fighting multiple people who are using weapons—by myself. I grabbed my knife, flicked out the blade, and asked, "Do you really want to fight with weapons?" But he decided to run away almost getting hit by a city bus in the process. I put my knife away, walked up to the brother and their friend that gave him the baton and asked if they wanted to have a go with me. None of them said anything and I said, "That's what I fucking thought." I said goodbye to the one neutral buddy who stood there with his little brother watching the fight, just caught in the crossfire of the whole situation and left.

I got on my board and proceeded to skate back home. Needless to say, I stopped hanging out with those three guys after that and still didn't have my money or the drugs that I wanted to numb myself with. There are so many habits I had to break free from, not just the love of the drug itself. In my opinion, this is where "Addiction is not a disease, it's a choice" makes sense. But to me, it's both,

I see it as a disease that causes an addictive, impulsive, self-destructive series of choices in order to get what you want. But to break the habit of the poor spontaneous decision making, then to break the impulses, then to still have to face breaking off the drug itself, only to then have to break off the relationships with all individuals associated with the drug or drug culture is a monumental amount of inner will and decision making that sometimes one does not want to face, or accept.

I started to think my life couldn't get any worse and knew I needed to get out of this endless loop of petty arrests, court dates, and meetings with the most horrid probation officer in existence. I was still getting angrier, more frustrated, and desperately needed to find a way to keep my sanity through all of it, which, at the time, was my girlfriend. But with the constant fighting and way I was living my life I didn't expect my life to last much longer as a single blow to the head could kill me. I again thought life couldn't get any worse, but I was more wrong than I've ever been.

Turning Martian

This chapter is dedicated to my uncle, father figure, and hero. To the late Anthony (Tony) Harrison, as well to all my Martian brothers and sisters out there who have been impacted by impaired driving. My deepest heartfelt condolences are with you, your family, and dearest loved ones. I'm terribly sorry for your unexpected and tragic loss. I'm even sorrier that you (likely) had to deal with a court system that was only there to make a profit off of that loss. It's time we share our stories to the world. It's time we shed light on the biggest, darkest, coldest, most immoral, broken, and unjust system in the world. It's time for a change for the better.

July 15th, 2012. I woke up on my buddy's couch as per usual for that time of my life. I grabbed my phone to see I had many missed calls and text messages. My first thought was 'Oh! Mr. Popular today.' Then I noticed it was all from my immediate family who I wasn't really in contact with at the time. I got up, stepped over my friend who crashed on the floor for the night, and went outside into the backyard to call my father. He told me that my uncle Tony had been killed by a drunk driver earlier that morning while he rode his motorcycle home. His words went into my ear, but they didn't register. I said, "What!?" hoping new words would come out of his mouth but he repeats that Tony was killed in the early morning hours by a drunk. The words I didn't want to register hit me, but I didn't want to believe it, I didn't want to accept it, nor did I want it to be true. How could the strongest being I know, someone who took a 9mm slug to the head and lived, just suddenly be gone? He couldn't die, he was so stupidly inhumanly strong that the thought of him being able to die didn't cross my mind. He had been a super human to me all these years. But he was still human, and humans inevitably die.

I got off the phone with my dad and immediately called my mother. We made plans to go out to my grandma's house as a family. I then called the bakery I was working at and let them know I wouldn't be coming in that day because of a family emergency. At this point, I was still in a state of shock and couldn't really feel or recognize what was going on. I headed over to my mother's before we went over to my grandmothers to see everyone. It wouldn't be until Tony's wake where I'd realize just who and what I had lost. I walked over to where Tony's lifeless body was peacefully laying in a casket. As I got closer, my feet started moving slower and slower. I wasn't intentionally trying to slow down but I think my brain recognized the situation and forced me to slow down because I wasn't at all ready for this. I got to the casket, looked inside, and there lay Tony's lifeless body. His entire body was swollen from hands to face. He looked very unnatural and un-human like. I stood there for maybe five or ten minutes just staring in disbelief. I then grabbed Tony's right hand and it was so swollen, cold, hard, and so lifeless it was the moment I broke like a tooth-pick and started crying my face off. I took off outside without saying a word to anyone and sat behind the funeral home under a tree and cried it out for a good half hour or hour nonstop before I got it together and went back inside. I don't think I've ever cried that much or that hard in my entire life. After the wake, we went and celebrated Tony's life at a family friend's house. We all gathered around for drinks and told funny stories about Tony's past. It was a blessing he had made it that far in life to begin with after being shot. I drank my rum and coke as we all laughed about the shenanigans him, and his friends caused over the years. Although we were smiling and laughing, we fought so hard to hold back tears.

Tony's killer was driving his minivan drunk on his third DUI and swerved over the centre yellow line. Flying down the highway, Tony laid his bike down trying to avoid the crash, but it was far too late. He hit Tony head on, killing him on impact. The coward then got out of his minivan and fled the scene on foot leaving Tony's lifeless now opened body cavity and motorcycle behind in the street with his van like it was all just trash. Witnesses called the police who happened to be in the area, and he was quickly found in a nearby field with his car keys still in his pocket and he was still three times over the legal driving limit when he was finally breathalyzed. He was arrested but shortly released on a two-thousand-dollar bail just a day or two after Tony's funeral. He was free to go back to his family a week after destroying mine. Freed on a bail that was less than mine for breaching a probation condition. It boggled my mind at how asshat backwards, pathetic, and useless the court system was. My logic says that someone who kills someone on their third charge should have a significantly higher bail than someone who was walking home and breached their probation conditions for the first time (as far as they knew).

I was so distraught that I didn't even realize it was my mother's birthday the day we buried Tony. The timing of it all was just horrific for my poor mother. The limo picked us up at my mom's before we all went to the funeral home again. There was a group of cars outside and a few motorcycles when we pulled up. With so many people there, they had to open an overflow section. When we walked inside, the hall was packed with people from the front row to the back. We walked down the middle isle and took a seat at the front with our family members. After the service, our family got back in the limo and the limo followed the hearse out of the parking lot and made a right onto the very road Tony was killed on. As we drove down the road, a trail of cars followed. As we came down 17th Avenue, Tony's friend came up on his motorcycle and led the convoy of vehicles. As we came down the hill of the valley my great-grandmother turned around and took a look out the back of the limo. "WOW! I've never seen anything like that before," she says as she sees the entire hill of 17th Avenue covered with motorcycles. I turned around to see all the westbound lanes of the hill covered with motorcycles. Two riders beside each other in each lane, two or three lanes across, stretched from the top of the hill all the way to the bottom.

Once we made it down the hill, we had to make a left turn onto Blackfoot trail. Only the light was not going to be long enough for everyone that came. Tony's friend who was leading everyone saw this and instead of making the left turn, he pulled up in front of the cop car that was first up waiting for the green light and he sat there. I had a laugh that the huge biker was just sitting sideways blocking the cop car so everyone could make the turn. We took Blackfoot all the way to the graveyard where Tony was to lay his head for the last time. From the moment we arrived to the moment we left, I had tears running down my face. As they lowered Tony's casket into the deep dark hole on top of my papa, I walked up to my mother and wrapped my arms around her. Squeezing her tight, we both cried it out for a few minutes. That was the last day anyone got to see my uncle, father figure, and hero.

The entire court process associated with the death of Tony was nothing but a vexatious atrocity. Every time my family would go in, they would have to re-experience the pain and suffering caused by the coward that killed him. Only to have a lawyer find the smallest thing to postpone the court to a further date and then the whole process would repeat. The murderer would go home free as my family was left grieving. It would be THREE agonizing Christmases, New Year's, birthdays, and crash anniversaries without Tony before we finally got a sentencing date. Three years later our entire family was there, I even showed up in my wheelchair ready to pounce on the loser that took Tony from us all. A few family members got to read their victim impact statements before he was sentenced. He was sentenced to six years in jail which was a huge deal and a hard sentence for his crime in Canada. However, he immediately started to apply for appeals and once again my poor mother, face-punching cousin, and grandmother had to go experience the pain again and again and again while arguing why he should stay in jail.

This killer's bail was a thousand dollars less than mine when I was arrested on my eighteenth and he was pretty much free for the entire three years till his sentencing. This whole process is just a huge stab in the back and slap to the face of my family, or any family that has been destroyed by someone's cowardly actions. We have our families horrifically torn to shreds, only to then be betrayed by the very court system that we are led to believe is there for the people's (society's) protection. But nope, to me it seems they just dig the knife in deeper and spin it a few times. It became abundantly clear to me that the courts are just here to help themselves to money in taxes, court fees, and lawyer bills. I horrifically realized we are solely there to be monetized even more when tragedy strikes, not helped. I think we should all take a page from their book and just start paying one third of our taxes if they're going to be releasing people after one third of their prison sentences. Whatever happened to that saying "you get what you paid for?" Well, we aren't getting anything from this broken system, so why are we paying them so much money?

I thought I was mad before, well Tony's death, followed by the unexpected court's betrayal, had me angrier and more upset than I've ever been. I now didn't only want to watch the world burn. I wanted to dump the gas, light the match, and be the one to make the world burn. It was an incredibly unhealthy mental state to be in. The stories I've heard from my Martian family are truly horrific and not something I would wish upon my best friend or worst enemy.

Some of the things they've had to go through include having perfectly fine, job-working, guitar-playing individuals kill their family members only to get off by "not being mentally fit to stand trial." The story that pisses me off and breaks my heart most was when my Martian sister watched her two-year-old child get killed in front of her as they sat eating at a patio. The drunk that drove through the patio was arrested and went to jail for four months and then was released. When my friend took that case all the way to Ottawa to the Supreme Courts the Courts said, "Sending him to jail longer than four months would cause him (the child killer) unjust harm." Now imagine the courts telling you that jailing the person that killed your child in front of you would be "unjust." This is why that piece of trash was kidnapped, beaten, and had his thumb cut off by people like me. I had nothing to do with any of that but if that happened to my family, I wouldn't hesitate to go vigilante-street-justice on someone. Especially if the courts just shit all over my family like they did. In my personal experience, there is no such thing as justice in the court system. Then the courts go and wonder why people go out of their way to take matters into their own hands. Personally, I don't understand why it doesn't happen more often with how useless and shameless the courts are.

Longboarding and music were my only healthy escapes from the mental entrapment I was in for years. When I had no drugs, alcohol, or paint, I found I would get on my board and go skate the pathways and listen to music all day. After an hour or two, I would forget what I was stressing about and just enjoy my freedom out in the vast beautiful peaceful space on my board. I found myself spending more and more time on my board in the provincial park and as the days went on, I found myself enjoying it more and more. The only problem was by now I was probably a borderline drug addict. I still craved the escape that drugs gave me so any chance, or opportunity I could, I was still doing them at my own will.

It didn't help that most of my friends were experimenting with them, buying them, and bringing them around too. That's when I realized the hardest part of quitting any addiction (for me) is kicking the people associated with them out as well. But when you spend most of your life with these people and know these people are always there for you no matter what, it makes it a hundred times harder to let them go. That was something I couldn't bring myself to do because I knew that at the end of the day these people have my back and most of them are actually decent individuals. There was no problem letting go of cowards (like the windmill guy) as you're much better off without them in your life. But now, I was that coward who gave up on everything in life. I gave up on school, I gave up trying, I truly believed I would never have a future and that I would be dead soon. I was in a constant state of self-destructing depression and still wanted to light the match and watch the world burn. I quickly realized there was no way I was going to be able to face my fear of death or benefit from being confined inside brick walls all day wondering if life's even worth living. So every day I could, I jumped on my longboard and I'd go explore neighbourhoods and parks all over the city.

I love Calgary for many things, one of them being the hundreds of kilometres of paved pathways that go all up and down the Bow River and throughout Fish Creek Provincial Park. Every day I would go skate and explore further and further away. Some days, friends would come with and we would take breaks in swim holes to cool off, we would sometimes climb as high as we could in the massive trees like a cat. Hilarity would arise when one of us got stuck or too scared to come down, paralyzed in fear. Our words of encouragement would be pelting them with acorns calling them names. Sometimes someone would get really frustrated trying to find the right way, break off from the group, and just go home. Eventually I'd run out of pathway at the end of the city limits and turn around to go back home or do another lap through the park.

I found and fell in love with this amazing scenic sixty-kilometre route from my mom's house to the west edge of the city limits to the reserve and back. I spent lots of my teen years longboarding this route in Fish Creek. I got to know all the sweet hang out spots where my friends and I would go relax from time to time. It would be here I would have my best and most frequent moments of happiness, peace, and clarity. I wasn't stressing if I was going to die or not because it was so fun, so peaceful, and beautiful. It was the only time I felt at peace and content without the use of drugs.

Skating deep into Fish Creek and far away from home was always risky though. I remember being out by the reserve with my friends, and all three of us biffed off our boards on the same corner. I ended up getting the worst of it after bouncing off the grass and back onto the cement. I was suddenly missing skin on my knees, hips, arms, elbows, sides, shoulders, and back, as well as my standard nosebleed. I then had to skate about twenty-five to thirty kilometres back home covered in blood and missing massive pieces of my skin everywhere. All-the-while baking in the hot sun. People would be walking by me and freak out more than I did, asking if I needed an ambulance or need them to call 9-1-1. I would just say, "Nope, I'm fine," and continue on in agonizing pain, just trying to get home. There, the emergency nurse could patch me up before I was off to do it all over again. It amazes me how resilient longboarders are. We would cheese grate massive portions of our skin on the pavement. Only to get back up and do it all over again the day they are healed, If not before then.

When I was thirteen or fourteen, I watched an hour-long documentary while my mother was off to work for a late-night shift. This documentary was about a psychiatrist who took a half-dozen terminal cancer patients facing death to a remote resort in the beautiful British Columbia area and gave them a dose of Lysergic acid otherwise known as LSD. Each of these patience explained how they experienced a profound peace. This peace forever changed their perspective and outlook on both their dire situations, and life. Each of them explained how their experience took away all stress, worry and anxiety. They each explained how they felt like "a normal person" and how they "felt like themselves" for the first time since their diagnosis.

Years later, this story came back to my mind after getting into a very in-depth conversation about psychedelic drugs with a friend. My fear of death after my second stroke had never been more real. This conversation made me think about self-dosing myself with LSD. As I lay down trying to sleep, I thought about it. My depression was at an all-time high with my goldfish of a probation officer still threatening me weekly, the suicidal thoughts came to me on a regular basis, and I was getting into fights all the time. Throw in mandatory court dates, mandatory dead-end jobs to work, and feeling like the world's biggest piece of shit and, after all that, losing the man that kept my family together. I felt incredibly suicidal. I was so sick of it all and I felt I should just end it. "I was a piece of garbage who was going nowhere and wasn't going to achieve anything in life" according to my probation officer and many others. So, if I died the world would be a lot better off, right? I again thought about ending my life as I tried to fall asleep that night. I then thought about my long-term girlfriend and my mother and what killing myself would do to them. I couldn't do it, leaving holes in their hearts and lives was not the answer to solving MY issues. However, I was so done with life that the urge to kill myself grew beyond just thoughts. 'What do you have to lose, worst case, I'll have a stroke and die peacefully. Best case scenario, "I feel like a person and get my life back again."

I concluded dying from drugs would be better than intentionally killing myself even though it could have done the same thing but I didn't care, I was done with it all so I asked my buddy to ask his guy if he could meet me the next day. Before I even looked at my phone the next morning, I woke to the thought of the world benefiting from my death, again. Was I going to die today? Was it going to be from LSD or was it going to be from jumping in front of a train? I was up early so I hung around until buddy text me. I was eager to meet this guy and grab the LSD. I was slightly weary, but my buddy vouched to me that it was good product, and he was reliable. Once I got the message, I grabbed my longboard and left to go meet this random guy and go skate in Fish Creek Park, just like any other day. I met the random guy at one of the train stations close to Fish Creek. Immediately after our hand-to-hand exchange I unfolded the tinfoil it came in and put a singular tab under my tongue as suggested and started skating. I can still remember the moment, feelings, and emotions like it was yesterday.

It was another beautiful day in the provincial park, the sun was shining bright which had me feeling good. It wasn't too hot and there wasn't a cloud in sight. I was skating my favourite twenty-kilometre loop and I got to the part where the head wind I was battling for an hour turned into a tail wind which was pushing me along at a nice steady cruise. The shuffle on my Blackberry was running into all my favourite Tupac songs and then out of nowhere when I least expected it, it hit me like a ton of bricks.

BAM. My life literally flashed before my eyes faster than the speed of light and I had this huge release of stress, anxiety, and worry. Suddenly encircled in a mental and physical place so beautiful, peaceful, and joyful I thought 'so what you might die.' You could go through life not smoking, you could eat healthy, and exercise regularly. But no matter what you do, at some point, you are still going to die. No matter what you do you're going to have to face, accept, and embrace it. I'm still at a loss as to how, but that's exactly what happened all within a nanosecond. It was like I was struck by lightning and when I was fried, I started to produce thoughts faster than the speed of light. Everything I went through, felt, done, caused, and lived through went vividly flashing through my mind all at once.

I thought, 'So what I might die now. I was diagnosed and given a twenty-five percent chance to live with cancer when I was two-and-a-half years old, and won. I should be dead. I was born and raised in Calgary, Alberta, which is one of the wealthiest, cleanest, and most peaceful places in the world. I had a hard-working single mother of three give her physical, mental, and social life to raise my brothers and myself. I always had food, clothing, and shelter. I was as blessed as they come.' I finally realized there was literally no reason for my self-destructing, cowardly-like actions. None at all. It was at that moment I realized how incredibly blessed I was to make it that far in the first place. In that moment, right then and there, I honestly couldn't have cared if I dropped dead or not, my peace with death was finally experienced for the first time and it was mostly majestic.

Not long after that experience, I found my thoughts quickly changed from being terrified of death, to being terrified of not achieving something or doing something great in my life before I faced it again, and lost. What would I do? What could I do? What is there to do? I knew what I wanted to achieve before I died as much as I knew what I wanted to be "when I grew up." I didn't have a fucking clue and, honestly, I don't think many people do when they first think about it. How am I to figure out where I want to go or what I want to do with life when I didn't even have a time-line? There was no way this was going to be an achievable task overnight. But how does one find direction in life? Now how does one find direction in life when they don't even know themselves?

From here on I used the fact that "I could die at any moment" to drive the motivation behind achieving something before I died. I didn't have the slightest clue as to what this was going to be, but it got me starting to think about it. I would tell myself everyday, "I can and would achieve something great before I died." I told myself, "I can and will change my life for the better before I die." I was still stuck in the same negative situation I got myself in. But now, for the first time in my life, I had finally started thinking of a way out instead of just doing nothing and feeling sorry for myself. I told myself this for days, weeks, and months on end. The only problem was, driving my life into the ground was the only thing I knew, it was the only thing I was any good at doing, and I had no idea how to break the cycle. I fought between letting my anger and pain continue my downward spiral of self-destruction and trying to think of a way out and a new path to take. My peace with death was made, however my anger was still there and it was the main fuel that drove my life into the ground. On top of it, my probation officer struck me as the kind of person that hated their life with a passion and used her power in a tyrannical way on other individuals to make herself feel superior, instead of self-improving, so the only help I had was useless to the entire situation. The whole thing continued to build and multiply my anger and rage in that time of my life.

Every single week it was the same cycle. I would leave my friend's house and longboard down the road that was ironically right across the train tracks from my probation officer's office. Every meeting I'd look at her office windows and think to myself 'I hope to God she doesn't see that this is me' as I'd have no explanation for being on that road, besides breaking my probation conditions. Luckily, on the west side of the road there was a high school so there was lots of foot traffic and I was sure I just blended in with the other students coming and going all morning and afternoon. Once I got to the train station, I'd walk out the emergency exit after making sure no trains or authorities were nearby. Next, I'd climb onto this electrical box, hook my longboard on the top of the fence before I'd hop the fence after unhooking my board and run across the CP rail tracks. After that, I would cut through a small opening in another fence at the bottle depot. I'd jump the fence and cut over the tracks instead of going around the entire train station because it would save me a few good minutes and being late was a guaranteed threat with jail. So I was breaking bi-laws, to risk not breaking laws, because that makes total sense.

After walking up a small hill and kicking down the road I'd get to her office and check in with the front desk before taking a seat and waiting. I'd usually wait way longer than my short cut was ever worth, but I didn't want to deal with me being the one that was late, and she was always dealing with other people so I would patiently wait and listen to music. Once she was ready, my probation officer would come get me, sit me down, and begin the interrogations. While talking to her, on occasion I'd be looking out the window right where I was longboarding five minutes before. She would ask me about my work schedule, collect my pay stubs to make sure I was working and if I was even one hour short of what was considered a full-time job, I would again have my freedom threatened. She would run my name and look for any new charges, sometimes bitching at me for other people's new charges thinking I'm them (like I said—goldfish). After that, she would confirm my next court dates for me which was the only consistent help I got from her. But then she would bring up my past and hold it over my head. She would tell me what a freeloading, never-going-anywhere, low-life loser I was. She never once asked me why I did the things I did, nor did she care enough about me or her job to look into it and ask. I was just another stock she had to temporarily monitor and was treated as such. After I was reminded if she caught me breaching probation conditions, she would report me to the judge and send me to jail. She would say, "Okay I'll see you next week," after confirming a date and time to come back when I wasn't working.

After months of this, I really started to get fed up with her, her negativity, her constant belittling, and threatening me. It was all making my mental health, motivation, and positivity toward getting my life together deteriorate faster than the fights and petty arrests did. Every time I would go see her, I would leave angrier, more upset, more frustrated with the system, and life in general. I still don't understand how she thinks bringing people down, belittling, and threatening them does any good. I couldn't help but think she got off on the little bit of power she will ever have in her life, and absolutely loved it. However, I never heard her story nor cared to ask either, so I suppose it goes both ways. I was just one sheep of thousands going through the system and I felt like less of a human and more like a number every single meeting and encounter with the police or court system. Which made feeling like I could have a purpose and make a change with my life much more difficult. Each week the anger and frustration built inside of me more and then was easily used as the fuel in the fights I got into.

For well over a year, I was catastrophically lost. I was going to the same dead-end job, jail, court, probation, and community service. It wasn't long before I had no idea who I was, where I wanted to go, or what I wanted to do in my life, let alone how to find my direction or myself. I wondered if I'll ever be able to escape this world of spiralling self-destruction, all the while wondering and hoping I could do it before I dropped dead without notice from the AVM in the centre of my brain that continued to be problematic. I had driven into the traffic circle of life and didn't know where to turn off. I just kept going around, and around, and around. I had no sense of hope or direction, not even the will to explore each turn off one by one. I just did what I knew, which was the continuous circle. It wasn't long before I really started to not only hate life but hate the coward I saw in the mirror every morning. As that person was responsible for this vicious circle of negativity. It reached its boiling point when I woke up one day and literally almost punched out the mirror in my friend's bathroom—I was so stressed, frustrated, angry, depressed, and done with life. I knew I needed to change my life around but was still completely clueless on how to shed this unlimited amount of anger, frustration, and hate I had for now not only the world, but myself. I tried to constantly remind myself, 'you can and will change your life for the better,' every single day all day no matter what this meditation routine had to be my mental focus.

Change of Direction

I started to ponder the meaning of life more than ever before and with probation conditions that I had to work full time it all wasn't sitting right with me. I honestly would rather die young than work dead-end, nine-to-five jobs for the rest of my life, although I was loving my job at the bakery. I felt I needed to do so many things at once. I had to find a way onto the right path, I had to achieve something great before I died because I felt life wasn't any good if you didn't do something with it. But we are modern day slaves. Solely bred to work, pay taxes, and be another brick in the wall. That was, and still is the furthest thing from living life in my mind. So, if I did survive long enough, I needed a positive direction to go as well. How an eighteen-year-old teenager was supposed to pull all of this off went well beyond my experience, expertise, and comprehension at the time. But I knew I had to do it.

For months and months, I was telling myself, "I would do something great with my life before I died." Then in the spring of 2012, I got up like any other day and was heading to work on my longboard with Tupac playing in my headphones. I suddenly remembered this Tupac quote I had seen on my friend's wall in his room. It said, "If you can't find something to live for, you best find something to die for." I fell in love with this quote the first time I saw it and as a constant reminder to find something in life worth dying for, I decided to get it tattooed on my left arm as there couldn't have been a truer statement applied to my life in that moment.

That very spring, I had booked my appointment with the tattoo shop. When the day finally came, I grabbed my longboard and skated a few blocks to the shop to get it done. The artist put the saying on my arm and asked how I liked it. I absolutely loved it so he began to make it permanent. As he was giving me ink, we started talking and I told him about my cancer, two strokes, and how I loved to longboard. He told me a bit about his longboarding days before I told him about how my longboarding adventures around Calgary kept me somewhat sane and grounded. He stopped tattooing my arm, turned to me, and as a joke said, "You should like, find a cause and longboard across Canada or something. Hahaha!" and proceeded to laugh it off like it was an impossible task and went back to work on my arm as I laughed it off as well.

Once he finished up, he covered my arm with plastic wrap and gave me a small bottle of cream to rub onto it. He told me not to take off the plastic wrap for a day or two to let it heal. After paying for the rest of the tattoo I started to longboard back to my buddy's place and as I was skating down the road, I couldn't help but think of the tattoo artist's joke about longboarding across the country for a cause. I didn't even stop to think about it realistically. I just shrugged it off and laughed like he did. But when I took a moment to think about it as I waited at a red light, it was a beautiful idea. I had more than enough "cause" and thought it could be my life altering event. The great thing I did before I died, that was if I made it that long without dying. I realized it could be my thing worth dying for. 'I have to do this or die trying,' I thought to myself as I crossed the street.

As I waited for the red light to change at my most popular arrest spot (Southland Drive and Haddon Road) I took out my phone and called my dad. I asked him what he thought about me longboarding across Canada for charity. His response was "whoa! That's big dude. Are you sure you would commit to something like that?" I told him how my life was going nowhere but down as I was still a homeless burden, working a dead-end, nine-to-five job, going back and forth between court and probation which after the fight with the brothers at the 7-Eleven got extended another year and moved from youth to adult probation, still with conditions I couldn't be anywhere near my friend I was still living with.

I think my dad could tell how desperate I was for a change in my life. My parents for years saw me driving my life into the ground and did everything they could to stop it and help. Only you can't help someone who doesn't want to help themselves. I FINALLY wanted to help myself, break the cycle, and change for the better. This was a way out of this loophole of self-destruction. I knew this would be the event in my life that forever changed it around, and make me a different person, so it just made sense for me to do it.

After I got off the phone with my dad, I was very excited about this new philosophical idea, so much that I went for a skate in my favourite Fish Creek location. I still had my arm wrapped up in the plastic covering my tattoo and didn't know if I should leave it on or not. But as I skated and started to sweat on the hot sunny day, I looked at my arm and I saw black ink was smudged all over the plastic wrap. I panicked thinking I ruined my tattoo, so I ripped off the plastic to see it was fine but some of the ink bled out making the wrap a mess. Ignoring the artist's words, I ripped it off and threw the wrap in my backpack to dispose of it properly later. As I pulled out the cream and rubbed it in, I skated through the woods. Once I finished my loop, I made a left turn to skate the twenty kilometres again before I went back home.

The next time my dad was in town, he asked me where a skate shop was. I told him the best one by far was Royal Board Shop. To me they seemed to be the most knowledgeable, friendly, experienced, dedicated, and loyal shop in the city. Plus, they had the best selection of gear in Calgary; you could never go wrong stopping by Royal. My father picked me up and we headed over there to see if they would support my mission. We got there, walked into the basement where the selection of boards were, and there stood the owner, Ryan, at one of the skate table shelving units.

We walked up to the kind, bearded man and told him about my medical stories, our plans and our mission before my dad asked if he would support us. Without saying a word Ryan looked at me, looked at my dad, before looking to his left where the phone was mounted on the wall. He picked it up, punches in some numbers, and calls "Rayne" Longboards in British Columbia and asks them if they would support our mission. They said they would without a doubt and Ryan hung up the phone before he picked it up again. This time calling "Landyatchz" longboards and asked them the same question. They gave the same answer. They were all more than happy to help, and just as eager to help, as they were happy to. Leaving Royal, for the first time in a long time I felt good.

Usually, people see you with a longboard and treat you like crap. My appearance of baggy, loose clothing, a hat, and dressing like a punk didn't help much. I was so used to being treated like a piece of shit by now that this blind faith Ryan had, was entirely alienated to me. Ryan took a look at me, the young punk, and he didn't see what everyone else saw. He didn't see the "low life piece of garbage" my probation officer saw. He took one look at me and believed in me. Unlike every single one of my case workers or probation officer he took a couple of minutes out of his busy day to listen to me and my story. He didn't judge me based on my clothing and appearance, he treated me with the upmost care and respect from the second I walked in. That was different to me, I wasn't ever treated like that. I was the kid everyone said would only ever amount to shit. I was the lost, rebellious, misunderstood teenager people avoided and tried to not bring around. Yet I walked into Royal and Ryan just believed in me, he believed in my cause, and he believed I would make it. It was a very unusual thing for me, but it made me feel great and also reaffirmed that this was the right thing to do with my time and with my life before I died.

A month or two later when my dad was in town again, he picked me up and we went over to Sayshun longboards which was in Calgary in the industrial area, very close to my tiny crack den apartment I was now living in. There we met with the owner and began to see if they could help us out with some longboard decks. The owner Matt showed us two proto-types they were working on at the time. He put down a thin foam mat on the concrete floor, then put the first one on top of the foam so I didn't mess up the bottom of the board when I stood on it. I felt good as I stood on the deck that had this amazing concave in it. The V-shape bubble covered almost the whole length of the deck and it felt very comfortable under my feet. Then he showed me the next board. The other deck had no concave in the wood but it was a drop deck so it was much closer to the ground which was ideal for a trip nearly seven-thousand kilometres long. I really liked them both, I loved the concave V in the first one and the lowness of the second one so I asked if he could combine the two so it was a drop deck with the V concave in it and to my surprise he said they could.

My dad and I then went on a tour of the factory, and we got to see all the industrial presses, sanders, saws, and computers that they had. After the tour my dad dropped me off at home. A month or two later my dad picked me up again and said he had something for me. He popped the trunk and there were two brand-new, "Drop Dead" custom-made Sayshun longboards. "Sweet! You got two boards for me," I said. I knew the trek would likely go through a handful, so I thought two was great. He then says, "Nope, one's for me," and said he was going to learn to ride and push the entire country with me. I thought he was kidding at first, but when I looked at him, he was dead serious. I thought he would have been a support driver or something like that, not longboard with me. 'You crazy ass old man,' I thought to myself when he told me this.

My father and I met at a Boston Pizza again a while later and he asked me what I wanted to call this longboarding thing. I thought back to my old "Skate for Life" internet profile name and decided to switch the skate (skateboard) for long (as in longboard) and said "Long for Life." Just like that "Long for Life" was born. The more I thought about the saying "Long for Life" the more I loved it and saw the multiple meanings and irony behind it. It discretely said what I was really doing—longing for my life. My dad began the legal work and started to assemble a team and to see what the longboarding community could do for charity he set up the first Long for Life event in Red Deer. With the help of the Heart and Stroke foundation and Allrose snow and skate, they worked together to create an awesome event. The longboarding event raised almost five-thousand dollars for the Heart and Stroke foundation. There were about fifty riders that came to ride and support the great cause. The weather was great and it was a beautiful sunny day which I was really glad about.

It looked like I was finally onto something. It looked like I may have found direction. It looked like my life was finally about to change forever. It looked like there was maybe some hope for this lost soul after all. The only problem with life is, right when you think things are finally getting better, it pulls down its pants and unleashes a long night of alcohol and terrible food all over you in the form of liquid diarrhea. The best part about this is, you can't do anything but take the shower and hope you come out smelling like roses and daisies.

Since the world doesn't stop spinning, I was on my longboard making my way to work one morning when my free (or so I thought and was led to believe) lawyer called me and asked why I wasn't at court yet. I told him I was on my way to work but I'd call work to let them know I must go to court first and I would be there as soon as I could. He then says to me, "Just go to work and I'll represent you in court today." I said, "Okay, cool thanks a lot," before I hung up the phone and went to work. It wasn't even a week later when I'm longboarding down Haddon Road going home from work when again "woop woop" the all too familiar red and blue lights and a siren is going off behind me. "Great now what," I said out loud. After thinking about it for a second, I had nothing to worry about this time. I had no warrants, I hadn't missed court or a probation meeting, my community service was done, I wasn't with my buddy, I had no knife, no drugs, and no drug paraphernalia so I knew I was going to be okay, but I wasn't.

I wasn't about to give them a reason to arrest me, so I complied with the officers. I stopped, got off my longboard, and walked over to the officer who asked me for some identification. I complied thinking I'm just being harassed for being on the empty road longboarding at night. The officer runs my name, then comes back to push me against the hood of the car and placed me under arrest. It turns out I had a warrant for missing court after all. Again, I was tossed in cuffs and taken downtown where I found out my legal aid lawyer did not represent me in court like he said and I was charged with missing my court date. It would be a few months later when I got a letter from legal aid saying I owe that lawyer over $1,200. I lost my mind upon receiving this letter. So I called them and told them to go do inappropriate things to themselves and their relatives before I said, "I'll die before I'll pay that stupid suit-monkey a cent of money. Who the hell do you think you guys are tricking kids into signing on the line thinking they get a free lawyer, then send them a bill for $1,200 after they fail to do their job." The lady started to explain something on how it works and I told her the system she works for is garbage, to go pound sand, and keep wasting money sending me letters and hung up the phone very pissed off. I just wanted this endless liquid defecation to end, but the courts continued to be the gift (shit) that kept on giving (shitting).

I went to meet my probation officer after work one afternoon. Over the phone she said she had some good news for me. I was filled with anxiety and worried because that very same morning I had quit my job (against my probation conditions) to train myself full time on my cross-Canada trek as it was coming up the following spring. But I couldn't tell her this because to me she was a power-tripping, untrustworthy, unreliable, miserable bitch that only seemed to enjoy threatening me and did not support me or help me in anyway and she was the last person I **took orders from**. So I went to my meeting and didn't tell her anything but now I had to hide another lie into the mix. It was there she told me she had found me "a cheap, safe, and secure place to live." I was super excited but super mad at the timing of everything as now I had no work or reliable income. I started the job search, found another job, and got back to work doing construction in southeast Calgary by my mom's new house. I finally moved out of my buddy's house into my own small one-bedroom, one-bath apartment. The housing charity that moved me in was great. They spent lots of money getting me stuff like a television, cooking supplies, cleaning supplies, towels and other miscellaneous household items to get me set up and I was incredibly grateful at first. I was there for maybe a few days when I decided to have some people over after tossing around concrete-covered plywood at work cribbing all day.

I had four or five friends over and we were hanging out having some gin, beers, and hoots. I met the guy next door down the hall and invited him over for some drinks, so he came over to hang out as well. A short time later my neighbour got a call from his girlfriend. As I am in the kitchen pouring another gin and juice he comes up and tells me, "I have to go talk to my girl, I'll be back in a few minutes." I said, "no worries, man, just come back in when you're done." So, he left and I'm standing there enjoying my drink thinking 'life's kind of nice right now. I have my own place, my new job is paying much more, and I was going on a crazy trip across the country in the spring that will hopefully give me some more direction in life.' I felt content with where things were going that night. But like I said, right when you think things are going well, life takes another squat over the toilet bowl that is your life and takes a good ol' dump.

As my friends and I were just hanging out chatting I heard a knock on the door. I assumed it was my neighbour coming back after talking with his girlfriend, which was another dumb assumption of mine. Without going to the door and looking out the peep hole I shouted out, "The door's open come in!" The door opened ever so slowly, and in walks this at least forty-plus-year-old, heavy-set, naked Indigenous lady. With boobs down to her stomach completely naked from head to toe, and she just stands ass-naked in my doorway shaking in fear.

My friends and I look at her, then we look at each other, then we look at her, and look at each other again and again wondering, 'Are you guys seeing this shit right now, is this actually happening?' All five of us must have taken a quadruple take wondering how the vibrations of our hang out suddenly got so weird. This strange naked lady is shaking in fear as she's saying, "He's got my child, he's got my child, he's got my child." Me, being half drunk, was like, "Well screw that guy, let's go get your child back." Ready for another fight, but definitely not ready for what was to come next. One of my friends threw his hoodie at the terrified lady to cover up, another went into my bathroom and got a towel.

Suddenly here are my friends and I comforting this terrified naked lady when out of nowhere I hear screaming from down the hall, "WHAT THE FUCK! THIS BITCH SHIT ON MY COUCH AND PISSED ON MY CARPET!" I thought, 'Oh Goodness, now what' so I run down the hall to where I hear this guy screaming mad. I got to his room which was directly next to mine and across the hall from the guy I invited over (who ended up being a druggie and stealing my things anyway). I took a look inside the stranger's place and he had a big wet spot on his carpet in the living room at least three feet in diameter. It looked like someone just dumped a bucket of water on his carpet. I then looked to my left to the bathroom to see he's got his couch upside down in his shower with the water running trying to wash poop off of it. Now I never saw the poop and I wasn't about to ask to see it either but with the couch upside down in his tub as he was scrubbing it while cursing, I took him for his word.

By now my friends are with me and I realized the naked stranger is still in my place, now alone. I ran back thinking, 'I swear to God if there's shit on my couch or piss on my floor, I'm going to lose it.' I got back to my place to see one of my friends was thankfully still there comforting the naked lady in my washroom. I asked my friend what we should do and she had no idea. My other friends came back and we had a little group meeting where we decided to call the police so they can deal with her. There was no child to be found anywhere so I'm not sure what the "he's got my child" was all about. There was no child with the man cleaning his poop couch nor was there one in the hallways, or in his place and she never entered my place with one, so I figured she must have been really high on drugs or something.

My friends and I got back into my apartment and talked about the events that just transpired now taking straight shots of gin, drinking more and trying to forget what we just saw. It was by far the most random, odd, weird, and disgusting thing all of us had ever encountered. The next day I went down and had a meeting with the people that run the housing program and told them what had happened. They were all in shock and disbelief, until they checked the security cameras to find that it happened. They saw her in the elevator with just my friend's hoodie on still half naked, but once she got off the elevator she was never seen again. The police came however they never found her, so who knows what happened.

It was at this moment I realized that moving from my friend's couch to this place wasn't at all a step up in the right level, but a massive step down. After that day I started to realize that there was nothing but a building full of crazies and drama. I'd notice it every time I walked the halls to take out the trash. Every single time I could hear people screaming and fighting. I could hear things being broken, things being thrown, doors slamming, all sorts of chaos, I was in a building full of freaks and scum. Apparently, my probation officer thought it was where I belonged. I decided I wanted out of there so I called my mom and made plans to come move in with her until my trek across Canada in a few months. Every job I was working at the time was within a few blocks of her new house so I thought it would be great.

My mother was okay with it, and very glad I was finally getting my life together. In the meantime, I needed some food after a check my boss gave me bounced. So after buying me a few handfuls of food she brought them over. I met her outside and grabbed a handful of stuff before I started to go back up the stairs. I got to the second floor where my apartment was and opened the stairwell door. I walked out to see three or four uniformed officers breaking into and raiding my neighbour's place (the one who went to talk to his girlfriend and stole my stuff). They say to me I can't pass them to the next door, so I would have to go down the stairs, down a long hall to the elevators before going up one floor, and back down the long hall again to get to my door. My short, little red-headed mom comes out the stairwell and just walks right through the group of cops not taking any of it. I went right behind my mom and walked right through them, and they didn't say a word to us. Mom then asks me what that was about. I told her, "I have no idea; probably something to do with gangs or drugs," (which seemed to be his only two subjects of interest the few times he came over). I think my mom also realized I needed out of the building as well. So, we made arrangements to move me to her new place as soon as possible.

Once I had a for-sure place to stay, I again quit my bounced-check job and found a new one while I waited for a check to come through for the housing program, but that wasn't my main concern. My main goal now was to focus and train on longboarding across Canada. So, from a new community even further from Cranston, I would skate to Fish Creek and go for a daily sixty-to-seventy kilometer skate. Some days, instead of staying in Fish Creek all day I would skate through Fish Creek before taking the roads into the west side of downtown then follow the pathways along the Bow River back to the streets that took me to Fish Creek and back through the valley to Auburn Bay. That trip was a bit over seventy kilometers there and back. Those sixty and seventy kilometer routes became my daily life when I wasn't working. With my newest boss getting into a fight and getting stabbed in the gut with a piece of a broken mirror, I had a lot of days off, so I spent every day I could on my board doing huge laps around the city.

Still struggling with the loss of my hero and father figure—my Uncle Tony—I had to continue to go see my probation officer to get belittled while I profusely tried to get a pass on our last two meetings so I could go on this cross-country charity mission. When I told her my plan and asked if I could miss our last two meetings so I could longboard across Canada for charity, she said to me, "No, if you miss our last two meetings ill report you to the judge and have you arrested." At one point when I went from youth to adult probation, I was incredibly happy I was going to be transferring probation officers, as from day one this one had treated me based on what the piece of paper said I was charged with. Which at the time was a co-charge, and nothing that I directly did. However, she felt obligated to make sure she got to manage my adult probation extension as well.

Not once did she ask me what had happened. She didn't know the assaults stemmed from a woman being hit and abused by a coward of a guy, over a dozen calls to the police changed nothing and she got no help. Instead, she tried to stress me out saying I could face seven to twenty-five years for every charge, I burst out laughing and said, "I never touched or hurt anyone with a weapon, so how would I do that much time if I never assaulted someone with a weapon?" She didn't reply and sent me home after that meeting. Here I was, months later, finally trying to get my life on the right track and she's there doing whatever she could to keep me on the wrong one with petty arrests while trying to continuously stress me out, hindering my abilities to move forward and on with my life. Not exactly the kind of person I wanted in my life, let alone be forced to see, or, alternatively, go to jail. Jail was honestly starting to seem like a better idea than dealing with this walking goldfish, but I had to stay focused on the mission ahead.

When I was telling her about the story of the naked lady that walked into my "safe and secure" (her exact words) apartment I referred to one of my friends as a "chick." She snapped at me cutting me off mid-sentence saying, "Don't you mean woman?" I was like, "Yeah, I guess so," not that my friend would have cared if I referred to her as a "chick." It's not like I meant to disrespect women at all. If it were not for two incredible women I would not be here today. I owe my life to two phenomenal women, however she didn't know that. Even though I was forced to see her after being arrested for trying to protect a woman, one I didn't even care much for. I probably have more genuine respect for women than most, but she did not know that, she didn't even know a woman saved my life when I had cancer as a child.

She didn't even know I had cancer as a kid or a stroke when I was fifteen either. After I told her I had a second stroke and that was why I had missed a court date, she didn't try to build any rapport and ask how a seventeen-year-old has a stroke, let alone two. But most of all, I questioned her sanity as I wondered how she could hear about an old, heavyset, naked, shaking Indigenous lady walking into the place *she* got me and all she could hear out of the story was the word "chick." This was just aggravating and reassured me the system and my probation officer was of absolutely of no help to me. If I wanted to change my life for the better, it was going to be on nobody but myself as the system has proven disgustingly useless to me again and again. With my PO not letting me pass on our last two meetings, my father and I had to postpone our trek by two weeks, so instead of leaving April 28th like my dad planned, we waited until the day I was off probation to be sure there was no funny business on the road.

However, before we left I wanted to make sure this trek wasn't going to kill me so I booked an appointment with my neurosurgeon to see if I was still at risk of having a stroke. I got up at six in the morning and spent two hours going to the hospital for my appointment. Only when I showed up I was told I didn't have an appointment. I guess there was yet another mix up with Alberta Health Services and I spent two hours going back home without the answer I needed to get on the road. On my way home, I contemplated calling my dad and telling him we need to postpone the trek, but then I started to think about the hole I was currently in. I needed to make a change with my life, and I needed to do it yesterday. Well really, I needed to do it years ago, but I had no idea how, and no plan to do it. Being one right turn away from a life in jail or a lifelong heroin addiction, I decided I was going to change my life or die trying. I figured I was going to end up dead if I didn't, so I felt like I didn't really have much of a choice.

Mission and the East Coast

This part of my book is dedicated to the Long for Life team and especially to my crazy-ass old man, Michael Floyd. Dad, it was one gnarly, eye-opening trip that I'll never be able to forget as long as I'm healthy and alive. Thank you for all the sweat, blood, hard work, time, money, organizing, logistical wizardry, more blood, and more sweat you put into making sure my dream and vision was a successful one. I wanted this trip to change my life, mind, and way of thinking for the better and it inevitably did just that; so, thank you. I love you, man.

This entire trek is also dedicated to all of the people in my magnificent, peaceful, clean, stupendous country. To my fellow Canadians, thank you for being there and treating us like family from coast to coast. I thank you all for ensuring my dream and goal became a success. This wouldn't have happened without you guys. I hope this will help bring some insight on how astounding, fantastic, generous, kind, and amazing we are. Even more so, how amazing we can be when we simply come together to lend a helping hand. Thank you for showing me without a reasonable doubt that everything happens for a reason, that good people do exist, and that I come from the most incredible country in the world. I am so incredibly blessed to call this outstanding country my home.

My dad chose to have us start at the furthest coast from home after reading about some guys that tried to longboard across Canada and started on the West Coast in British Columbia but after they got close to their hometown in Alberta they got lured by the temptations of their beds and gave up. This way, we had no other option but to push all the way back home. The only problem going east to west were the natural trade winds blow from west to east across Canada, but it was still the right call.

At nineteen-years-old On May 14th 2013 (the day I was officially off probation), we took a five- or six-hour flight to the East Coast. Riddled with anxiety and emotions we finally landed. I couldn't help but think 'holy shit, am I really about to do this?' As I tried to cope with the shock of it all. From the St. John's airport, we caught a cab and went straight to Middle Cove Beach. There, a reporter from the Telegram newspaper was going to meet us and take pictures of my dad and I dipping our boards in the Atlantic Ocean to have the story of our mission in the paper the next morning. Right after we did the interview, we came across a young couple that had come to the beach that day.

The kind man started to ask my dad why the media was there with our mountain of suitcases and longboarding gear relaxing on the beach getting their tan on. My dad tells Alby and his wife Vanessa the story about what were up to and they're blown away. My dad then asked Alby if he knew of a motel nearby that they could possibly take us to. Without skipping a beat Alby says something like, "Yeah there is, we have something to do real quick, but we'll be back in half an hour or so and take you right to one." I was thrilled about the generous ride these two strangers we randomly came across at the beach offered us, and it was only the beginning of the amazing people, moments, and generosity to come. I spent the next fifteen or twenty minutes bombing the big half pipe like hill that went down to the rocky beach, but I was too chicken to bomb down the one whole side so new into the trek. Meanwhile my dad walked around the rocky coastline and we both soaked up the beautiful view for a while.

As promised, Alby and Vanessa returned a short time later. Alby comes back over to us and says, "Alright we got steaks for the barbeque, the fridge is full of beer, your beds are made up, and you guys are staying with us." Again, we were blown away by the generosity of this amazing couple. What was going on? We literally just landed and there were people that wanted to actually help, this was still a new concept to me. Before we went to their house, they took us out to a few places. The first was called "Signal Hill." At the top of the hill was a beautiful lookout spot that overlooked the city of St. John's and the Atlantic Ocean. Where the land met with the sea there were big, beautiful, light-brown cliff faces with a small, white lighthouse and what looked like a white church at the bottom of the protruding rocky ground near the cove. As we hung out there, we took a few pictures and had a short chat where I believe Alby said something about that place being the furthest Northeastern point of North America. It was so windy up there at the time I had to keep my hand on my custom "Long for Life" hat to keep it from flying off of my head. After the sights, we went to a small local underground pub owned by a lady named Linda. Linda briefly talked about how she was there at Middle Cove Beach the day the legendary Terry Fox was there dipping his leg in the ocean at the start of his monumental journey. She claims to be one of the first people to give him a donation of ten dollars after asking the young man why he was sticking his leg in the cold Atlantic water. I thought about the odds she would meet the legendary Terry Fox and the assholey punk of a kid at the very beginning of our journeys. I thought that was pretty cool and wondered how many others she would meet at the start of their own personal journeys in the future.

Linda's bar was full of all sorts of cool knick-knacks. There were small pictures everywhere, parts of boats here and there, little ships, and all sorts of miscellaneous East Coast, ocean-travelling items from abroad; it was pretty neat. After a chat and a beer or two on the house with Linda we said goodbye and gave her a hug as she wished us good luck on our cross-country mission before we headed over to Alby and Vanessa's place for dinner. As were all sitting around the table eating dinner, Alby looked across the table to where I'm shovelling steak, potatoes, and salad down my gullet and asks, "So have you boys ever been screeched in before?" I replied with, "No, what is that?" Alby suddenly gets a shocked look on his face like I just punched a baby. His eyes opened wide almost bulging out of his face as he says, "Oh! We gotta go out and get you boys screeched in tonight!" And he doesn't explain anything further. So, after dinner we all got into their car and went for a short drive.

They have a street in St. Johns that has bar after bar after bar. So we went to have a drink at a bar before we walked down the street and then had a few drinks at another bar. Then we proceeded to walk over to the next bar to have a drink and listen to music for a while before we wandered to the next bar and got screeched in and had a few more drinks. To get "screeched in," we had to say some saying that my brain couldn't process. For the life of me, I could not understand the handful of words and had no idea what to say before we kissed the fish and took a shot of screech—in this case, a Newfoundland rum. That was the tradition of being "screeched in." The saying was "Long may yer big jib draw" meaning "May the wind always be in your sails." But between the thick heavy Newfoundlander accent and my new alcoholic buzz I couldn't understand a word the bartender was saying.

For some reason I've always had trouble hearing through thick accents. The Draper family knows how many times I've had to ask them to repeat words or sentences for me during dinner with them when I was dating their amazing daughter after they moved from the heart of London, England to Canada. I swear almost every other sentence they said I had to say, "Sorry, pardon, what, come again, what was that?" It was quite embarrassing for me but comical for Emma and her brother who would just smack their faces, shake their heads, and repeat the words ever so slowly so I could understand, it made me feel like quite the illiterate, non-English-speaking dumbass, just like this.

The bartender was going around the bar making sure everyone who was getting screeched in was saying the sentence I can't even process through my brain, let alone say. So as everyone else around me was saying it, I was just sitting there moving my lips so it looked like I was saying something and hoped nobody would catch on. The big, bearded bartender gets to me and immediately stops going around the bar. He looks at me mumbling absolutely nothing and says, "TERRIBLE, OH JUST TERRIBLE!" and that was something I couldn't even try to deny or argue with. The bartender then had us kiss a cod before we took our shot of screech. After that, he gave all the participants a signed certificate with our names saying we are now honorary Newfoundlanders.

After our shot and another beer or two, we left. Next thing I know it's four in the morning, I'm piss drunk, and were all going through the McDonald's drive-through in a taxi getting some late-night munchies. We then went back over to Alby's house. When we got back, I got to have a nice heart to heart chat with Vanessa in the garage before we ate our late-night chow down and went to bed. Suddenly, it's now nine or ten in the morning and my dad is shaking me and waking me up so we could pack our bags and get on the road. We all looked at the article in the Telegram before Alby kindly drove us to the highway in his white truck so we could begin our two-day journey across "The Rock."

Alby pulled over on the right side of the highway and my dad and I thanked him kindly, jumped out, then started to push down the road against the cold, spine-shivering wind, getting rained on, and going uphill. With every kick my stomach wanted to empty its remaining late-night contents as I was hungover like I was fourteen in the Dominican with the Lloyds again feeling like absolute steamy-hot garbage. It was the very first day of so many to come and I was already contemplating why the hell I signed up to do this. The whole day I had to remember it wasn't just for me, but it was for all the people that never got the second or third chance to live after they have been affected by stroke or cancer. But as much as it was for them, it was also for a positive change of direction in my life. At the same time giving back to the world before I passed as it could be my last moment of life at any given second. I had to remind myself that THIS was my purpose, and THIS was why I've survived all I have.

However, after only a few hours in the cold rain longboarding on the highway I was fed up and done with it and it quickly turned into, "Screw this, this is fucking dumb," I said, cussing and cursing at the wind that blew directly in our faces. I saw a big downhill up ahead after some time and I got excited to bomb down it. I saw the big hill coming around a right bend on the road. When the road turned back left, it descended and I started to kick like a mad man trying to get speed for the hill. Only the head wind was so strong I had to forcefully kick down the entire huge hill. Needless to say, I was not very happy. Not to mention we were left to push on a tiny, almost non-existent shoulder. The ditch was maybe a couple inches from our right wheels, then our boards, and then the rumble strips were only inches from our left wheels. The white line was just on the left side of those rumble strips. With the right wheels almost in the ditch and the left wheels inches from the rumble strip, it made it a bit difficult to stay within the space I had as I kicked the ground and came around the left downhill corner.

Despite the technical challenges, the island itself was very beautiful and incredibly rocky. Everywhere you looked, there was rock protruding from the ground. I suppose that's how the island got its nick-name "the Rock." Even when I got off the highway to take a pee like a dog on a tree in the middle of nowhere, I was walking on rock that was covered with moss which had grown for millennia.

As I walked off the roads, my foot would often slip on a slanted rock and reveal, beneath the moss, the dark-black rock glistening like a diamond when I moved my foot and looked back to make sure I didn't step in some animal's excrement. The island was only a two-day push, so my father and I lived out of our backpacks for those two days. Day one we had no problems, other than the regret of having too much to drink the night before, the rain, the head wind, the cold, and uphill. However, on day two we ran out of sunlight and were longboarding in the dark on the side of the highway nearing our destination. We were wearing headlamps so we could see where we were going and be at least a little visible to traffic in the dark.

All of a sudden, "Woop woop!" The red and blue lights came on. 'Oh great, here we go again, I swear to God if I get arrested for a missed court date or something stupid I'm going to be pissed.' I wanted to believe I was going to be fine, but I made that assumption before, and it was not fine at all. My head automatically went to 'I'm getting arrested' with my recent past. The officer got out of his vehicle and says "what the heck are you guys doing out here in the middle of the night?" my dad told him our mission and he was certainly impressed, however with the lack of sun light we had to get off the road as we were not only a danger to ourselves, but a danger to the people driving on the highway as well. The officer asks for our ID's, ran our names, and then put us and our gear into the back seat of the police car. He then drove us down a small hill and around a right-hand corner where he dropped us off at our motel for the night. I couldn't help but think how that was the first time I was put into a cop car not in cuffs, not going to jail, and not having to worry about charges, court, and especially that god-awful probation officer. It was great.

'Well, that's a first,' I thought to myself as I was getting let out of the police cruiser. I can only imagine how weird it must have looked to anyone that saw us. To see a police cruiser pull up to a motel, have an officer let out the two occupants in the back, shake their hands, wish them luck, then leave, would be strange to say the least. If I saw that, I would have questioned if the cop just helped them escape from jail. The officer's, "good luck, gentlemen," at the end would have compounded that. At minimum I'd be thinking those two people were just released from jail and to stay the heck away. But oh, how looks can be deceiving.

From Placentia (the west side of the island) we were supposed to get on a ferry and take it over to Halifax on the mainland but there was a little issue. Massive icebergs were still coming through the channel we had to cross, so the ferries where not running yet. With no way to get across the channel, we now had to go back across the island we just finished pushing across to St. Johns and get on a short flight to Halifax. With no idea on what to do we sat in our motel and tried to figure out a game plan. We spent the next day trying to hitchhike with a sign on the side of the road, but nobody wanted to pick up the two guy longboarders. The sun quickly set on us that afternoon and it again got dark. There was a gas station beside our motel just off the highway, so I walked over there and started to ask strangers if they were going to St. Johns. About ten- or fifteen-minutes went by and I had no luck getting us a ride. However, the woman inside working at the gas station had seen me asking people and came outside to make sure that I was okay. I told her I was fine before

I told her what my father and I were up to, and she was stunned. I told her how we now had to get back to St. John's so we could get on a plane to get to Halifax and continue our journey.

About another half hour went by and I still had no luck getting a ride. Now it's completely dark out aside from the surrounding street and store lights. Just as I'm about to go back to the motel where my father was, a black truck pulled up beside me and the passenger side window rolled down. "Hey, are you guys those long boarders?" I was asked. I said, "Yes, sir," and he replies with, "I'm here to give you guys a ride." I asked him, "Where?" to make sure there was no confusion and he said, "to St. Johns." I then asked if he could wait for a couple minutes as I ran back to the motel to get my dad. I burst through the door of our motel room. "We got a ride waiting, let's go!" I quickly blurt out. My dad closed his computer and packed a few things before we walked over to the gas station and got in the back of this kind man's truck. With his teenage son in the front passenger seat, the four of us drove back to the other side of the island and went to Alby and Vanessa's house for one more night.

As we were driving, my dad asked the kind man how he heard about us. He said, "Someone called the local radio station and said what you guys were up to and that you needed a ride." I can only assume it was the sweetheart working at the gas station who called it in because she was the only one that took a minute to get the full story of what we were doing. As we drove down the road, I sat in the back seat absolutely silent. I was too completely mind-blown over everyone's generosity, it was unlike anything I've ever seen or experienced. Since when did the stars in my universe start to align like this?

Once safely back at Alby and Vanessa's my dad and I said, **Thanks for the** ride" to the father-son duo before we went inside and relaxed for the rest of the night. My father and I got to meet their beautiful little boy who was at grandma's the day and evening before. As I lay there trying to sleep I couldn't help but think , 'What if Alby and Vanessa didn't go to the beach that day? What if that kind woman at the gas station didn't take a few minutes to listen to me and make that phone call? What if the father-son duo didn't have the radio tuned into that station? What if they had already past the gas station or just didn't have the time or patience for the five-minute, gas station pit stop? Where would we be?' My mind was drawing a blank on why the stars in my life were suddenly aligning. This kind of stuff didn't happen to me, heck I spent the last nineteen years having life shit all over me until eventually that's what life to me became; shit. However, I was feeling better than I had in a very long time. I was so happy, grateful, and so thankful for this sudden astronomical alignment of stars, and it felt unbelievably good.

When we got up the next morning, we got our bags packed, grabbed our boards and Alby kindly drove us straight to the airport. We joyfully went through airport security and got on the plane for our very short flight to Halifax. Once we landed, my dad set up his computer at a small coffee shop and began reaching out to the Halifax longboarding community. I was full of good feels, excitement, and energy so I grabbed my board and went for a skate while we waited. There wasn't much but a tiny slip of a road to ride out front of the airport and that was it, not the fun adventure I had hoped for. Across the street there was a tiny dirt hill and, in the back, I saw a few C-cans. I got off my board, walked across the small field of grass, and went to see if there was any graffiti art on the C-cans. Some graffiti writers like to paint those so I always took a gander at them if I could.

After finding no art to admire and nothing to skate I went back to skating slowly on the sidewalks avoiding people as I span in circles on my deck, just longboard dancing to pass some time. I went back inside after a bit and my dad said, "Our ride is out front." I was still energized so I grabbed my board and started to skate it through the airport to the furthest door away like we used to do back in school to get teachers to chase us. I thought I had the GoPro on and started filming the quick skate. I went coasting by a group of people and ducked down to average height, so a gentleman just saw this head floating on by and I think I broke his brain because I got the weirdest look I've ever received in my life; it was like I had five heads. I got to my exit and turned my board sideways to slow down and stop, only I forgot how slippery longboarding wheels are on tile floors and I fell off my board thinking 'sick moves jackass' as I ran out of the door and over to the taxi my dad was putting his things into. I quickly piled mine into the back and we took off to Wayne and Stephanie's place for the weekend.

Wayne was a tremendous contributor to the Halifax longboarding community and organized a little cruise for us to go on in town with several other riders. We all met at a local basketball/tennis court area. When we got there, I was asking for some tips on sliding because it was entirely new to me and was something I never learned but desperately needed to. My dad did an interview with Global News before we all rode over to the Olympic Oval, just a few blocks away. There, I would do my interview with Global and longboard danced around for a bit. We had a little barbeque and skated around before it started to pour rain again and got incredibly windy. Skating one way around the oval, you were fighting and struggling to push, whereas the other way, the wind just pushed you flying around the corners so fast you had to slow down or you would hydroplane, wipe out, and hit the cement hard. Once the rain stopped, some of the guys set up a jumping stick to see who could jump over the stick the highest while still landing on their board and riding away without falling off and eating the pavement of the oval for dessert. I was still full from the BBQ and didn't feel like eating the pavement of the oval as I knew how terrible I was at doing that, so I sat back and watched the locals go at it, hoping to learn a thing or two. My feet leaving my board was something I never liked and was very uncomfortable about. So I nibbled on some snacks and skated around in peace, just longboard dancing while watching the other guys do it.

Some riders made it the first try, and some didn't. Some had done really well and they raised the bar to another higher level to go at it again. When they couldn't go any higher without knocking it off, they started to do one-eighty and three-sixty-degree spins over the bar before they landed on their board and rode away. Some of that didn't go over to well and a few started to fall off their boards after leaping and spinning into the air. Others did pretty good. As I pushed around, I tried it around the corner, and my first try only a foot off my board I almost ate it. I thought to myself 'oh yeah that's why you don't do that'. Its a good thing we all had helmets on because there were a few clicks here and there which was the sounds of heads hitting the concrete ground. Between the wet grounds, jumping the stick, and longboard dancing the clicks of heads meeting pavement continued on for a while.

We ended up finding some plywood lying between some sheds and used it to make a wooden ramp that connected the Olympic Oval to the paved path that was a few metres away across some grass. We threw one piece down and made it flush to the end of the oval then put another down with the far end of the previous piece lifted onto the next one. We did the same with another piece or two until the overlapped ramp was complete. One by one, we all started to skate it hoping for the best. Most of us made it with no problems, then one guy's trucks got caught between the two pieces of plywood when they separated as the last rider in front of him hit it. He made it off the oval onto the first piece of wood and rode it to the second but when he went to ride onto the third piece his front trucks and wheels dropped between the two pieces and immediately stopped his board from continuing to move. However, he was pushing hard up to it across the oval and his momentum didn't want to stop at all. His feet lifted off the board one at a time as physics took over. He began to take flight through the air like a 747. Only he took off more like a helicopter than a plane. I'm not sure if he was trying to jump but his vertical lift seemed to be much greater than his forward momentum. Luckily it was only a short flight and when he hit the ground, he hit grass and rolled out of it like a boss missing the paved pathway by a few feet. He, his friends, and I had a good laugh as he quickly pops back up to his feet with no injuries. After we were all satisfied with the skate session, my dad and I went back to Wayne's house for the weekend. There he had a little, yellow bearded dragon and a small snake that we took turns holding and hanging out with.

That weekend when I wasn't hanging around the house with everyone and the reptiles, I was off skating and exploring Halifax. I went down to the harbour that wasn't too far away and sat by the edge of the water looking off into the distance, reflecting in silence. There were a few massive cargo ships in the harbour and not too far down the water line I could see the massive loading docks, cranes, trucks, and all the heavy equipment needed for an immense operational import/export dock. I sat there in the sun listening to the small waves hit the sea wall and splash around before I saw a tunnel that led somewhere.

I got up, grabbed my board, and pushed over to check it out. It was only a pedestrian tunnel that went underneath a road. When I came out of the end, I recognized that I had skated right by it when I was adventuring around. I began to skate in the general direction of Wayne's house when I got distracted by the short steep hills in the downtown area. Block by block, street by street, I began ripping down the hills before going to the next block. The way down the hill was always fun but the walk back up wasn't my forte. However, I was thoroughly enjoying my little side adventure. That was until I got myself turned around and got lost. I thought I was almost back at their place then I realized that I now had no idea where I was.

I was circling the same few blocks trying to find my way when I realized the water would take me to a place I would recognize. I threw my board under my feet; only now, instead of zigzagging through the blocks like I was, I kept bombing down the hills of downtown Halifax eventually getting to the water. Once I found the water, I followed it towards the shipping yards knowing I'd eventually get to the spot I was reflecting at earlier. Once I got there, I made my way through the tunnel and began to skate the streets hoping I didn't make another wrong turn and get lost. Thankfully, I found my left turn and made my way back safely.

After our reptilian hang out with Wayne and Steph for the weekend, we had to meet our volunteer support driver who would be with us for the rest of the way across the country. Only when we met him at the nearby grocery store, the trailer was in a state of unbelievable, uninhabitable chaos. It looked like someone had rolled the trailer a few times, then it got hit by a tornado, before it was juggled by a giant. The contents of the trailer even the cupboards and cabinets were everywhere but where they should be. Everything was broken, fallen off, and smashed all over the place after travelling through, "some rough roads through Quebec," our shelter for the rest of the trip was a dump, sweet. After an extensive few-hours of clean-up and going through what we could salvage, we got back on the road going west bound. My father and I were supposed to be on our boards all day going an average of about sixty kilometres a day on the side of the highway and the driver was supposed to park where we would meet him down the road, and set up camp for the night. However, it proved to be too much for him and only a week or two in, we were being left in some terrible situations and the arguments began with the driver and my dad.

Another day and another mission. Today the goal was to make it over to Fredericton. It was a beautiful sunny day skating through some woods. Because there was zero shoulder on the roads my dad and I had to jump on and off the roads every time a car came by. At some point, I saw this road sign on the right side of the highway that I had never seen before, and I didn't have a clue as to what it meant. It was a green sign with a backwards white round spiral swirl that was also kind of like a question mark with what looked like three sailboat sails coming out of the bottom in spikes so I jumped off my board while my dad took a picture of me standing beside it, pondering its existence for a second. We then continued down the road that still didn't have an adequate shoulder for us to ride on until off in the distance on the right side we could see a big metal bridge that crossed the St. John River.

I stood on the right side of the road while my dad took a picture of me with the big bridge in the background. After he took the picture, we began to push towards the bridge to cross over it. We got there, crossed it, and once we neared the other side of the bridge we stopped and took a look to our right over the edge of the bridge. We finally got to see the scope of how much water was dumped on us over the first two weeks of the trip. The nonstop rain that was happening had catastrophically flooded the river. It looked doubled maybe even tripled in size. Millions of gallons of water swallowed the trees, bushes, and land.

We continued on through New Brunswick and along the way we met incredible people everywhere. Convenience store owners, a young couple and their dog, an amazing mother and daughter who came to our trailer and donated to us a huge stockpile of food to help us out, and gas station employees. Every single person we met did nothing but support us and help us get to the next city or town. And by the time we got to that next city or town, the news that we were on the way had spread and there were more amazing people that continued to give us this inconceivable, unconditional love, care, and respect. It was one of the most beautiful things I had ever experienced. To see community after community, stranger after stranger provide my father and I with everything and anything we needed was completely estranged from my mind. Who were all these people? Why did they all treat us like their family? They treated us as if we were their own flesh and blood. They did absolutely everything in their abilities to get us food, water, shelter, equipment, showered, cleaned up, and back on the road.

My dad and I were skating all day as per usual and just got to our small-town destination where we ran into a convenience store as we got caught in another nasty thunderstorm. My dad started to talk with "Skippy" who was working at the counter as we hid out from the rain that was coming down sideways. It wasn't normal rain. I looked out the window and it was like gravity didn't go up and down in a vertical direction, but horizontally. I was so happy and grateful we had gotten to the store when we did and we were not currently stuck in the sideways rain, again. It had been nonstop rain for the last two weeks now and I was beyond over it.

After a few hours in this store waiting out the storm my dad finally got our support driver on the phone who told him he was lost. Skippy then tells my dad to put him on speakerphone, which he does, and Skippy tells him to describe his last known settings. The driver says something incredibly vague like "Ugh, I came down this gravel road, over a hill, and now I'm at a church." Skippy says, "Okay I know where he is. Let's go; I'll drive you over to him." I then got in the back seat behind Skippy while my dad got in the front passenger seat, and we drove off in this kind stranger's red pickup truck, down a gravel road, into the middle of a forest, now in complete darkness. It was something you'd scream "don't do it!" at the TV in a horror film. We could have easily been shot and pushed out the door never to be seen again, but luckily for us Skippy was yet another good, kind, caring, genuine man the universe directed our way.

After a short ride we turned right off the gravel road and into the yard of a small white church that was hidden in the deep depths of the Canadian forest. We thanked Skippy for uniting us with our very unsupportive support driver, and I headed to bed for the night. But the arguments between my dad and the driver only continued. My dad argued how we were left in a very vulnerable position while the driver sat back drinking.

The Driver couldn't handle his job and wanted to trade my dad positions. He wanted to be the one on the highway and see if my dad could drive sixty kilometres down the road, park, and set up for the night. He just laughed like, 'yeah, okay buddy.' With a cup of summer warm straight Wild Turkey in his hand he insisted he's not a heavy drinker and he only drank when he was "stressed out." Now it was a matter of what do we do with this guy that's too stressed out by driving sixty kilometres a day? So stressed he had a bottle of booze hidden everywhere. In the bed of his truck, in his computer bag, and beside his bed in the back but continuously insisted he wasn't "a heavy drinker" eventually things settled down as I tried to sleep, and they also went to bed.

The next morning, I was excited when I woke up. I was stoked because as we waited in the convenience store for hours, Skippy asked us, "What are you guys going to do when you get to the big hill a mile down the road?" I replied to him, "just bomb down it then go back to the top to do it again." Back on the road and about one or two hours later (about ten or twenty kilometres, definitely more than 'a mile down the road'), we came around a right bend that then turns back left into the forest. On the right side of the highway was a yellow downhill sign that reads "10 percent grade for 1.3 kilometres." I got off my board to take a picture of the sign and the GoPro dramatically beeped at me to let me know it died just as I went to take the picture. I called my dad over and he took one for me before I got back on my board and went for the hill.

The hill had a bit of a slight bend in it. A quick right, then left before going straight down with a nice run out that then made a hard left turn into the forest about a kilometre away. I took the top easy and slow dragging my foot on the road. I had a quick look for traffic in the remote woods and saw no reason I should have to slow down so I picked up my left foot and ripped down the middle of the empty road. As I got closer to the bottom of the hill, I noticed there was a van ahead on the left side of the highway in the oncoming lane, pulled over on the shoulder. As I went flying by the two guys standing there, I gave them a man-nod before coasting around the left turn into the woods. As I continued to ride out the momentum from the hill, I waited for my dad to pop out behind me, but he was not there.

I waited for a bit before I made my way back around the corner half expecting him to be laying dead in the road, or on the side recovering from a fall. But when I turned the corner, I saw him on the right side of the road standing there talking to the two guys standing by the van. Turns out those two guys were Skippy and his buddy who sat there all morning, (for who knows how long) and waited while drinking their Tim Horton coffees to see what would happen when we rode down the big hill. I flew by them so fast I didn't even recognize that it was Skippy until I came back.

Once I got back over to everyone, Skippy kindly offered me a ride back to the top so I could do it again, even though it probably would have been done again after a short chat with my dad and a walk back up the hill. But now that I knew the feel of the nice smooth road and didn't see any holes or anything to be worried about. I didn't do much foot breaking and just went for it. With everyone else in the van behind tailing me and checking my speed I flew down the hill. I got to the bottom and coasted back around the left corner into the woods and once I slowed down a bit I stood on the road while my dad and Skippy came out to tell me I was only going about seventy-five-kilometres-an-hour down the hill. He then began to tell us about the "Four Mile Woods" we were about to enter.

As we entered the "Four Mile Woods" the bugs came out hard. It was incredibly bad with mosquitoes and we were literally getting eaten alive by them. I just hoped the "Four Mile Woods" wasn't four times longer than his ten-plus-kilometre "mile to the hill." In the Four Mile Woods, you better have had your mouth closed because as you came flying down hills and corners or even pushing on the flat ground you would hit a big patch of mosquitoes hovering in clusters by the thousands and if your mouth or eyes were open you were getting bugs in them. I remember I got one big mouthful of bugs and as I was coughing and spitting out bugs, I got another mosquito in my eye and I could feel it fighting for its life on my eyeball as it moved around. My eye started to profusely water and when I rubbed my tear out of my eye, I wiped out some of the bug as well. With what remained of the mosquito on my finger I wiped it on my jeans and hoped the other parts of the bug were no longer in my eye. We eventually came around a right corner in the woods and the road went straight for a few kilometres. As we pushed the flat empty road, a small purple pickup truck pulled over to the right side and a very tall, skinny man popped out and told us he's a local reporter for the area and asked if we could do a quick interview. The three of us then stood on the side of the road in the Four Mile Woods getting eaten by more mosquitoes than you had the ability to kill or count. After our quick interview, the reporter apologized for getting us eaten alive, thanked us for stopping, and he goes back on his way while we get back on the road still being eaten by thousands of mosquitoes. It was terrible. But they were good in the sense they made sure we kept up a good pace because if you went to slow, they could get you. Our only defence was speed and the thick coating of useless bug dope (insect repellent) we had on.

Still three weeks into the trek, it's been nothing but rain. Every day we would get up, pack our bags, and get on the road in the cold, wet rain. All of my life I hated being wet and wearing clothes. It was incredibly uncomfortable to me and I hated it with a passion. However, after a week or two we began to do things like wrap our feet in plastic bags and then tape them around the ankle before putting our shoes on to keep our feet dry. But no matter what we did. We had endless hours of longboarding in the rain that would eventually have us soaking wet, head to ankle. The rain gear we had on did a mild job of keeping you dry from the rain, however they kept your body heat and sweat inside as well. As we jumped on and off the road for passing traffic, we would take off our raincoats to expose our bodies to the rain and both get a much needed cool down and a quick wash off of the nasty amounts of sweat on our bodies.

Flying downhill in the rain, our four wheels spat up water, dirt, mud, and road gunk. By the end of the hill, you were covered waist-high in tiny microscopic-sized pieces of mud, dirt, water, squished worms, and debris from the road, and I hated that too. Every day I was cursing and screaming at Mother Nature. My dad on the other hand had a different opinion as he noticed on rainy days the wind tended to be a bit in our favour, but with the resistance of so much water on the roads I personally didn't think it was of much or any benefit.

Within the first two weeks, my brand-new converse I had bought before leaving Calgary were already worn out and I needed some new shoes. My dad and I stopped into a small skate shop in the East Coast, and they were generous enough to donate me a pair of red Vans to keep me going which I was super stoked about and grateful for. My holey shoes were terrible at keeping the endless water out and they were losing their ability to slow me down and act as a break so my new Vans felt heavenly hugging my plastic-wrapped feet.

My dad and I both made the mistake of drinking our waters too fast on the road one afternoon. Standardly, our "support" driver was nowhere to be found, and we were again alone in the middle of the isolated back woods. After being on the road for hours without water we finally started to see houses again. At one of the first few houses we came across, there were some people sitting outside hanging out. My father and I got off our boards and walked up to the group of three or four guys. "Excuse me gentleman, would you guys be able to fill our water bottles for us?" my dad politely asked. Without hesitation, "Ugh, do you guys want a beer?" one of the guys replied. On a beautiful sunny day, in the back woods, exerting stupid amounts of energy, an ice-cold beer was not only a wonderful privilege, but a sure thing. We walked up to the strangers, stepped up a few stairs onto their deck, and they handed each of us an ice-cold beer. We cracked our beers, sat down, and chatted with the guys about what we were doing.

After our first beer, they offered us more, but we really just needed water and with the beer dehydrating the body, we really needed water now. One of the guys grabbed our bottles from my dad and went inside for a minute. The one guy sitting on the red cooler stood up and opened it one more time to show the stash of beer and ice beneath him and asked again, "You guys sure you don't want another?" My dad said, "I wish we could, but we really have to get back on the road," just as the man with our full water bottles came back out of the side door and handed them to us. We threw them into our bags, thanked the gentleman for the chats, ice-cold beverage, and for filling our waters before we got back to pushing down the road.

As we pushed on, I couldn't help but reminisce and love the random people we had been coming across. More people wanted to help than not. This concept was entirely atypical for me, especially being a skater. I wasn't the person people helped. I was the person people put down so they could feel superior in some way. People don't usually stop to just help a longboarder, believe it or not usually it's the other way around, the longboarder generally stops to help others. But every stranger we met was more than excited, thrilled, grateful, and willing to help. It was a beautiful journey until I had to again experience the most uncomfortable thing in my life when skating through the woods. That was taking a shit without a washroom. The first time it was about a week into the trek. I told my dad I'd be a few minutes, got off the highway with the toiletry bag, and walked into the woods. I wasn't at all excited for this first of my life and wondered how one even takes a dump in the woods. Luckily for me I came across three trees that had fallen down in a triangular pattern and it made for a perfect sitting spot to drop a roast.

I perched up on one of the trees and did my business but when I went to jump down my pants caught on the tree and I almost stepped back under my squatting tree into my own steamy dung. I was hoping that was going to be the end of my shitting in the woods experience but here I was, walking back off the highway into the woods. This time I found an old oil barrel. The thing was half sunk into the ground and the rim on it was bend inward which made for a middle of the wood's toilet. As I sat there not far off the highway, I hoped no little child driving by playing "I spy" or something pointed me out going, "Mommy, look at the guy in the woods with his pants down taking a dump," as they drove by. It was very awkward and weird being in the forest going to the washroom. I felt like a barbarian or like some sort of animal. I couldn't help but think how I'd hate to have to do that every day. I then pondered life in countries without running water and toilets and thought about how lucky I am to have those simple things in my life before I finished up and got back on the road.

I had made the huge mistake of packing lots of silk boxers for the trip simply because they are more "comfortable" but that was really the dumbest thing to do because, well for one they don't stretch, and for two, they don't breathe. I forget who mentioned it but we were in the East Coast near the Stanfield's Underwear Factory in Truro, Nova Scotia with a donation request letter in hand to see if they could help me with my ripping-three-pairs-of-underwear-a-week problem. The driver and I walked inside, and I had a chat with the lady at the front desk about what we were doing that summer and asked if they would be able to help. She made a call to John Stanfield or his grandson (the current owner of the factory) then asked us if we could come back in a half hour. So we took off and found my dad at Subway to grab supper. While my dad was there, he told the kind ladies our story and mission. Deedles and Loraine kindly hooked us up with a meal on the house before my dad took a picture of myself and the two lovely "sandwich artists" that hooked us up. We ate our delicious, much-needed subs then headed back over to Stanfield's. I walked in and the receptionist pointed me towards two big boxes resting on a nearby counter and said, "those are for you guys." Not only did they hook me up with underwear for weeks, but they also threw in some thermal leggings, shirts, socks, as well as a bunch of lightweight athletic gear for both my father and myself. They hooked us up big time; it was awesome.

Longboarding through the woods in the East Coast was as cool, as it was kind of freaky. The really cool awesome part about it was riding the waves of cement roads through the woods, it was like the land was water that rippled on a lake, only this was in the middle of the forest not on a body of water. It was like surfing on the land. Once you got to the top of a crest you stood on your board and let gravity do the rest. Flying down hills in the middle of the forest surrounded by complete silence and peace made for some awesome hill-bombing experiences. The freaky part was being in the dense woods. With the impenetrable woods all around you, you couldn't tell what was coming next around a corner. You could just see the roads slightly turn corners but as soon as you got to the corner, if you were flying, you had mere seconds to react and ride according to what popped up around that corner. But there was usually enough room and time for us to stop when needed. All I could do was hope I didn't fly around a corner and hit a moose or have a scary encounter with a bear or something.

It was especially scary when you turned a corner blind into the trees then lost the tiny shoulder you had to ride on. Suddenly being forced onto the road, with unexpected or unanticipated traffic jams made for some intense rides and unexpected stops. We had to really be on our game and pay attention or we'd go into the ditch, wipe out, cause an accident, or get hit by a car or semi-truck. My new favourite times were now riding the hills in the isolated woods of Canada, it was like Fish Creek Park back home but on steroids. It was just my father, myself and the road. There was nothing else I could focus on besides my surroundings, and my surroundings were incredibly quiet, peaceful, beautiful, and joyful. Most of the time anyway.

Every once in a while, Mother Nature would remind you that she was ultimately the one in control and would unleash a downpour that felt like you were standing directly under a cold shower. That whole downpour, while you're in the middle of the woods dressed in jeans and a shirt was never enjoyable as there aren't many places to hide from Mother Nature in the middle of the woods, or on the highway. With our support driver being a huge lack of, well, support, it was just us and the elements, day in and day out. As much as it drove me crazy, made me mad, and caused a rapid river of cuss words to flow forth from my mouth, I couldn't help but know and feel it in my soul that I'd rather be there getting drenched, cold, angry, and cussing like I was the product of a sailor and trucker that had a child together, than sitting in a classroom or at a dead-end job just going through the motions like I was doing for the last few years of my life. This was more living life to me, and as much as I hated it, I absolutely loved it. The endless rain was a reminder that there are some things in life that we can't control and we as humans can do nothing but adapt to any change that may come and continue to positively progress forward.

Somewhere along the highway my father, the driver, and myself stopped at a truck stop to take a break for lunch. As I was longboarding around the big parking lot full of semi-trucks being an idiot, tucking down and riding underneath some of the parked trailers I met one of the truckers. This older woman, Donna, and I had a nice heartfelt conversation and traded stories. She was also touched by cancer in her life. She was diagnosed with terminal cancer and was only given a few months to live. This was when she suddenly got sucker punched in the face by the thought of death like I did when I was fifteen. That's when she abruptly realized that there was still so much in her life that she wanted to do, particularly travel across Canada.

She had always dreamt about travelling across Canada and seeing our incredible country, but now her dream was suddenly in jeopardy. With only a few months given to live she realized there was no better time than right now. To be able to live her dreams, it was now or never. She sprang into action with a drive unlike any other and got her trucker licence, became a long-haul trucker, and began to travel the country like she always aspired to do. The few months the doctors gave her turned into a year and she was loving driving across the country so much she continued to do it. After two years of shoving her doctors' opinions down their throats, she was right there standing in front of me, still very much alive, well, and happy. I couldn't help but immediately hypothesize that there is some sort of a profound connection between one following their heart and their passions which allows humans the ability to heal, power on, and persevere even in the face of something like cancer and death. I feel as though there is some powerful connection between following your heart and passions, and the abundance of natural healing properties for one's soul, mind, and body that comes with it.

After another day of pushing, we finished in the Moncton area. There we got our support driver to meet us at the local sports arena. We went inside and asked if we could park out back and use a power outlet for the night, and they kindly let us. The next morning, we were all getting our gear together for another day on the road in the rain and the caretaker for the building stumbled upon us in the back and struck up a conversation. He asked what we were doing there and why, so we told him. He was flabbergasted to hear what we were up to and wanted to help us anyway that he could, so he kindly offered to let us have a hot shower in the referee rooms. A nice hot shower wasn't something we were going to pass up on after days without having one. He probably caught a whiff of us and almost passed out before he made his generous offer. The gentleman took us through the back entrance and my father and I took turns having a nice hot shower. Then after our showers the kind caretaker took us into the back staff area and let us have some complementary hot chocolate and coffee out of the machine before we took off to push in the rain. He wished us luck and we thanked him kindly for his generosity and took off on the road again.

My dad and I were on the highway coming out of the Fredericton area when we decided to fill our waters and take a break at the Kenwick pharmacy. After we filled our waters, we went outside to the front deck with a wooden bench. Mavis, who was working at the time, heard our story and my brush with cancer as a young child then proceeded to tell us about the local three-and-a-half-year-old baby girl Mikaela who was currently battling the same kind of cancer that I had as a young child. As we sat outside on the bench drinking our water and taking a short break, two young teenage girls came up and struck up a conversation with us. After a short chat, one of them told my dad they happened to know where this young child and her family lived.

We wanted to go give our love and support to the family, so we got on our boards and headed over to their house. We arrived and my dad knocked on the door, rang the bell, but unfortunately nobody was there to answer. My dad took out a pen and paper then wrote them a nice note and left his contact information to get a hold of him when they could. While talking to Mavis and the two young girls outside the pharmacy, it was beautiful to see how the entire community rallied around this sick little girl and her family. It was touching to see everyone come together like they did. It reminds me of how the other families supported my mom when she was told I had cancer at the children's hospital.

Travelling on the 104 highway was amazing. We met nothing but the kindest, most caring, positive, and supportive individuals all the way down. Every small mom and pop shop or convenience store we stopped in was full of people that wanted to help out with what they could. Not only the people working at the stores but the people coming in and out that overheard our story wanted to help out. From food, water, equipment, to mental and moral support they all helped us every way they could, it was spectacular to experience.

A short time later my dad and I got up and hit the road. The mission that day was to make it to Hartland in New Brunswick. We said goodbye to the driver and took off. After pushing all day, we made it to Hartland, and to our surprise the driver was not only there but he had gone to the local school, talked to some people about what we were doing, and got some of the local kids who wanted to meet and skate with us together. Once we arrived to town, we met the driver at the local grocery store before we headed over to the school to see if anyone was still waiting around, and there were a few of them. A couple skateboarders, a kid with a scooter, and a couple of longboarders. A few of their friends all hung around and waited for us as they wanted to skate the world's longest covered bridge with my dad and myself which ran across the river only a block or two away. As I was in the parking lot of the school, I was still trying to teach myself how to slide and passing on what I did know to some of the young boys and girls there. After a while we headed down the street and over to the big, brown, wooden bridge that crossed the Saint John River. Once we all got to the end we had to wait because there was only one car allowed on the bridge at a time. The old wooden bridge only had one lane so you had to stop and wait for the car on the other side to get across and off the bridge before you could cross the other way.

We patiently stood there waiting for the car to finish crossing the bridge and as soon as it cleared, all of us took off on our boards and started to push across the rickety old bridge. With big gaps between the planks of wood it made for a very loud, bumpy, and rough ride to the other side. Once we crossed the 1,282-foot-long covered bridge we turned right and pushed down the road. That road came to a large concrete bridge a kilometre or two down that also crossed the river. The big concrete bridge had a lane in each direction for traffic, as well as sidewalks for us to safely ride on, however with no traffic, I opted to ride on the road and dodge the one or two straggly cars that might drive by. Once we made it back onto the other side of the river we turned right again and began to skate back down the road to the school where we all started. It was a fun little ride with the local kids and all happened because of the driver. We spent that night in the parking lot of the grocery store where we met our driver earlier that evening.

A short time later in the Edmundston area, my father and I put on our Stanfield gear and hit the road as always. It was there we decided to let our support driver go for his lack of, well support. He had the one good day in the three weeks of the trip thus far. It was clear not only was he a huge lack of support, but apparently also trying to scam us on top of it.

As my dad and I were walking through the parking lot of a Tim Hortons an older age gentleman rolls up to us in his small black car and stops. He then rolls down his window and asks, "What are you guys, some sort of professionals?" Looking so fresh in our athletic Stanfield gear, were now apparently "professional" looking. We stopped for a chat with him and told him what we were up to. The story really hit home with this older man as he then started to tell us how his dad was in his mid eighties when he was diagnosed with cancer. Instead of fighting the horrendous disease in his older years, the man opted to grab his gun, go into their back yard, and ended his life on his own terms fast and painless. My dad and I were incredibly heartbroken to hear this man's family's brush with cancer in their life. It was the same heartbreaking, gut wrenching, life-altering story I've heard time and time again throughout my short existence on this planet.

Now that we were nearing Quebec, we had to have a chat about the trek. More specifically, what to do about our route through Quebec. The original plan was to follow the St. Lawrence River for the whole seven-hundred-and fifty to eight-hundred kilometres but after a thorough discussion, it was decided we wouldn't push through Quebec for a few reasons. A big reason came after we got pulled over by the police a short time before.

As we were hiking up a hill, an officer put on his lights and siren to pull us over and have a chat. The officer was okay with our mission and supported us but gave us some of his advice. He highly recommended that we didn't even go through Quebec at all. He said, "The police in Quebec are not nearly as friendly and cooperative as they are in the rest of the country." This was coming from the police themselves, which had me more concerned. The officer then asked, "What are you guys going to do when you get to the mountain at the top of the hill?" As soon as the word "mountain" come out of his mouth I got excited and went to walk up the hill instead of standing there talking.

Another reason for cutting Quebec was the distant memory of what had happened to our trailer when it went through the Quebec roads. The road conditions were apparently horrendous. However, the number one and two reasons were because we now had no support driver or shelter, and my dad nor I could speak French to communicate or even attempt to adequately communicate with anyone. The communication with random people, in random locations seemed to be what was keeping us alive and moving from one town to the next more than our driver was. By cutting out that line of communication we would have no way to ask for help if we needed it, and that was going to leave us incredibly vulnerable. However not all the police we encountered would drop bombs on us like this.

Once we got to the top of the "mountain" the officer had mentioned, I got on my board and started to push away. It was definitely not a "mountain" to me as I was born and raised beside the Canadian Rockies. It was more like back-to-back massive hills to ride down. The first one was really scary as the shoulder we had to ride on was again only a few inches bigger than the width of our boards. We had the rumble strip on our left and the ditch to our right, if we moved over just a few inches we were on the strips or in the ditch so there wasn't much margin for error. As I came around this long, slow left-hand turn that went downhill, I moved over onto the rumble strips while going pretty fast and it almost caused me to biff into the ditch. But luckily after I looked for cars and saw none I shot over onto the road and regained control. After the first big hill we got to a truck stop, turning around a long right corner there were big semi-trucks lined up in every lane at what looked like a border crossing. With big trucks all around us, my dad and I just kicked along through the traffic jam and continued down the road.

Once we got to the second of the big hills the kind officer told us about, I looked down and could see the massive hill had a slight right curve in it but you could clearly see the hill from top to bottom, including the nice straight run out. At the bottom you could see a small, thin bridge that crossed over the highway. With the truck stop behind us, there wasn't much traffic. But I took a quick look behind me and saw nothing, so I quickly crossed over from between the rumble strips and the ditch onto the road. Only as soon as I did, a big rig came around the corner and was approaching fast so I moved over to the empty oncoming lane to let the driver pass. I came flying down the hill at full speed in the empty lane. As the semi driver slowly passed me on my right in the outgoing lane, he gives me a little honk on the way by, probably to say, 'get the hell off the road, you crazy bastard.' It was my first time ever ripping down a hill that big, going that fast, in the oncoming lane, and having a big truck within a few arms' lengths away beside me—it was a tad freaky. Just the driver passing me or driving beside me threw me off balance from the wind it created.

I wanted to rip the whole hill without stopping but it was both the beginning of the trek and the beginning of the longboarding season, so I always started the hills off slowly before going full speed. I always took it easy at the beginning of the longboarding season because when you try and pick up where you left off at the end of last season, more often than not, you're just asking for the road to shed your skin like a cheese grater, to break some bones, and go to the hospital. I've done it, I've seen many of my friends do it, and I've heard more stories than I'd like so I always took it easy the first few months on my board until I felt the profound connection with it, like I somehow became one with it. Once I hit that stage I don't stop or bother to slow down, and I ride down the hills like a speed demon. It's great.

One of the coolest experiences of my life happened on the highway in the East Coast of Canada. I don't remember which day or exactly where it was, but we were on the highway just skating along when out of nowhere I hear, "Woop Woop!" the sounds of the police with red and blue lights flashing right behind us. My first thought was 'for fuck sakes' as until this trek every time I've been in this spot, I've been warned, frisked, harassed, fined, arrested, and continued to loop that traffic circle of self-destruction. So, my mind always immediately went to that head space with every unexpected police encounter. But this was different. This was for a cause, this was me doing some good before I died, and this couldn't possibly end with me in the back of the car arrested, could it? My dad and I jumped off our boards and walked over to the officer as he got out of his car. He then asks what we're doing on the side of the highway in the middle of nowhere. My father tells him our mission, and my story before the officer kindly asked for some identification. We gave him our IDs and the officer goes back to his car to run our names following the usual police procedure.

As he's in the car running our names my hands got all sweaty and clammy from my nervousness as I half expected to be arrested for another unknown reason. Maybe it was because of all the fights, maybe it was because my probation officer wasn't done making my life miserable, or maybe it was because of something I had completely forgotten about, like another fine. My mind's now racing with the worst-case scenario which is causing my body to transpire and shake. A few minutes later, the officer emerges from his vehicle then comes back over to us, and as he's handing us our identification back he says, "Well you know, I'm kind of a sucker for causes, guys." I wasn't quite sure where the officer was going with this. My first thought was 'maybe he's going to write a check for one of the foundations we were supporting.' Then the officer asked, "How would you guys like an escort into town?"

My mind exploded in disbelief while thinking, 'hopefully it's not another escort to jail,' as I scream out "HECK YEAH!" My father then replied with a more subtle, adult-like answer before we got back on our boards and began longboarding down the road again. For the first time since we took off on this trek, I was able to put both my headphones in and tune out the traffic as we now had a police officer behind us with the lights flashing giving us an escort and could ignore the traffic.

He did tell us if he got a call, he would have to take off so we may lose him any time, which was understandable, but this was way too awesome and I knew I had to enjoy it while it lasted.

Now I'm kicking down the road thinking 'this is way too cool' and 'it's funny how things can change if you want them to.' One of my songs ended and as I was waiting for the next one to come on, I heard a car honking at us as it drove by. A bit further down the road another car came honking as it was driving by. This time there was an arm out the passenger window waving at us and giving us a thumbs up in support. That was a huge first for me. Apart from this mission, most people seeing longboarders on the road just honk and tell us we are number one by giving us the middle finger. Before this journey, not a single person ever waved and gave a thumbs up in support. But now that's changed. What in the heck was going on in the world? People are being kind, courteous, and supportive even when they're just driving by with no clue on what was going on. Like the people driving by, I was in a mental state of 'what the hell is going on?' probably as much, if not more than they were.

I had spent the last nineteen years having life, the government, courts, and police shit all over me. Suddenly people I didn't even know (police included) did whatever they could to help, support, and be sure that my dream and mission became a success. All of it was beginning to pull on my heart strings and touched my soul with something it never had felt before. This new joy, happiness, hope, and positive reinforcements my soul was receiving from every person that came our way was beginning to change me, shape me, and enamour me with the hopes of a successful dream and even a future.

It was definitely one of the coolest experiences of my life. It was in that moment I realized without a reasonable doubt that I was finally on the right path in life. Because to me, when an officer takes time out of his busy day not to harass, frisk, or bother you, but instead to help ensure your dreams get achieved safely was a pretty amazing feeling. This trek was the first and only time I felt the enveloping love, respect, and care from a police officer given my recent history. This experience confirmed I was on the right path in life. I was no longer aimlessly lost on that traffic circle. I had finally taken a turn off and it turned out to be the best decision I've ever made, even if the road after the turn off was nearly 7,000-kilometres long. It was long sure, but it was also right. For the first time I felt like I had purpose, like life was worth something. It was like I had direction in life and not just travelling west in physical form, but like it had direction in the mental and spiritual form as well. As well as unleashing my unfathomable, pent-up rage and anger in a good positive way, life wasn't as shitty as I once previously thought; life was actually pretty beautiful.

Once we got to the Quebec boarder, we took a bus into Montreal where we then had to wait for a bus to take us to the Ontario boarder. We had some time to kill in Montreal, so I went for a little skate and adventure hoping to see some graffiti as I've heard good things about the street art in Montreal. I grabbed my board, walked outside, and went left out of the doors onto the sidewalk. I put my board down and started to skate. I got maybe fifty feet when the brick wall on my left side indented and as I coasted by the indent of this little nook, there was a guy sticking a needle in his left arm. I saw that and kept skating along. Just the thought of sticking myself with a needle made me quiver and feel sick but I continued on hoping I wasn't going to come into a sketchy part of town. But after seeing needle man in the little nook, I figured I was already there so I continued on, minding my own business.

I took my next left and started to skate down the street and saw some decent graffiti pieces on my right side, high up on some walls. There were also some C-cans there, so I went to investigate them as well. After checking out the cool graffiti pieces all over the walls and C-cans I continued to skate down a few more streets before making another left and skating back towards the main street the heroin-infested bus station was on. I got back to the main street and made another left to come around the building where I began and went back inside to wait. It was only a short ten- to fifteen-minute cruise around a few blocks, but still a small side adventure for me.

As I got back, I was noticing police, closed off roads, and lots of cyclists riding through downtown. They had some sort of big bike event going on that day. I was tempted to go out to join for a bit and push my longboard around with the cyclists, but after the warning about the French police and looking incredibly out of place, I decided against it.

To make up for the missed 750-kilometres through Quebec we decided we would take a little 750-kilometre detour across Ontario. This detour would only include the most amazing time of my life, spark a series of events that would travel thousands of kilometres across Canada, completely restore my faith in humanity, begin friendships that will last a lifetime, and prove to me without a reasonable doubt, that everything happens for a reason.

The Big Beautiful O

Once we got to the Ontario boarder, we were back on the road pushing again and maybe five minutes after getting to the big Ontario sign, I saw a big bag in the ditch on the right side of the road. I skated up to it in the outbound lane and as I got closer, I started to make out the contents of the big, clear Ziplock bag. Inside the big Ziplock bag were two smaller sandwich bags. One of the smaller bags I could tell had multiple packs of different types of rolling papers and the other I didn't really quite identify completely, however from the green colour I could only assume an excessive amount of smoke clouds were the contents. As soon as I saw the big green bag inside, I was tempted to grab it, however I quickly started to reminisce about the dozens of times we've already been pulled over. The last thing we needed on us was a big stinky bag of the Devil's lettuce on top of the portioned-out bags of white protein powder that already look a little suspicious. Plus, we were on a mission, a charity mission. I don't think we would have been making it very far if we were in the ditch giggling at the clouds. So breaking the heart of fourteen-year-old me, the big bag of bags stayed on the side of the road in the ditch and we continued on. From the Quebec/Ontario boarder, our first major city we hit was going to be Ottawa, however we had a couple small towns to go through first.

As my father and I were going against traffic in the oncoming lane coming into a small town I was pushing along when one of my headphones fell out (one of the reasons I like the oncoming lane is that I could see everything coming and cut out the sounds of approaching traffic and listen to music); however, my new musicless ear opened up violently to the sounds of passing traffic. Just as my headphone fell out, a big semi-truck let out a tremendous blast from their air horn on the other side of the highway in the outgoing lane. Just as the truck driver let out this colossal roar from his air horn a tiny little pebble jammed the front right wheel on my board which produced an awful screeching noise and the sudden stop almost tossed me off the front of my board. Between the sudden, loud noises from the truck's horn, my wheel screaming against the ground, and my body being suddenly thrown forward from the unexpected stop of my wheel, it genuinely scared the shit out of me. I literally jolted into the air off my board before I almost ate the pavement of the highway for the first time on the trek. Luckily, I caught my balance and ran it out after I flew forward, and didn't nosedive into the pavement, that time. I just let out one or two cuss words, kicked the rock that jammed my wheel, grabbed my board, and continued pushing into the small town with soiled pants and my heart now racing.

We saw a rest stop area on the right side of the highway when we got to the small town and decided to stop there, take a short break, and have a coffee. As my father and I rested our feet and were enjoying our nice, hot burnt-bean juice outside, a middle-aged man came up to us and asked us why we were on the highway. Turns out he was the trucker that honked his horn and scared the pants off of me. I told him how his horn and my jammed wheel at the same time scared the pants off of me, and all three of us had a good laugh. Once he heard what we were doing the kind gentleman reached into his back pocket and pulled out five bucks and gave it to us saying, "Coffee is on me, gentleman." He then told us he was going to radio the other truckers on the road and send out a message to watch for us.

We thanked him for the coffee money and the radio shout out before we got back on the road through the small town. After a short skate through town, we came across a picnic bench on the right side of the highway. It was right before the uphill leaving town that we had to walk up. It was our last chance to take a break and rest our feet so we grabbed our waters and sat at the bench to have a sip. We sat there debating whether or not to get ice cream from the ice cream shack conveniently located beside us across a small patch of grass. Meanwhile, an older man came around the corner of a nearby building, walked up to us and we started to chat. This man said he was living in a half-burnt-down church just around the corner and he was slowly fixing it up and restoring it day by day. Once he heard our mission, he was astonished and pulled out his wallet to give us twenty of his last forty dollars so that we could eat a meal and get closer to our final destination. After a short chat, we thanked him for his generosity and got back on the road walking up the hill that exited the small town.

Once again, I was amazed at how every single person that heard what we're doing did whatever they could on the spot, and even more after our presence was gone to help us complete our mission. It kept reassuring me that this was the right thing to do with my life and with my time. Before this trip, my life was like an empty, blank canvas, and every single person we met along the way was a colourful brush stroke that slowly started to change that blank empty canvas into a beautiful, intricate, complex piece of art. Day by day, person by person, kilometre by kilometre the canvas of my life was beginning to take shape. It slowly began to have depth, it began to have meaning, and for the first time in my life it began to hold value. I no longer saw life as disgusting and unfair.

I started to see how incredible, meaningful, purposeful, and magnificent life could be if one just simply chose to make the most of it.

Once we left the small town we were in, it was back to being in the woods and only in the woods. There was nothing but tall trees and one lonely road that twisted through them. It was incredibly peaceful, quiet, and very beautiful. Until out of nowhere the dead silence was broken by the blast of another air horn. I looked to my right and saw a semi-truck driver looking and waving at us in the outgoing lane, so we smiled and waved back. For the rest of the day almost every semi-truck driver gave us lots of room by moving over for us as they passed us. They honked, they waved, and they gave us big smiles and thumbs up out their windows all in support of our mission. The truck driver's message over the radio was noticeably heard loud and clear by the others. It was really nice to see the long-haul, big-rig family have such loving and caring hearts. Their hearts seemed to be as big as the rigs they drove. It was like the blast of every air horn wasn't just a loud ear-piercing noise that recently nearly had me crap my pants, but more of a reminder to keep going forward on our mission and not to give up. The blasts from the air horns became somewhat of a motivation booster and kept me going throughout the day. Each one was another person letting us know they approved of our mission and, every time they let me know, it hit that emotional heart string that I wasn't used to having so many people hit. The frequency of these magnificent individuals hitting that string was so incredibly overwhelming I had no idea how to take it all in and process it.

Once we hit the edge of Ottawa, my dad's buddy, Kevin picked us up and we stayed at his place for the weekend. With the success of another city under our belts, dad and I decided to go have a beer at the local pub with his old buddy, accompanied by his girlfriend. After I had my beer, I was hungry, so I took a look at the food menu which was around twenty bucks for a basic meal. So, I convinced my dad to let me use his bank card so I could go to the McDonalds I remember seeing not too far away; there I could eat for cheap instead of spending five times as much at the pub and he agreed.

I got the card from my dad, grabbed my board, left the bar, and started pushing along. Only I started to go the wrong way. After skating for a bit I came across an outdoor market area so I got off and carried my longboard around as I walked around checking things out. Then I saw the parliament buildings off in the background. I had only ever seen pictures of it, so I skated over to it, then skated around the brick castle-like building to give it a look before ending up back at the market. After my short loop, I was still aimlessly skating around. Then I saw a hill that went into the downtown core part of town and couldn't resist the urge to bomb down it.

Now, with the sun almost gone, I was aimlessly skating around in the downtown core area with no idea where I was going as I tried to find some cheap food, hoping for the best. On top of that, I had no phone after the pockets in my rain pants filled up with water and drowned it. I finally came across a McDonald's and ordered a couple burgers off the cheap menu before I scarfed them down.

Now I just had to make my way back to the bar by King Edward Ave. That's all I knew about where we were staying; but I knew once I found King Edward Ave, I could find my dad's friend's place from there. But after leaving the McDonald's I started to go the wrong way, again. I skated around looking for the hill into downtown that I came down on. It wasn't too far so how hard could it be to find? After an hour of aimlessly skating around I finally realized I was super lost, had no idea where I was, what way is what, what the time was, or what way I needed to be going. All I knew was that I needed to find "King Edward Ave." As I'm in this thought process, I saw a guy in a white muscle shirt and blue jeans covered in tattoos having a cigarette, so I approached him and asked the buff man if he had any idea where King Edward Ave was. The guy looks at me, then just laughs, and says, "ha! that's far, man." Those were definitely not the words I wanted to hear, but it was just his opinion.

That's when I told him, "I just skated here with my dad from St. John's and were heading all the way to the West Coast, now that's far." He, like most people who heard the story said, "Holy fuck, no kidding, that's one hell of a trip man." I then asked, "Do you know what way I need to be going to get to King Edward Ave?" He then says to me, "You're on the complete opposite side of downtown, buddy." How I got that far just pushing around, I have no idea. He then says, "You need to go that way," and points off in a general direction. He follows up and says, "You have to go that way until you get to the river, then go over the bridge at the river, across the university grounds, and keep going that way until you hit King Edward Ave." I repeated the instructions to be sure I got it right and he confirmed I did. I thanked him for his help before he wished my dad and I the best of luck on our trek. I got back on my way, now in the complete darkness of night praying that the stranger didn't send me into the Canadian equivalent of Compton Avenue which I've heard lots about in movies and rap music over the years. With a movie quote from Menace to Society that says, "Hope you can find your way down Compton Avenue, mother fucker," running through my mind, I went around the corner and skated through the dimly lit streets until I got to the small, brick bridge that crossed the river the man was talking about.

I then got off my board and began to walk across the bridge, stopping in the middle to watch and listen to the water running underneath me and enjoying the peace and tranquility of the moment. I was feeling very content with life more than ever these recent few weeks. It was also a beautiful summer night. There were no clouds, no wind, and it was the perfect temperature for a nighttime longboarding adventure. With the sun gone, it was dark but with the streetlights on combined with the natural moonlight, I could see where I was going, and I could tell if I was going to hit a big crack in the roads or sidewalks.

After the bridge I had to find the university grounds which wasn't too far, but I had no idea how big the university grounds were or where I had to go to get through them. Luckily it was fairly easy as there were students walking around everywhere on that beautiful, warm night. After asking a few students for directions I got to the other side of the relatively small university grounds. From there I didn't know where to go as I only had "that way" and nothing else to go off. I patiently stood around spinning my board with the top end in my palm and the back end resting on the ground waiting for another person to ask for directions and after about five minutes, I had found one. The young man pointed me the way I had to go, and I started to skate in that direction. After about five or ten minutes of skating I got to an intersection and on the road sign I was relieved to see it said "King Edward Ave."

I finally had a general idea on where I was and what way I needed to go for the first time in hours. I took a left onto King Edward Ave and started to push down the empty streets avoiding the odd car here and there. I skated and skated only to realize I skated too far, and I turned back. This time I decided to take the side street I remembered everyone walked down to get to the bar, trying to retrace our steps. I got a block or two down that side street when I saw a few people coming my way on the sidewalk. As I got closer, I could swear these people looked familiar. As I got even closer to them, I noticed it was my dad, his friend, and his friend's girlfriend. The timing of it all was impeccable. I got off my board and walked with them the half block back to his house. I again skated too far and rode past the house. As I came up to them, I said, "Man, am I ever glad to see you guys. I've been lost for hours." They thought I had just gone back to his friend's house and decided to come see if I was alive. When we got back, I gave my dad his debit card back with the receipt before I went to bed and crashed hard as I was tired from my random unexpected trip around downtown Ottawa after skating all day to get there. I remember thinking 'good thing it was a tiny downtown and not one like New York, Boston, Los Angeles, or other huge cities like that.'

From Ottawa, we headed south down towards Kemptville, Ontario where we stayed with some incredible "couch surfers" for the night. The next morning, we were up and, on the road, again when we came across a little convenience store called "Moose Mart" on the left side of the road we were on. We decided to stop there, grab a coffee, and take a short break. My dad was talking to the store owner and Kevin was kind enough to give us the much-wanted morning coffees on the house. As we grabbed our coffees a young couple came into the store and overheard the story of what we were doing while my dad talked with Kevin. They were amazed and asked if they could help us. My father kindly asked if they could take our heavy backpacks and drive them to the next town where we were going to stop for the night. Nina and James had nothing going on for the day, so without hesitation they offered to be our support driver and drive behind us to be sure we were safe from any crazy drivers on the road.

All morning and into the afternoon, in the on-and-off rain Nina and James followed us in their minivan on the side of the roadway with their four ways flashing. For hours on end, they slowly tailed us just to make sure we were safe and got to our destination that day. After hours and hours on the road we finally arrived at the town where we were to stay for the night. My dad and I got off our boards to have another chat with Nina and James and to thank them for their kind generosity. While James drove behind us all day, Nina got a call from her mother who asked what she was up to on her day off. Nina told her mom what they were doing before going into our mission and what we were doing that summer. Nina's mother was so blown away by our mission that unknown to my father and myself, she booked us a hotel room in town for the night to help us out. We had no idea until we got there which was an incredible surprise. Again, my father and I were awestruck by the ripple effect caused by the amazing people we came across. My father and I were not only riding the ripple-like waves in the stunning land, but we were also riding the waves of people's generosity in between and it was such a beautiful thing to watch unfold before our eyes as we went from town to town and city to city.

With so many random strangers that went out of their way to help us, I started to realize that I wasn't in a country full of strangers. Sure, I may not know them personally, know their names, their background stories, or past. But to me, it was like being lost and travelling in a country full of family, not strangers. Every single person we came across just wanted to help and offered their services. With each individual's act of unconditional care, love and kindness, the canvas of my life was becoming clearer. It was becoming more colourful, beautiful, spectacular, and more unlike anything I've ever seen in my life. My dad and I took a picture with the amazing couple for the Facebook page before we checked into our room and relaxed. 'This is unbelievably amazing,' I couldn't help but think to myself as my father and I rested in bed for the night after a much-needed shower and change of clothes. Getting to our destination then finally changing out of our soaking-wet clothing and into fresh clean, dry stuff was the absolute best feeling in the world. Top it off with a soft, fresh, clean, and warm bed to lay in after a few thousand one-legged squats and pushes, I don't think there was anything more enjoyable than that.

The next day, we began our way farther south to Kingston and as my father and I were on the side of the highway, a man driving a blue Ford Explorer pulling a small trailer pulled over. It's not very often you come across two random people on the side of the road in the isolated Canadian woods. Cory got out of his SUV, introduced himself, and asked if we were okay before he asked what we were doing in the middle of nowhere. My dad introduced the both of us before telling him our mission. Cory was amazed and asked my dad, "Where are you guys heading today?" My father told him, and Cory said, "You will be passing my house as soon as you get into town." We only had one road to skate that day, one very long road, which would consume the next five or six hours of our day.

Cory asked if there was anything he could do to help before my father asked if he could take our fifty-pound bags for us into town where we were going to be staying. Cory said he was more than happy to do that for us. He also said he would be outside all day working on his front yard so when we get to town keep an eye out for him and be sure to stop and say hello. After several hours of skating, we came around a right turn through the woods where I saw houses coming up on the right side. I saw Cory on his front lawn right away. He came running over to me then said, "I brought your things to the hotel in town." Before he adds, "Open this when you get there," as he hands me a small brown envelope. I put it into my hoodie pocket thinking nothing of it before we thanked him for his help and kept on pushing through town. Every once in a while, I would put my right hand in my hoodie and feel the envelope in my pocket. The suspense of what might be inside had me guessing. I was assuming it was another check for one of the foundations we were supporting but had no idea. We got to town and went to our hotel to spend the night. Once there, my father and I opened the small brown envelope from Cory. Inside was a reservation number on a note. The reservation number was for a room he paid for, to put us up for the night.

The generosity from the strangers we met was just unfathomable, my father and I were once again blown away by it. We gave the reservation number to the guy at the front desk of the hotel, and it came up with nothing. He also had no idea where our backpacks with everything we owned were. The kind man at the desk picked up the phone, called the hotel next door, got a matching reservation code for us, and confirmed our belongings were there safely secured. We grabbed our boards and pushed through a parking lot over to the other hotel, got our belongings and settled in for the night. I really struggled to sleep that night which was something I was well accustomed to. The thought of death had kept me up late at night for years, but this was entirely different. The thought of death hadn't crossed my mind in weeks other than the close calls with cars and ditches. I was now kept up by reminiscing over the overwhelming generosity, kindness, love, and respect everyone had given us, literally from day one.

It was the most beautiful life experience I have ever lived. I also couldn't help but think about the previous four years of downward spiralling I had done in my life. I couldn't help but wonder how I had become such an asshole in a country with so much genuine love and compassion. I had no excuse for any of it. Sure, I felt life had shit all over me but even that was no excuse for not being a caring, compassionate, and genuine person. I couldn't help but shake my head in disgust while reminiscing about my past trying to fall asleep that night.

The next day it was get up, shower, pack our bags, and push on the road for another day. After a few hours on the road, we decided to take a break in a Tim Hortons. We walked into the Tim's and there at one of the tables sat a group of four or five OPP (Ontario Provincial Police) officers. Thinking ahead, my dad began to talk to them to let them know we would be on the highway around town that day. Once one of the officers heard our story he said, "Holy! Longboarding across Canada, hey, You must have lost a lot of weight." My dad doesn't even take a second and replies with, "Yeah. When we started, I looked like this guy," as he points to the officer at the table with the biggest gut and build. The officers all burst out laughing meanwhile I'm standing there trying so hard to keep a straight face, but I couldn't. I had to turn around because I couldn't keep my composure. While laughing hysterically I was thinking, 'oh shots (insults) fired by my dad at the OPP.' By the end, they didn't care about us being on the road, they just told us to be safe and not to obstruct traffic. Later on, one of the cops passed us in his marked car and gave a little "woop woop" with his lights and siren as a "hello" as he drove by. I couldn't help but think 'that must have not been the officer my dad insulted as he probably would have just run him over' and had a good laugh thinking about the situation again.

A few days later, we had another break at a Tim Hortons. Tim's was doing a promotion on the Keurig coffee machines where if you bought an eighty pack of the Keurig cups, they would give you a free Keurig coffee machine and we just happened to be there that day at eleven in the morning. We got there at around ten thirty or quarter too eleven and stood in line to place our order before we sat down. As we stood in line, my dad and this woman who was at the tables started talking and told us about the promo. We ate our meals and right at eleven the place was suddenly packed with people there for the promotion. My dad got in line and the lady said she would pay for my dad's Keurig pods and they both got a coffee machine. I thought my dad was an idiot for getting it as he now had a huge box to skate with, but then he donated it back to her and suggested she gift it to someone she mentioned would love one. So, they put the machines in the back of her car, and after she wished us good luck on the rest of our journey, we got back on the road. The few minutes we stood in line and had a chat with this woman would later benefit us when she sent us a generous donation to keep us going.

With all the rain in the East Coast, I was praying for some nice sunny ones, and got them. But if there's one thing I learned about life, it's that you better be careful what you wish for. One morning I would get my wish. When we first got on the road, it was a nice sunny day to start but after an hour or two the temperature dropped ten degrees, the moisture in the air was felt, the dark clouds rolled in, and we got dumped on by rain. When it started to pour on us, we jumped off the road and tried to hide under a big tree just off to the right side of the road. We sat on our boards under the big tree and hid out the nasty storm for five or ten minutes before it past. After the worst of it was over, we climbed out from under the tree and got back on the road. That's when the sun came out with a burning vengeance. The sun quickly evaporated the huge amounts of water everywhere and it got incredibly humid and hot at the same time. The extreme humidity of southern Ontario was something I had never felt in my life before. It felt worse than the humidity I felt in the Dominican with the Lloyd family, which blew my mind. Once I started longboarding, I started to overheat, once I started to overheat, I started to slam back my water, as did my father. It wasn't long before we both had no water and continued on in the incredibly hot humidity. I'm from Calgary where its super dry most of the time so skating in the humidity was completely new to me and I got uncomfortably hot and didn't like it at all. I was just glad I didn't have silk boxer shorts on.

I quickly realized how dumb it was to slam back all my water after thirty minutes with it still super-hot and humid outside. Now I was uncomfortably hot, sweating like crazy, while wishing I didn't drink all my water. With my dad's water supply also depleted, I couldn't steal any of his. We needed to stop and find a place to fill up. But we were in the middle of nowhere, trapped in the abundant, endless Canadian woods, on a random road. No houses, no stores, or anywhere we could see to fill up. Even if we had Life Straws (or something like it), we couldn't find a big enough body of water to drink from as the hot sun had dried everything up, compounding the humidity to the unbearable level. It was the first time in my life I felt like I was physically melting without legal or illegal drugs in my system. I was high, but not on drugs, what was going on? I continued on with my dad slowly getting further and further ahead as I felt like I was about to drop and pass out. "RAIN! PLEASE RAIN OR SOMETHING!" I screamed out to the sky before having a laugh at the irony of me screaming for the rain to stop for three straight weeks and I was now begging for it.

After an hour or so of melting in this incredibly uncomfortable humid heat we finally came across a house that had some people outside on their deck enjoying the hot summer day. We walked off the main road, down a gravel road, and over to them where my dad kindly asked if they could fill up our water bottles. We sat outside and had a short chat about our mission with this nice family as they filled up our bottles with water and ice. The kind lady came out, handed me my water bottle, and I drank it all in about five seconds flat. She looked at me and said, "Holy! You must have been thirsty." I replied, "Yeah, you have no idea." She then took my bottle and kindly filled it up with some more water and ice. We thanked the family of strangers and headed out, as they wished us good luck with the rest of our trip.

We got back on the road, turned a left corner into the woods, and were now facing a massive uphill. We began walking up and I started to get tired and thirsty again so I took a very small sip of water to try and conserve as much of the precious commodity as I could. Once we got to the top of the hill we began to skate down the now flat roadway, and after one or two minutes of skating down the road, a small silver car pulls over onto the left side of the road on the median. A very tall, skinny man jumped out and flagged me down. He asked, "Hey, are you the ones longboarding across Canada?" I replied, "Yeah buddy." He then tells me to hold on and wait a minute as he rummages through his car. I stood there as my dad came up to us and after a few minutes the tall, thin man came back over and he handed me some change and says, "Sorry I thought I had more, I wish I could give you guys more, but that's all I could find." I told him, "Don't even worry, man, every penny counts, thank you," as I put the change in my small jean pocket. My dad asked him how he heard about us and he said, "Facebook." Then it was back on the road continuing on our detour south across Ontario. After some time, we got to Kingston. I got off my board and my dad took a picture of me and the "Welcome to Kingston" sign on the beautiful sunny day.

There we stayed with another awesome couch surfer who had a nice big house that backed onto the St. Lawrence River just before it entered Lake Ontario. On his second story back deck he built a ramp that went from the back deck down to the end of his dock, with a jump at the end. He and his friends would take their bikes down on it and launch into the water on the hot summer days. I was incredibly tempted to try it on my longboard but knew it wasn't worth losing or destroying a complete longboard, so I had to hold myself back and just dreamt of doing it. Although, a roll of black and white polly and a garden hose could have made things very interesting.

From there, our next major city was Oshawa where my dad had a relative, Barb. She generously put us up for a few days as we came through town. This is where I would have my first longboarding tumble of the trip. But first, as soon as we got into town, we stopped at the local West 49 so they could re-grip my board. The kind associate, Jake, put fresh grip tape on my board before we stopped by the dollar store to grab a handful of items, then went over to Barb's who conveniently lived at the top of a little hill.

I thought it would be cool to mount the GoPro on my board and go for a ride down the hill that Barb lived on and see how the video went. I traced the outline of the GoPro mount just above my front truck, then cut out the small piece of fresh grip tape and pulled it off so the mount would stick right to the longboard deck. I pulled off the piece that covers the adhesive on the mount and stuck it on my board before I stood on it for a few minutes. Once I was satisfied, I stood on it for a sufficient amount of time, I got off and pulled on it a bit just to make sure it was on the board snug and secure. I then clipped the camera onto it, got on my board, and walked down the few steps before jumping on my board, gaining speed down the driveway at the top of the hill. I went down the driveway onto the street before I slightly carved left and took off down the hill.

Only problem was the vibrations from the road made the camera fall forward. The camera kept vibrating down, so it was either looking down at the road, or up so it was looking at the bright blue sky. I had to keep bending over and looking down so that I could reposition the camera. As I was looking down repositioning it, I looked back up and saw the front end of a silver Ford SUV heading right for me. I cut right hard to avoid the head-on collision. As we passed each other I shouted out, "SORRY!" to the guy driving who was shaking his head.

Narrowly avoiding the head-on collision, I started to gain some speed, so I started to carve left and right, then left and right, feeling the board and road under my feet getting ready to do a slide. After my quick 180-degree slide, I turned my body around on my board, so I was again riding my preferred way. After riding past another few houses, I got enough speed to do another slide. I gave one big momentum kick and did another little 180-degree slide. As my wheels screeched against the road the vibrations made the camera fall again. I turned my body around again and coasted through the T-intersection, across the street, and onto the sidewalk before I turned right following a small loop around to the benches at a small rest area. I bent down and turned off the camera before I walked back to the top of the hill.

Once I got to the top, I turned around and started to push down the hill again. This time I wanted to go faster as I did a slide, so I rode further down the hill and gave a few extra kicks to really get going. I then did my usual 180-degree slide, but I spun around way too fast. Now I was going too fast for my abilities to ride switch down the hill. I noticed there was a right turn onto another street that looked flat. So, I turned right. But it wasn't all flat, it was flat for a few houses then went down like the hill I was previously on. I started to go even faster, and I knew I wasn't going to be able to ride out the small hill going backwards. I then went into full-on desperation panic mode and looked to my right where I saw a big grass lawn. I figured a soft grass lawn would be my safest bet to crash onto, so I hesitantly turned towards this person's lawn until I hit the curb. My board made a dead stop as I went flying into the grass and across the entire lawn, just barely missing the small tree in the front yard after I took an awkward bounce. I got up, dusted myself off, and took a quick look around to see if anyone saw what just happened. Thankfully I didn't have an audience that I could see, so I tucked my head down, grabbed my board, and did the walk of shame back up the hill. I turned left off that street and headed back up the hill to Barb's house, to do it all again. I thought I had gotten my fall onto the stranger's yard on film so as soon as I got back, I went to watch it. However, I forgot to turn it on and got genuinely chapped I couldn't re-watch it and laugh at myself.

After not being able to watch myself fly off my board, I went down the hill one more time to try and slide faster without the summersaults across people's lawns. I came down Barb's driveway at the top of the hill then started to push as hard as I could to get some speed and once I thought I was going a bit faster than the last time, I put my right hand down and did a much slower slide and lost most of my speed. I quickly did a 180-degree jump on my board really wishing I took the time to learn how to slide before the trek. After jumping and spinning around so I was standing my preferred way I kept on going to the bottom of the hill and did another slow 180- degree slide and another 180-degree jump so I could keep pushing. As I turned right onto the street, I took a few big kicks to get some momentum again. I started to come up to a T-intersection with a stop sign. Just as I was approaching the stop sign a black Chevy turned left at it and was coming my way. I looked at the driver and passenger to see it was my dad and Barb. I put my right hand down and did a slide to lose some speed before I jumped off my board. I went up to Barb who was driving, and she said they were going to take me to a bigger hill around town.

I had been asking Barb about some big hills to ride all night since we got to town, so she kindly took the time to take me for another small side adventure. I put my longboard wheels up in the bed of the truck and jumped into the back seat. It was only a short five- or ten-minute ride until we got there. I was dropped off at the top, and they drove back down to the bottom to pull over and try to record my speed. I put the camera back on my board to see if it worked on that road. I pressed record, put my right foot on the front on my board, pushed it back and forth a few times to get the feels and then got on my board just as a small Chevy car came up the hill in the oncoming lane. I gave a few light pushes taking it easy on the first run to see how the road conditions were. I then hit a huge crack in the road. As soon as I hit it, the GoPro went face down towards the road. I took a quick look and saw a blueish green Chevy truck coming my way, so I moved over to let the truck and small white car following it pass. After traffic was clear I bent down to fix the camera. Just as I started to get going faster, I hit another crack in the road and the camera again went pointing down towards the ground. I bent down and fixed it again just as a small white Toyota car went by me in the oncoming lane. I took another quick peek behind for traffic and saw nothing, again I bent down to fix the camera, only I was now going so fast the vibrations just had it fall right back down to the road. It obviously wasn't working, so I just left it alone until I slowed down a little.

I came flying by my dad and Barb standing on the right side of the road as I bent down to fix the camera hoping it would stand on the smoother part of the road, only to have it fall over again. I repositioned it yet again and it fell so I completely gave up. Instead, I did a quick slide to lose some of my speed before heading back to the truck for a lift to the top so I could rip down the hill again. I got out at the top as they drove back down the hill. I wasn't having this GoPro issue again, so I took it off my board and put it on my helmet before I started to skate for the hill. I passed a big house on my right that sat on the crest of the hill before I took a few big kicks and started off down it.

I noticed a car coming in the oncoming lane, so I looked behind me to see nothing in mine and I came down the middle of the outgoing lane, hitting the cracks in the road harder than I did before. A white Honda drove by, followed by a motorcycle, then a Pontiac SUV in the oncoming lane as I flew by the house at the bottom of the hill that was on my right followed by Barb and my father standing on the side of the road. As I got to the bottom, I looked around and only saw one car in the oncoming lane so once it had past me, I turned my board and did a little slide then my usual 180-degree rotation and a hard U-turn before I headed back to the truck for another ride to the top.

This time I wasn't going to take it easy, so after a quick look around for traffic and seeing none, I passed the white 60 kmph sign before floating by the big houses on the right and left sides of the street. I looked around to see a small, grey Pontiac car in the oncoming lane. After it past me, I took another look around and saw nothing so I tucked down as low as I could to reduce the drag from the wind and went straight down the hill in the outbound lane. I looked behind me again to see a black jeep slowly approaching, so I moved over as much as I could, and he slowly trickled by. After he past me, I looked for more traffic to see an empty road and I did my usual slide before I headed back to my dad and Barb who reported to me that I was breaking the speed limit on the short hill. After the few runs on the hill, we headed back to Barb's for supper, and for dessert, we had a scoop of vanilla ice cream with a shot of maple flavoured rum poured on it before heading to bed.

The next day, we were to ride from Oshawa into Toronto and Barb decided to join us on the sixty-kilometre day. It was a nice ride in the trees and along lots of water. As I came riding through the trees, I came around a right corner way too fast. I saw the pathway dip down and then back up with a huge puddle of water that filled the entire dip. I came around the corner so fast I had no time to even try and stop, I just had to brace for impact. I hit the water and a wall of it came over my board and crashed like a wave over my feet and lower legs. Now my feet, my board, and lower legs were soaking wet. However, on the nice hot and sunny day, it only took a few kilometres for me to completely dry off. I wasn't very happy about my soggy feet, but I was sure glad I didn't fall into the water or fly over the water and eat the pavement like I almost did. I barely had enough momentum to make it through the foot-deep puddle that was two or three feet across. That puddle was the puddle that gave me my one and only rule for bombing fast in populated areas. That rule was. If I couldn't see around a corner, I needed to assume there was a brick wall or something around the blind corner I may need to stop for, just in case. Because if that puddle was a family, I would have turned myself into the trees or have taken them all out.

My only problem was I still sucked at sliding and didn't know how to slide to a quick stop. I couldn't quickly drop and slide to a stop in case of an emergency. Every time I did one, I just naturally did a 180-degree spin and lost a little speed then I would be stuck riding switch which I was terrible at despite riding lots of it in the East Coast to balance the muscle mass growing in my legs. I had to switch and alternate pushing legs when the muscle mass in my right thigh got so big it started to pull my hip out of place. I knew I would figure out sliding eventually, but would I be able to do it in time? We had experienced many blind corners through the woods on the East Coast, but we were on a highway so for one, there was usually more than enough room to react and two, there was nobody around. This was the first time that I didn't have the room or the time to react and I needed to be prepared for it if and when it happened again.

As we were riding on the paved trail heading into Toronto, we ended up coming across another two longboarders. As it turns out, one of them was Jake (the same guy that put the new grip tape on my board at the local West 49 a day or two before). With nearly three million people in Toronto, we just so happened to run into him in the middle of our skate that day. I found it funny how small the world was beginning to appear. After our ride into Toronto, we caught a train and headed back to Barb's for another night. We ended up getting some white paint and stencils at the dollar store when we got to town which I used to write "love life" on my new black grip tape and my dad wrote "Long for Life" on his.

While we were in the Toronto area, there was a "Skate for Kids" longboarding event that we went to attend. The next day we got up and drove into downtown Toronto for the event. Only problem with that was the parking lot of traffic the whole way. It was probably only a half-hour to forty-five-minute drive away, but it took us what seemed like 2 or 3 hours to get there and we missed the start of the event. When we arrived, I could see a big stage set up with white pop-up tents set up everywhere like a little outdoor market. We got very short general directions to skate across a street, around the marina, then down the channel, and to turn back after we got to a spot on the path. Being late, my dad and I quickly got on our boards, and got going hoping to catch up with everyone else.

I put the GoPro on the GoPro stick that was a ski pole someone in Halifax altered for us when we were hanging out with Wayne and the Halifax longboarding society getting ready for the mainland. Looking back, that seemed like an entire lifetime ago, and not in the very recent past. As we headed across the street, I saw volunteers guiding people the right way and looking out for cars. We got to the marina area, and it had a nice, paved path that ran along the water which we skated down. It wasn't long before I started to notice some riders were already heading back, so I started to give them high-fives as we skated by each other. This one guy was riding pretty fast, and I was going the other way also skating pretty fast and we high fived. He swung his hand really hard into mine. With my hard plastic slide gloves smacking his bare hand he shouted out in pain, "ouch!" I shout back, "Sorry, man!" I stopped skating so fast and high fiving people after that. I wasn't willing to take the hard pucks off because I wanted to find a place to learn to slide around.

The pathway I rode broke left and right in a Y-shape. With my dad now behind me, or ahead of me, I had no idea where to go so I decided to follow the water and go left. After skating down the paved path for a bit longer I came across a group of riders and went to say hello. When I got there, I realized they were all arguing about where the turnaround point was. Some argued it was up ahead, while others were saying we were well beyond it. The argument was resolved when one of the kids remembered he had a map in his backpack. He pulled it out to show everyone we were well beyond the turnaround point by a kilometre or two. The arguments ended, everyone grabbed their stuff, and we all started to head back. On the way back, I had a slight idea on where to go, so when I got to the spot where the path broke into a Y-formation, instead of staying with the water, I wanted to go left to see what that way was like.

I went left, and it went uphill, and I was thinking 'oh yeah go the hard way' but it wasn't long before I got to the top of the tiny hill to see it go right back down. It first had a short-left curve before it had a longer right curve that descended, connecting to the path at the bottom of the hill. At the bottom, it had a left and right turn at the end which connected it to the waterfront pathway. There were already a few kids there trying to slide the hill. One of the riders at the very top tried to slide the little left curve and couldn't pull it off with their lack of speed and the tilted path. Another one of the riders pushed until he got going fast enough to slide on the long, slow, gradual right turn that went down to the waterfront. I pushed down the little slight curve at the top then gave a few hard kicks around the long bend while struggling to keep my balance on the steady right turn all the while balancing on my right leg. Once I got to the bottom, I put my glove down and slid around the right turn. Now I was facing the way I first went to the turnaround point, so I got off my board and walked up the side of the grass hill to do it again. Once I ripped down to the bottom of the hill, I did the same thing, but I ended up kicking out my left leg too hard and did a 180-degree slide before riding out on the grass and almost did a tumble. Luckily, I caught my footing, so I didn't go onto the pavement or over the edge of the barrier and into the water of the channel.

I grabbed my board thinking about one more run as the hand and foot positioning on my first run had me do a perfect right slide. Remembering how late we were, I decided against it as I headed back down the path still wondering where my dad was. I came down the path with the water now on my right side and eventually got back to the marina area. I noticed you could either skate around the waterfront going around the building or get off and walk through on the left side and take a few stairs on a wooden staircase and cut through the building. I saw kids cutting through the building that way when I came around the marina the first time. I went for the leisurely skate around the waterfront as it was more scenic. I was half tempted to ride for the wooden stairs and launch off of them, but I couldn't see around the big white building that was on the corner, and not being able to see anyone coming deterred me from doing so. I then spotted the big stage surrounded by tent city and rode over. When I got back, I still had no idea where my dad was as I lost him on the cruise maybe five- or ten-minutes in. I could only hope he didn't get lost like the other riders and myself, or like my dumb ass did in Ottawa.

I started to walk around looking for my dad in his white "Long for Life" t-shirt. After about five minutes, I spotted him talking to a lady at one of the tents. I walked over and he introduced me to the amazing woman who organized the whole event. Shortly after, I found the Monster energy drink tent, got a monster energy drink, and a sticker for my helmet.

Then it was picture time. All the riders gathered, most of the hundred or so riders wearing the blue 'skate for kids' event shirts. I decided to go to the very back while my dad took a picture, but with so many riders in front of me I couldn't see him. So, I put my longboard in my right hand and stood it straight up and held it up as high as I could, hoping he could at least get my Landyachz Switch-40 protruding in the air. It worked, popping out behind all the kids is my red longboard being held high in front of the big white apartment buildings. After that I took off the camera and walked around to take a few pictures of the area. The open fake green grass and walking area was surrounded by a medium-sized concrete wall with a few stairs leading from the grass to the top of the concrete walkway which went through and around the apartment building.

After the pictures, a young kid got on the stage and started to tell everyone his story. He was born with a disease that gave him a very bad stuttering problem. It was difficult for me to understand him as he talked about his story and what he was saying for a bit, then he said he was going to rap for us. At first, I was a little hesitant about that, as it was hard to just hear him talk. But then the beat came on and he started to rap. When he started rapping it was like he flicked a switch in his brain and his stuttering problem vanished into thin air. I was astonished how he was just able to go from hardly speaking, to rapping more clearly than he could talk. After his song, he started to explain how when he raps his stuttering problem just went away. I thought my connection to music and finding knowledge, peace, gratitude, and freedom within it was awesome. However, it didn't even come close in comparison to what music did for this young kid. I thought music was a huge mental escape for me over the years but for someone like that, my mind just went blank. I was really intrigued and impressed all at once, also for a fifteen-year-old kid he wasn't bad at rapping. I'm quite confident we've all heard much worse music on the radio. I gave and continue to give much respect to the young man when he finished his show.

After the cruise and show we headed back to Barb's, which took no time at all without any rush hour traffic, and relaxed, hung out, and chatted for the night. My dad and I were going to meet with his mom and drive south to Windsor to visit family for a few days. Once my grandmother got to town, the three of us piled into her small, red sports car and drove down south. It was a few hours drive, so I tried to get some sleep in the back seat. But there wasn't much room in the back seat of her small red sports car filled with boxes, longboarding gear, and lots of luggage.

Once we got there, we said hello to everyone before we had a barbeque in the back yard that rested on the water of a large channel. On the other side of the channel was Detroit, we were as far south as you could possibly go in Canada. We hung out, chatted for hours, and after the delicious barbeque, we had a few beers. I assumed we were staying there, but I was wrong. Instead, we got onto the speed boat and caught a ride over to the marina where we got onto a bigger boat that had rooms and beds which is where we spent the night. I remember being a little claustrophobic as I shimmied into a little crawl space where my bed was. Once I got inside, it opened up and I had a lot more room, but it was still freaking me out knowing I'm in a little hole in the belly of a boat, my anxiety didn't like that too much. I had never slept on a boat before and my mind went racing with the thoughts of possibly getting seasick as I've heard some not so pleasant stories throughout my life. But for me, I loved it. The boat gently rocking side to side was very relaxing to me. It was like a mother gently rocking her baby to bed.

The next morning, I got up and went to the washroom at the marina. Then we got on our longboards and skated through the town of Leamington down the road that paralleled the channel until we got to where we had our barbeque with family the day before. There, the party, entertaining chats, and beers kept on going for the afternoon. It was nice to get to catch up and have a fantastic time with family I rarely got to see. Right before sundown, I found out there was a wakeboard I could ride. I put on a life jacket, jumped in the boat, and we got away from shore into deeper water before I climbed onto the stern of the boat and put my feet in the wakeboard, well, tried. I struggled trying to get my giant fat feet into them for about five or ten minutes, questioning my abilities to even ride the thing. Once I finally got my fat feet in the board I plopped backwards into the water, getting a nose-full of it in the process. I came bobbing back up coughing out nose water before they tossed me the tow rope and we were off, well they were, I hadn't been on a wake board in probably eight-plus years and when they took off, the rope slipped out of my hand as I was attempting to get up.

They did a big circle around me, brought me the rope to try again, and I almost got up, but not quite. So, another circle, another attempt, and another failure to get standing. Another try and I almost got up but then fell over. The three or four people in the boat came around again to bring me the rope to give it another shot, and I failed again. Now I was getting frustrated. They came back around and I tried again, this time I was able to get up, but only for a few seconds. I had no idea how I could be longboarding across Canada, yet I couldn't even stand on a wakeboard. I was always a natural at anything board. whether it was a skateboard, snowboard, or a wakeboard, I could always ride them comfortably and easily. I was always pretty good at it, until now apparently. I could imagine the people in the boat were also getting frustrated. I got the rope, and they took off, I got up standing for maybe five seconds before they watched me fall back into the water. This time I got a bunch of water up my nose and in my mouth. I choked on more water for a bit as they just sat in the boat. I wondered if they were at the end of their patience rope, I had already long surpassed mine so I wouldn't be surprised. I also wondered if I couldn't get up because I was drunk or because I just sucked at wakeboarding. I couldn't help but sum it up to the combination of the alcohol and the many years I haven't been on a wakeboard.

They were just sitting in the water as I floated around in my red, grey, and white life jacket coughing up water from my last fall. After a few minutes of wondering what was going on, my cousin pulled up on a Seadoo. They disconnected the rope from the boat and attached it to the Sea-Doo instead. They had called into shore to get it because "it's easier to get up on" and I clearly needed all the assistance I could get, so it was a good call.

By now the sun was setting and the westward sky was turning a nice yellowy-orange colour. My cousin came around on the Sea-Doo and she brought me the tow rope wearing her bright-orange life vest. I gave her a thumbs up and she took off. This time I popped up rather easily, and I was staying up. She began to ride north down the channel as I started to carve left and right, going up and down the wave, trying to get a feel for it. She then started to turn in a big counterclockwise circle before doing a big clockwise rotation. Somehow, I managed to stay up and ride the circles with her. She then went across the channel a bit just after a huge cargo ship went by. I tried to ride the waves of the massive ship, but she began to go back to the shoreline once we got close to it.

She then did a few more circles and I caught an edge doing a face plant into the water getting even more water up my nose, gagging on it for a minute. She came back to give me the rope again and after losing the slack I gave the "okay" thumbs up still coughing up nose water. She took off and I came back up easily. We rode south down the channel for a bit, and I noticed the sky and clouds were getting a lot darker. I started to carve on the wake this time trying out the right side going up and down. She did a big half circle and we started going back north up the channel as I rode the right side of the wake in the calm water. I then told her to go faster and that she did, pinning the throttle. I almost fell a few times and let out a "whoa" as I got wobbly while going, but fully regained my balance. We kept on cruising around until she started to rip along closer to the docks. I started to carve in the middle of the wake but as I went over the right side of it, I took a spill into the water. I now sat in the water, bobbing up and down like a buoy in the waves. As I sat in the water, I looked to my left. With the sun still setting, the westward sky was still lit up in a beautiful bright-orange colour. I turned around to look south and it was nothing but ugly. Big, black, stormy death clouds were on the way, and fast. My cousin came back with the rope and pulled me over to our dock that was just a house or two away and we got off the water for the night. I dried off as we hung out around the fire in the big backyard for a while before the storm came in. Then my father and I got dropped off at the marina for the night. I got on deck, went down the stairs, and got in my little cubbyhole bed area and fell asleep as I listened to it raining outside.

The next morning it was a few hours drive north up to Toronto to continue our cross-country mission after a fun weekend off. Once we got to Toronto, we had to take Yonge Street going straight north. Yonge Street wasn't just a little street either, Guinness Book of World Records once dubbed Yonge Street the longest street in the world, and some argue it still is. Once we got back, we got on the sidewalks and skated north on them for hours until we ran out of sidewalk and had to go onto the highway. As we skated down the road on the highway against traffic, I noticed a massive turtle coming through the guardrail and start slowly heading for certain death. It was attempting to go across at least four lanes of highway traffic that was going to kill it or possibly cause a crash, so I stopped.

As I waited for my dad to come up, I tried to use my board to get the turtle to turn around and walk the other way, but he snapped and hissed at me which caught me entirely off guard because I never heard a reptile hiss or snap at me before. Once my dad got there, we took a look at the big guy. First, we tried to use our boards to push him in the direction from which he came but he wasn't happy and continued to hiss and snap at us more. My dad being the owner of a massive snapping turtle years before, bent over, grabbed it on the left and right side of his shell, and gently lifted the massive snapping turtle back over the rail and placed him in the grass going downhill back towards the water. Satisfied the massive dinosaur like reptile wasn't going to go back on the road we took off down the highway again. Till then, I had never seen a wild turtle before. We don't have any in Alberta, so seeing this reptile that had a circumference bigger than a beach ball come squeezing through the rails in front of me was kind of neat. I'm just glad we caught him before it got run over. I recall skating by many turtles in southern Ontario. But they were all squished, exploded, flattened, deceased turtles on the side of highways. After passing dozens of dead ones over the last few weeks,

I finally got to see one that was alive, and it was pretty neat. The designs on its hard, protective shell I thought were pretty cool. He had an attitude with a hiss and a snap that said, "Touch me and millions of years of evolution will take off your finger with ease." It was definitely not the kind of cuddly pet you bring home to your wife. Unless you're trying to prank her and or get a divorce of course.

After another long day on the road, we got to Bradford, Ontario. There, we stayed at a local motel for the evening. We didn't have the prettiest of places. It kind of looked like a motel you'd go to for the last night of your life. But it didn't matter, a shower and clean bed to sleep on was all we really cared about. After showering and changing, my dad and I relaxed on our beds and watched television while chugging down our protein shakes. The next morning, we stopped at a local skate shop called Bare Beaunz. There, my dad and I got to talk to Beau about what we were up to. He was impressed with our cross-country longboarding charity mission and pulled out a few binders. The first one was full of pictures of a charity longboarding barbeque event that he put together with the locals. After showing us his own longboarding charity work, he opened the second binder which was full of stickers. The binder was filled with the clear plastic sheets for pictures but instead of pictures in each slot, he had stickers. Page after page, Beau flipped through the binder pulling out the odd sticker for my dad and myself. He eventually got to a page then stopped. He reached into one of the slots and pulled out a few of his custom Bare Beaunz stickers for my father and I.

As my father and Beau had a chat, I walked around the store checking out the selection of goods. Beau then asked my father if we needed any gear so my dad drops a quick list. He said, "Yeah, we need gloves, wheels, bearings, and shoes." Beau walked over to one of his stands and grabbed a couple pairs of socks before he came back over and asked, "Have you guys tried these kinds of socks before?" They had a rubber grip on the bottom of them that kept your feet from sliding in your shoes, which was what caused blisters. We thought it couldn't hurt to give them a try. Beau saw the state of my longboard and told me I should start riding it backwards. So as a reminder to do so he cut off a small piece of Vicious grip tape and put it on my board at an angle. We put our new comfy socks on our feet, took a picture with Beau outside the store, and then got back on the road. At first, my dad and I had a laugh about the socks. But after a few kilometres, we could totally feel the difference. My foot was secure in what remained of my shoe giving me firm, solid kicks and as a bonus they were incredibly comfortable as well.

We came across a coffee shop in Bradford and decided to get a coffee and take a much-needed leg break. Outside the coffee shop was a pic-nick table to the right, and to the left leaning against the fence, right before the door stood the legendary "Log Board." It was a massive ten-foot-tall log that stood taller than the fence it leaned on. They had attached a pair of skateboarding trucks to the bottom of it for fun and rode it down some hills every now and then at events. Only problems with that were that it was a massive log, and it was incredibly heavy. The log was so heavy that the axils on the trucks were bent in a V-formation. When you looked at them, it looked like a pair of trucks that had been run over by a car they were so grossly mis-shaped. Also, the log weighing so much made it nearly impossible to stop in a short distance and took several grown men to slow it down and stop it.

My dad was inside talking with an older woman as I was checking it out. After I looked at the log board, I went inside where the lady my dad was talking to told me she "loved the Long for Life name" I had chosen. After a short chat with the nice woman and a delicious coffee we got back on the road heading to Orillia

After skating down the highway for hours we got to a small city where we stayed with Deborah, another amazing couch surfer in Barrie who put us up for the night. When we got to her place, I called my mom, gave her an update on things with the trek and how incredible it has been before she filled me in on things back home in Calgary. Once my mom and I had a nice long chat I went inside, and we all sat down for supper. After dinner, I got a little adventurous and wanted to go skate and explore the area like I always did. So, Deborah's son Doug got on his bike, I grabbed my longboard, and he showed me a nice little ride around. As I skated down his block and around the corner, we were losing the remaining glow of sunlight we had left. I skated the streets for a short distance before we got onto a paved pathway that went around a lake. As I was skating through the trees coming down a small hill it got even darker. The trees cut out the surrounding streetlights and now I could hardly see the pathway.

All of a sudden, I found myself flying through the air after hitting a drift of sand that took over my side of the pathway. Because I didn't see it coming, I wasn't prepared to hit it and I went flying. Luckily, I caught my balance at the last second as I let out a "holy shit." We continued on the nice, paved path in the silence of the dark night, and it was getting hard to see the ground let alone what was going to come next, so I started to go a bit slower. I told Doug about my sand trap experience, and he said, "Yeah, there's a few of those around here." Starting to get tired, I suggested we should turn around as we still had to go back around the lake, through the community, then back to his house, and he agreed. Once we got back to his place, I went straight to bed as I was incredibly exhausted.

The next morning, we were up and at it again. After we packed up our stuff we got back on the road. While we were travelling on the highway, we were going right passed the casino in Orillia where Deborah worked so we decided to take a quick break to say thanks before we continued out of town.

When we got out of town onto the highway, we eventually came to the top of a massive hill where we saw a cyclist just reaching the top as we were about to go down. He was huffing and puffing like the Big Bad Wolf and his thighs where the size of tree trunks with muscle that had just been put to the ultimate vertical test. After a quick man-nod to the cyclist, we continued towards the hill. I was a little paranoid about the first rough-looking steep part at the top but saw that it had a very nice long run out for a kilometre or so. I took the first bit a little slow feeling the road conditions before I picked up my foot and ripped the rest of the way down. I got my dad to wait once he got to the bottom as I went up for another run. I set the camera up for my dad to take a video of me, and I hiked my way back up on the right side of the road. The one-foot-wide, flat dirt shoulder turned into grass for a few metres before it turned into a wall of trees that ran all the way down both sides of the highway.

Once I got back to the top of the hill, I put my board down, looked for cars, and after seeing none, I gave a few hard kicks heading straight down the hill in the outgoing lane. Just as I started down the hill, I could see a few cars coming up in the oncoming lane, so I made sure there were still no cars coming in mine as I started to really fly down the hill. Once I passed the light-brown-and-white minivans coming up the hill, I took another look both ways for cars as the hill flattened out and I continued to cruise. I flew by my dad who was standing on the left side of the street with the GoPro filming me. Or so I thought, turns out I left it on picture mode by accident when I gave it to him, so it wasn't a video, just pictures every few seconds.

After skating on the road for hours we took a right turn off the highway and headed down this road that eventually turned into a tunnel of trees. A natural canopy of trees covered over the entire road. As we skated on through the shade, we carefully watched for traffic to move over out of their way. About half-way down the tree tunnel, we had a huge red dump truck pass us in the oncoming lane, after a few more minutes of skating in the tree tunnel we came out and there were houses on the right side of the roadway, backed into the forest of trees.

After the two or three houses on the right side of the street they vanished and turned back into the bushes and trees as the road started to descend and turned slightly to the right into the bushes. Once I turned the slight right bend, I could see another slight left and right bend in the hill as it continued to descend, then at the very bottom of the hill was a hard left turn. As the road took the hard left at the bottom you could see the water from the bay touched the right side of the road. At the time I could have sworn the water was coming over the small barrier onto the roadway, so I took the hill carefully. However, as I came around the corners, I could see the road continued and was dry, so I flew down the rest of the hill and went by a small, white house on my left before riding out my speed on the right turn that went around the edge of the bay.

I got off my longboard, kicked it up, and waited for my dad. When I saw him get to the bottom of the hill he walked over to the white building I thought was a house and stood outside talking to someone that sat at a picnic bench, so I rode over to say "hello" when I got there I realized it was Deborah outside the small convenience store who got off work to meet us at Carthew Bay and take our heavy bags to our final destination. I grabbed a drink from the convenience store I thought was a house then stepped back outside to see my dad was now on the phone. I walked around as my dad chatted away for what seemed like forever. So, as he chatted, I walked around and explored the wooded areas and pathways behind the store. They led nowhere, so after I took a quick pee in the back woods I went to sit down in the grass and rest while I waited for my dad to finish his call.

We got back on the road pushing to Gravenhurst where we stayed at a bed and breakfast called the "Tuktaway-Inn" which was owned and managed by a wonderful local couple. The house rested on an incredibly beautiful lake and had a huge backyard with a path from the back of their house, through their yard and garden, and down to their dock where their boat was tied up. The lake reflected the green trees that surrounded the water and the bright blue sky above it. There were no waves, no ripples, and no imperfections in the water at all. It didn't even look like water; it was like a giant mirror that rested in the back yard. Only when the wind picked up could you see ripples appear in the water. Robbin offered us a boat ride, but I was so sweaty and gross after our long skate I decided to have a nice cold shower and relax in the big, peaceful, beautiful backyard. As I had a cold shower and changed out of my dirty clothes, my dad went on a quick boat ride on the lake. When everyone got back, we sat down and had a delicious dinner. After dinner everyone was hanging out, relaxing, and chatting away. Meanwhile I was full of energy and feeling adventurous, so I went for a late-night skate and explore through town.

I walked out the front door, grabbed my board that rested along the wall to the right before walking down the pathway to the street. I turned right and started to skate on the incredibly rocky, and rough road. Once I got to the next street, I turned left towards the main drag that ran through town. I headed to the street where I saw all the stores to see what was there and if any of them were still open. But by now the sun was long gone and it was pretty dark. I got off my board and turned left down an alley to walk around and get to the front of all the stores. The rocky alley wasn't rideable, but I could see the back door to one of the stores was open and I could hear a few people talking in the back as I walked by. I exited the alley and turned right onto the sidewalk of the main drag.

I started lightly pushing down the sidewalk and saw no stores that were open except the one pizza shop where I heard the guys in the back alley talking. I looked around and there were no cars or traffic of any kind, so I moved from the sidewalk onto the street. By now it must have been pretty late because it was like a quiet ghost town. No people, no cars, and no open stores. It was like I had the town to myself after a plague. Down the road, I came to a tiny hill just after the stores running down the left and right sides of the street turned into houses. With no one around and a tiny bit of speed from the hill, I put my right hand down and did a slow 180-degree spin before rotating my body around, so I was riding my preferred way. I put my left foot on the ground and dragged it on the pavement to slow down and stop before I picked up my board and walked back up the hill to do it again.

I was still riding my Landyachtz Switch-40 board, and it had been nearly un-rideable for weeks now. The three weeks of rain in the East Coast and the 1,200 plus kilometres of riding started to delaminate the eight layers of compressed wood. It was so bent out of shape you could see sideways right through the layers. At the end of my board, the flat spot the back trucks attached to was nearly pointing straight up, when it should be flat. The back end of my board got so low to the ground, Beau from the skate shop in Bradford, Ontario told me I should start riding it backwards, which I did. I continued trying to slide to a stop playing with hand and foot positions, but for some reason I was still doing 180-degree spins from my slick wheels. After a few more attempts to stop, I got frustrated and gave up, so I went back up the hill, down the street, past most of the closed stores, then turned left down the side street, and turned right back onto the rough road until I got back to the bed and breakfast. I leaned my longboard up outside where it was before and quietly went inside, down the hall to my room on the left and passed out for the night.

The next morning a local reporter came over to interview us before we hit the road again. When she heard about my late-night skate after I was skating all day, she thought I was absolutely batshit crazy. Her words didn't exactly say it like that, but the tone in her voice when she asked, "You went out boarding after you spent all day pushing to get here?" most definitely did. I told her how I loved to skate, explore new places, and adventure around. After our short interview, we got back on the road heading to Huntsville. After several hours, we got off the highway and arrived to the small town. As soon as we arrived in town, there was a school with about 100 kids outside just standing around waiting for something. I came flying up to the sidewalk with no way to stop as I was missing most of the bottom of my shoe, so I slid to lose most of my speed. Now slowly riding backwards along the sidewalk I jumped off my board slightly pushing it away from me in the process, so it would stop before I took one step over to it, picked it up, and waited for my dad on the side of the road. As we walked down the street, one of the students at the school saw the "love life" I painted in white on my grip tape. When he saw it, he shouted out to me "love life, man!" I gave the young lad a thumbs up in agreement and we continued on through town until we got to the house of a local schoolteacher who put us up that night. After dinner, my father was chatting away with the kind lady while we waited for her husband to get home. With a full belly of great food, I got on my board and went for my usual side adventure to see what was around town.

It was already getting dark when I left and once I found my way back to the main drag I noticed there were no stores open. After skating through the small town for a while, I realized I forgot to bring some water and I was getting thirsty. I eventually came across a convenience store, so I went inside and got a small Slurpee to cool off. With everything closed and dark I slowly skated around while drinking my ice-cold Slurpee on the warm summer night. After skating through the dark, dead, quiet streets for a while and seeing nothing of any interest I decided to make my way back. Trying to remember my way back I was hoping I didn't have another Ottawa incident but luckily, it's much harder to get lost in a small town like this one. I finished my ice-cold drink just as I got back to the house where I got to meet the teacher that was putting us up. He was over at the school where all of the kids were for some school event all afternoon and into the evening. I sat down and started to tell my dad about my shoe that was now essentially a top piece of fabric held together by a tiny strip of rubber going from the left side of my shoe to the right side on the base. I told him, "I desperately need to get another pair of shoes when we can because I can't even foot break to stop." As I showed everyone the lack of bottom on my shoe I said, "and it doesn't really do a good job at keeping the water out."

The next morning, we got up and headed over to Algonquin Outfitters where both the store and the teacher we stayed with joined forces to get me a new pair of comfy shoes. I had now worn through my second or third pair of shoes just from foot breaking and we haven't even gotten to the big hills in the country yet, which was another reason I needed to learn to slide to a stop. We got a quick picture with the girls that were working at the store, thanked them kindly for my new comfy hole-less shoes, then we got back on the road and continued to head north. Now this is where the real mind-boggling craziness would begin. If I had thought the stars were aligning for my father and I before, well this is where entire galaxies started to align for us creating astronomical alignments in the cosmos never before seen by humankind. The kind of alignments in the cosmos that would make a professional astrophysicist like Neil deGrasse Tyson go a little off script while doing a show or lecture and say something he never would like, "what in the gentle Jesus astrological fuck, I've never seen something so magnificent."

We were heading north up to North Bay when my dad and I came across a small convenience store. We were in the absolute middle of butt-fuck nowhere, in the thick Canadian woods and thought we should stop to grab a drink. After we got our drinks from the fridge, my dad paid for them, then began talking to the man at the counter about our mission and what we were doing. With dead legs, I headed outside to sit on the bench and rest them for a bit, on the way out of the store I held the door for another man who was entering.

After a few minutes, my father came back out of the store, so I quickly had another sip of water before I threw the bottle in my heavy backpack and zipped it up. As my dad was having a sip of water and getting his bag ready, the other man came back out of the store and asks, "What the heck are you guys doing?" My dad then gave him the story before the kind man immediately asked if there was any way he could help us. Little did we know us meeting was the collision and shifting of multiple tectonic plates which created the tsunami that would ripple over thousands of kilometres across our spectacular country.

My father asked Josh if he would be able to bring our fifty-pound backpacks to the town we had to hit to get halfway to North Bay. It turns out he just happened to live in that small town, and he said it wouldn't be a problem as he pulled out his wallet and gave my dad a business card and told him to call him when we got to the Tim Hortons just off the highway on the edge of town. We threw our bags in the back of his silver SUV and as Josh went to close the back hatch, I remembered something I was going to want and screamed, "WAIT! I almost forgot something!" He let the hatch open up again and I grabbed the full water bottle out of my bag before I zipped it up and put it back. We thanked Josh then took off down the road again. After hours of skating through the endless tranquil woods, we saw the Tim Hortons coming up on the right side of the highway, so we stopped, gave Josh a call, and grabbed a cold drink while he drove over to get us.

Upon picking us up, Josh told us that he and his wife, Lisa, decided to put us up for the night and cook us a delicious home-cooked dinner as we came through town. As we headed over to their house, I couldn't help but think, 'Wow the people in my country are so generous, loving, and caring.' Upon our arrival, Josh drove up his driveway and just as we went to get out of the vehicle he says, "Oh no, wait, wait, wait a second guys. Shut your doors." So, we closed the doors. He then put the car in reverse, reversed down his driveway, put it in park, then got out to grab his newspaper before he got back in the car and drove back up the driveway again. As he parked, the reality of what he just did hit him and he said, "WOW! I feel incredibly lazy. Here you guys are longboarding across Canada, and I just reversed my car to get my newspaper." We all had a good laugh as we walked around to the backyard to meet his wonderful wife, Lisa, and their beautiful son, Joel. At the back of their house was a big beautiful, enclosed gazebo where we sat to eat dinner and enjoy the rest of the beautiful sunny day. As the wind came through the screen windows it provided a nice breeze that cooled you down which was a great escape from the crazy heat. Once our wonderful dinner in the gazebo was done, we had a chance to have a shower and get cleaned up. After that we all hung out, chatted, and relaxed for the evening.

Another day, the same mission. We got up, packed, and started heading north towards North Bay. We were about halfway there when my dad got a phone call from a woman named Kathleen in North Bay saying she got an e-mail from her co-worker, Lisa (Josh's wife), that said what we were up to, and she too wanted to help us any way she could. She offered to put us up for the night and told us to stop at the Tim Hortons on the highway when we got to town, and she would meet us there. We were almost to North Bay when we got caught in one heck of a rainstorm. The gods decided to give us another shower on the side of the highway in the middle of the thick Canadian woods. Luckily for us, we just past a little hut off the side of the road just as it began to storm. We grabbed our boards and dashed back to the hut already soaking from head to toe after mere seconds of exposure to the rain. As it poured, my dad got a phone call and I decided to record the downpour, so I took the camera off my head to record a short video of it. After we hid out the storm, we got back on the now soaking-wet, puddle-filled road finally arriving at the Tim Hortons to give Kathleen a call.

Kathleen picked us up as promised and after a short drive into the woods we arrived at her home where she introduced us to her family. I had a much-needed shower to wash the sweat, dirt, rain, and road gunk off of me, then changed into some dry, clean clothes before I put my dirty clothes in the wash and went upstairs for supper. While we all sat around having another delicious supper, Kathleen dropped a bomb of a question on us, she asks, "What are you guys going to do between Sault Ste. Marie and Thunder Bay?" Between there, there is next to nothing in civilization or big populated areas, it's just small towns, provincial parks, and endless wilderness. We had no support driver, no camper to stay in, and had no idea what we were going to do. She then told us how she was in the process of planning a five-week vacation with her family at all the provincial parks between the two cities and suggested we should stay with her and her family between Sault Ste. Marie and Thunder Bay. She said they could get us on and off the road, to and from basecamp, make sure we were clothed, fed, and safe. With no other option and completely baffled by her generosity we happily accepted her offer. So, from there, Kathleen and my dad started to plan when and where we would meet them.

However, before we left North Bay, we had to go to one of the most wonderful places in the existence of the world. It combined two of my most favourite things in life, which are pizza and coffee. I thought that they were all just joking with me until we got into the truck and drove over to Twiggs Coffee Co. It was a nice, quiet, clean, and comfortable place where my dad posted up on one of the long, white benches along the window and turned on his computer, continuing his logistical wizardry before he ordered a couple delicious coffees for us. Once we had our coffees, he ordered a pizza that was just as amazing as the cup of hot bean water. I honestly didn't want to leave but after an hour or two of hanging around and chatting we got outside for a picture with one of the girls who was working that day. After we took a picture out front of the majestic place my dad and I got back on the road.

If I didn't lose my phone to the rain in the East Coast, I probably would have lost it to the nasty storm just outside North Bay. My pockets got so wet from the few seconds we were in the storm it fried my iPod, and I was pissed. Within an hour or two of being on the road again I was noticeably losing my mental battle with the cross-country trek. Without music I lacked a huge portion of the motivation I needed for the daily push down the long highway roads. As much as I enjoyed the tranquil peace and quiet of the woods, I enjoyed my loud, underground hip hop and rap music flowing through my neurons at very high decibels.

From North Bay, we were finally heading west again, the next stop was Sudbury. Leaving North Bay heading to Sudbury there was a nice long stretch of highway that was freshly paved. However, it didn't have lines painted on it, so it was still closed off to traffic. My dad and I walked over the meridian to the oncoming side of the highway and got to have the entire freshly paved road to ourselves over the rolling hills that where like ripples in the land for endless miles. We would walk up a hill then bomb down it on our boards, walk up, and bomb down. All day it was walking up hills, bombing down the other side, before skating over to the next hill, and repeating the cycle. Out of pure musicless boredom I was using the pylons on the closed road as objects to carve through, and around. I came ripping down the hills like it was a slalom course. It was kind of fun, but I was quickly getting lethargic and slow. After a while I had to bomb down the hills as fast as I could to catch up with my dad as he was slowly getting farther and farther away.

After losing my mind all day not having my music in my ears to inspire me and keep me motivated, I put out a request online in the Sudbury area to see if anyone had and old iPod or music playing device they wouldn't miss if they donated and I put why I felt I really needed one. To my surprise, right before we got to Sudbury, I got a message from a kind young woman named Janelle saying she had an old iPod touch she could throw my way. When we reached the city of Sudbury sign on the side of the highway, I ran down the ditch, over to it and held my board high above my head as my dad took a picture before we skated over to the local sports store—Pinnacle Sports—for a chat and a look around. My dad spoke with the store manager as I checked out their stuff until some time later, we took a picture outside as Janelle pulled up in her small, green car. Janelle and I drove over to her place to hang out and relax for a bit while dad continued to his relatives' place where we were to stay the night.

I had just started to watch YouTube videos of a comedian who she never heard of, so I put some YouTube videos on and we watched and chuckled while I had a few hoots and chilled out before she drove me to the house of my dad's relatives. I went inside, put my things down, and said hello to everyone before I was shown to my room and took my things down. Then, as I opened my computer, I saw the iTunes program open, and I completely forgot to ask Janelle for the iPod while I was there. Incredibly disappointed in my stoner moment from my few hoots I gave Janelle a message to see if she could meet me in the morning before we took off. But by now it was late in the evening, and everyone was heading to bed. I was still wide awake and not tired at all, so I hatched a plan to sneak out and have her pick me up down the road.

I grabbed my backpack then slowly walked up the stairs hoping everyone was still in bed sleeping. I got to the door and couldn't help but wonder if there was an alarm set. I guess I was about to find out. I slowly twisted the door handle praying to the house-alarm gods and opened the door. To my great relief, there was no alarm, so I grabbed my board, walked down the steps, across the driveway, and to the road. Trying to be quiet and sneaky, I walked down the road for a bit before putting my board down and began to push down the dark, empty street in the rural area. I hoped I wouldn't come across any dangerous animals now by myself in the middle of nowhere and couldn't help but sense the eeriness of it all. I got to the end of the road where Janelle said she would be and

I climbed into her car thanking her for coming to get me, again. She asked why I got her to pick me up down the street and laughed at me after I told her, "Well I kinda just snuck out."

I still wasn't tired at all, so we went back over to her place and hung out with her roommate who made us poutine before she went to bed. After a while, I looked at the clock and it was around two or three in the morning. I figured I should probably get going and asked Janelle for the iPod so I didn't forget. I told her I would trade my hoodie she liked for it so she wasn't walking away with nothing, but she politely declined and said it was okay before she went and got the old iPod she never used. Again, I tried to trade it for my hoodie, but she insisted it was fine and declined. However, I knew she liked the hoodie more than the device whereas it was the other way around for me, so before giving me a ride back I put the hoodie on a chair for her to find when she got home as some sort of memento.

The entire way back through town I couldn't help but worry that I would set off an alarm when I got there. I was riddled with the anxiety of being that asshole that woke everyone up at 3 a.m. by setting one off. Everyone was sleeping when I left, nonetheless I still couldn't help but worry someone may have gotten up and set it while I was gone, which made the drive back seem very short. I got dropped off down the street, thanked my new friend for the iPod and gave her a big hug, before I skated down the empty dark road in the middle of the night, again hoping I wouldn't get attacked by any wild animals. I picked up my board, made a right onto the property, and then walked up the few steps as quietly as I could before I put my board down. With my heart racing and full of anxiety, I felt like I was thirteen- or fourteen-year's-old sneaking out again. I couldn't help but chuckle as I was now nineteen and could do whatever I wanted as an adult. But I was still worried I was going to wake someone up, so I quietly and slowly tried to open the door, but it was now locked. As a young teen, there's no worse feeling in the world than sneaking out, only to come home to a locked door and being stuck outside. Normally I'd just throw little rocks at my brother's window to get him to let me in, but I was at a stranger's house in the middle of nowhere thousands of kilometres away from home. Overwhelmed with anxiety and panic, I thought I was pretty much screwed. I messaged Janelle and told her I was now locked out, so she offered to come get me for the night. I told her I'd message her in a bit if I couldn't get in as I crept around the house to the back door. I got to the back door hoping it was open and there wasn't an alarm set. I grabbed the doorknob and, as quietly as I could, twisted the handle.

Only when you're trying to be quiet, the quietest thing sounds like a rock band. As I was twisting the doorknob, just the tension of the spring inside the door handle winding sounded like a sword fight to me. Ting ting ting. The spring of the doorknob tightens as I thought to myself, 'Damn, I hope nobody heard that,' which was then followed by, 'I hope there's no alarm.' Again, praying to the house-alarm gods, I crept inside. My light footsteps sounded like a heard of horses stomping their feet to me. No alarm sounded. I went back downstairs to my room, opened my computer, plugged in the iPod, and started downloading my music onto it. I told Janelle I got in safely and then went to bed after thanking her for saving me, and from a catastrophic meltdown on the highway.

Tired as ever, I got up the next morning and got ready for another day on the road. I packed up my bag, made sure the music was on the iPod, and did a quick sound check before we took off. With music in my ears again I was happier and more motivated than ever. From Sudbury, we made our way to Iron Bridge, Ontario which is where my dad's grandmother lived. After a few days of pushing, we finally got there. Once there, we were taking the weekend off to spend some time with family that I had not seen since grade two. For supper, we had some good food at the chicken restaurant. The restaurant even had a chicken costume I thought about putting on and skating around in, but it was so hot out I didn't even want to be in my skin, let alone in a thick chicken costume over my clothes. After dinner at the chicken place just off the highway, we headed back to my great grandma's and relaxed for the night, and as it got later into the evening, everyone started to go to bed one by one.

The next morning, I woke up in the upstairs spare bedroom and as I came downstairs, I saw everyone huddled around the television. I walked down the stairs, into the living room, and over to the television where everyone stood glued to it. Once I saw what everyone was looking at my jaw dropped and I couldn't help but say, "Holy shit." On the television was aerial helicopter footage of my home city, and downtown Calgary was completely flooded with millions of gallons of water. I immediately started to think and worry about all my friends and family that were there, so I started to contact them over Facebook and thanks to Janelle's old iPod I didn't have to run upstairs and bust open my computer. I pulled the iPod out of my pocket and opened Facebook where my jaw continued to drop. My Facebook feed was bombarded with pictures and videos of the colossal flooding. I couldn't help but think, 'Well, so much for the Calgary stampede this year,' which was only weeks away. I also couldn't help but think, 'I'm going to be coming home to a disaster in my city,' and I knew the old bakery in the basement I worked at, only a few streets away from the flooded river was gone as I saw roadways turned into fast, white rapid rivers.

We were taking that weekend off pushing, but being me, I wanted to go skate, explore new areas, and find some hills to bomb. So, I asked around and I was given some directions to what seemed to be the only hill in town. I grabbed my board, took off down the highway, skated by the chicken restaurant before finding my left turn into the woods that I had to take. I started skating down the road off into the woods with my music playing in my ears and the nice hot sun beating down on me as it was setting. I skated down the twisty road in the isolated woods for about fifteen or twenty minutes. The whole time sending all the love, happiness, and positive vibes to everyone back in Calgary.

After coming around a turn I finally started to see the bottom of a hill. After I skated over to it, I started walking up the short, steep hill and after a few minutes of walking uphill it levelled out then made a right and left turn. Just as I was coming up to the left turn, I noticed something move on the right side of the street in the distance. My curiosity got the best of me, so I put my board down and started to skate across from the left side of the road to the right as I came around the corner, which was a colossal mistake. **What** I thought was a small animal turned out to be a massive black bear. I came walking around the corner and it walked out of the trees onto the road right in front of me. My initial thought was 'I hope to God there are no cubs, so it doesn't perceive me as a threat.' But luckily, it was just one big, scary-looking, hairy bear, by itself.

The massive bear just stood there looking at me as I looked back standing frozen in fear for an intense few second that felt like minutes. The bear was close enough I could hear its breathing as it exhaled. The creature stared at me as I looked back at him studying each other. When I looked him in his big brown eyes, I got shivers that ran down my spine and made the hair on the back of my neck stand up. That was when I said to myself, "Well, it's time to get the fuck out of here." I turned around, ran the other way, threw my board down, and started to kick as fast and as hard as I could. I turned around to see the big, black, furry beast still standing there with a half-turned head looking confused like he's wondering where I was going. He had no desire to follow me and walked back into the trees from which he came just as I came around the right-hand turn with a huge rock wall on my right. The road then turned left and went straight down the hill. I gave a few more hard kicks when I got to the top of the hill before tucking into a little ball and flying down the middle of the secluded empty road.

The hill was fun with a nice run out so I decided to walk back up to ride it again. I walked back up to the top and slowly creeped to the corner where I saw the bear and thought I should stop and go from there in case it was still lurking around the area. I put my board down and started to kick the road with my left leg. As I came flying down the hill, I noticed three strangers walking down the road with longboards. I did a big slide to reduce some speed on the now-flat ground still frustrated with my variations of hand and foot positionings not helping me stop. The three kids turned around, saw me, and waved. I waved back at them as I skated over to say hello. There were two young guys and a young girl all in their early teens just out and about for a ride on the nice evening. I told them the hill was pretty fun and asked if they wanted to come to the top and ride down it which they decided to. All four of us walked to the top of the hill and started to walk around the right turn at the top.

I walked on the right side of the road so I had a nice line of sight around the left corner, and I would be further away from the bear if it was still around. Once the road started to go left, I mentioned to them we should probably stop and go from there as I just saw a big black bear on the road just around the corner. The poor teenage girl then had a catastrophic meltdown of epic proportions and started to panic. I told her it was just standing there not doing anything before I told her I'd go check if he was still there. The three teens all stood there as I slowly walked around the corner on the right side of the road. I saw nothing but an empty roadway, so I shouted out to them that the coast was clear. The two young guys started to walk over carrying their boards, but the poor young girl stood there petrified in fear and couldn't get her legs to move. The other boys and I couldn't help but laugh. They tried to assure her it was okay, but she just got on her longboard and went back down the hill from where she was. The two young boys continued to come up and we all walked down the road a bit before they put their boards on the ground and slowly began to push down the hill after their friend. I took a few running steps, threw my board down, and jumped on it before I started to boot the road like crazy. By the time I got around the right bend, I had caught up to the two guys and by the time I got around the left turn and halfway down the hill I was caught up to the young girl too. I coasted down the straight road and once I slowed down a bit, I turned my board sideways and did a slide. Only it was much harder to do on my Sayshun drop dead custom longboard my grandma brought from Alberta to Iron Bridge. My Landyatchz Switch-40 was completely ruined after the eighteen straight days of rain and the (approximately) three-thousand-kilometres I put on it from St. John's, Newfoundland to Iron Bridge, Ontario. I was honestly impressed that the board made it that far, I thought I would have been through two or three longboards by now but thankfully I was wrong.

    I did a little 180-degree slide spinning very slow with the soft red wheels gripping the road more than my old, harder green ones. I then got off my board and waited for the youngsters to come over. Once they got over to me one of the young teens wanted to know how to slide so I gave him some tips that I knew as I told him, "But I'm not any good at sliding yet, I'm just starting to learn myself." I asked if he wanted to put on my slide gloves and give it a try, which he happily accepted. The kid gave it a try and it didn't go over so well, he threw his body down like he was trying to tuck and roll out of a moving car and rolled on the road once before popping back up onto his feet. He tried again and I noticed he was going to slow, so I told him to get more speed on his board first. Once he did, he finally got a screech from his wheels sliding on the pavement. He then cracked a big smile of enjoyment that I could instantly relate to, and he tried it again going even faster.

    Once the young man came back over still grinning from his first time sliding, the three of them asked me some questions like where I was from, what I was doing, why I was there, and all those curious teenager questions. So, I gave them the whole story about my cancer and stroke life before going into my current mission with my dad. When I finished telling them all my story and how I got there, all three of the teenagers collectively said the same thing at the same time. "Holy shit." "That's intense," one of them added. I couldn't help but ask if they had rehearsed that response together as we all had a laugh how they all said the same thing, at the same time, with the same tone of voice. They asked me a few more questions before I gave them details about my battle with cancer and what it was like having a stroke before I gave each of them a card to follow the rest of my journey. After a long chat with the youngsters, they went towards the bottom of the hill but went left on the road that crossed it at the bottom going home. I didn't want to run into any more furry, four-legged surprises, especially in the dark so I decided I should probably get going too. I still had to skate through the woods and the sun had been setting for a while now. But first I walked up the hill for one last rip down. After I got back up to the flat spot at the top I slowly walked by where I saw the bear. As I walked by the spot where the bear stood looking at me, my eyes and ears were glued to the tree line looking and listening for anything that may be around. Once I was the furthest I've gone down the road I turned around and started to ferociously kick the pavement. My mission was to go as fast as I could to ride out the hill as far as I could to reduce my kicking for the way back, though it took much longer to get to the top now that I was getting tired and slowing down.

However, it was a decent fun and fast hill that I couldn't resist riding one more time. I came flying around the corner at the top. As I tucked down low, I kept my eyes peeled for traffic at the four-way intersection at the bottom as well kept a look out for any animals. It was all clear so I continued to stay as low as I could to get going as fast as I could. I rode down the hill and, with the momentum and speed I had, I probably coasted for a good kilometre down the road. Once I slowed down enough, I started to spin and dance in enjoyment on my board as I listened to music. I began to kick the road and make my way back through the forest, but the mosquitoes were now out, and I was getting eaten alive, again. Of course, I didn't think to bring any bug spray, so my only line of defence was speed. I skated faster and faster with swarms of the tiny bugs all over the place for a few kilometres. At last, I reached the main highway and made a right turn then skated by the chicken place before I finally got to my great grandmother's street where I turned left onto the rough road and skated back to her house.

Once I got back, I got on my computer and started to talk to my friends about the devastation of the flood that had happened. I also called my mom on Skype to check on her and the family to be sure they were all okay. One of my mom's doctor friends in High River had his house completely flooded and they were going to go help him clean the eight feet of water and mud out of the basement that week. After I knew everything was okay, I closed my computer and went to bed. I remember seeing something about the Calgary mayor saying, "Come hell or high water we are going to have stampede," and I couldn't help but think how awesome it was that I was crossing Canada preaching a message to "never give up" and my mayor was back home doing the same thing **after a devastating tragedy**.

The next day, my dad and I had to do a ride out and back in to catch up on some kilometres. Back on the road, we kicked past the chicken restaurant on our right and kept on going down the road. I pointed out the left turn to my dad as we rode down the highway and told him that way was where I went to "bear hill" the night before. I decided to name the hill after my run in with the big, furry animal. After hours of skating, we got to a T-intersection and turned left down another highway continuing to skate for a while before we made a right turn on another highway that went into a small town which was our halfway turn around destination. On the edge of the town, we saw a Tim Hortons and decided to take a break there before heading back.

I walked into the Tim Hortons and right away an older woman came up to me and asked, "Are you the young man longboarding across Canada with your father?" Incredibly confused on how this stranger in the middle of the woods would know this, I replied, "Yes, how did you know that?" She then told me that she's Kathleen's mother and Kathleen had been talking about us for the last two weeks since we stayed with her in North Bay, and she started to plan with my dad where we were going to re-connect over 300 kilometres back. I couldn't help but think 'wow, what are the odds of that' and 'what a small world.' My view of the world was continuously shrinking as the trek went on. We then went outside where my dad and I met with Kathleen's dad who was also there. While we were outside talking, Kathleen's mom stopped talking mid-sentence, looked me in the eyes and said, "Well aren't you a very handsome young man. If you were a bit older, I'd take you around the block once or twice." I busted out laughing so hard. I was shocked, stunned, in disbelief and kind of flattered that a sweet, old lady—old enough to be my grandmother—just threw that at me out of nowhere. I was so embarrassed, I had to turn my tomato-red face away for a minute or two. After our chat with Kathleen's parents, we said our goodbyes as they wished us the best of luck on the rest of our trip, and we got back on the road heading back to my great-grandmother's house in Iron Bridge.

On the way back, I was getting annoyed with my dad for something stupid enough that I can't even remember why, so I put in my headphones and started to kick the road harder and harder, faster and faster. I only stopped kicking when I turned around and could no longer see him. With him behind me somewhere I sat on a fence and waited for ten or fifteen minutes before I decided I'd just meet him back at grandmas. I remembered the way back as it was only the one turn, past Elliot Lake, a right onto the other highway, then a skate down the road through the forest down to Iron Bridge, past the turn off to "bear hill" followed by the delicious chicken place on the left and through town to my grandmother's.

I got back on the road with my tunes playing, enjoying the peace and tranquility of being in the middle of nowhere while appreciating my passions for music, longboarding, and nature in a state of total bliss which was suddenly broken when a small yellow school bus came flying by me on my right side as I rode in the oncoming lane that was empty. I looked at the bus and saw probably eight to twelve girls all have their heads turn at the same time looking at me as they drove by, probably wondering why there's a dude longboarding down the highway in the middle of the woods by himself. After some time, I got back to my great grandmother's where I sat on the couch and relaxed while I listened to music. There I waited for my dad who arrived about fifteen to twenty minutes later. Shortly after we got back, we all headed over to the chicken restaurant to enjoy a much-needed supper, followed by a cone of scrumptious soft serve vanilla ice cream. The next day, my dad and I were up early to pack up and get ready for the next gnarly portion of the trek, Lake Superior.

Lake Superior

Our next leg of the trip was with Kathleen and her amazing family. Together we began the gruelling task of conquering the stupendous terrain of Lake Superior. My grandmother gave us a ride out to our first base camp at the beautiful "Agawa Bay" camping grounds. I was really excited because it had been a few years since I went camping, at the same time I was nervous as I heard this part of the country around Lake Superior was the most dangerous and isolated part out of the entire country. Agawa Bay was absolutely beautiful though, our camp was only a few metres from the white sandy beach overlooking the massive, ocean-size body of water. All night I listened to the wave's crash as I lay cozied up inside a sleeping bag in my tent trying to fall asleep. The sound of water is something I have always loved. Hanging out by a beach, river, or lake I've always found relaxing, calming, and peaceful. So, the sounds of the waves crashing put me to sleep like a baby that night.

At some point in the middle of the night I woke up and had to go to the bathroom. I opened my sleeping bag, got up, climbed out of my tent, and walked down the pathway along the silent empty beach until I found a tree or washroom. I went pee on a tree a bit off the pathway before I started to walk back to my tent. On my way back, I realized it was very bright out for being the middle of the night. That's when I looked around and saw the most incredible, jaw dropping, mind-boggling sight I have ever witnessed with my own two eyes. I looked to my left in the direction of the colossal lake and above it I saw more stars than one could count. I stopped and took a moment to look up and for the first time in my life, I could see our Milky Way Galaxy. I had only ever seen it on television, movies, or in books and magazines. But this was different, this was in real life. No telescope, no television, no computer, no magazine or even a way to connect to the internet, I was witnessing it in real life with my naked eyes.

Millions upon millions of stars were visible in every direction as I looked up. The colours, the complex intricate design, the brightness, and how vivid it was, was something so literally out of this world, it instantly froze me in my tracks. Being enveloped in its stunning beauty, I sat there for five or ten minutes in complete awe of the magnitude of its gorgeousness. After ten minutes or so, I went to go back to my tent, but I couldn't help but stand there and stare at our galaxy for another ten or fifteen minutes. It was something I'll never be able to forget. It was something I feel incredibly blessed to have seen, and it was something so beautiful and so peaceful it seemed to almost stop time itself. As I was standing there, I couldn't help but think, 'I should be dead right now.' I thought, 'My mind, body, and soul should be one with everything that I was currently seeing,' and how, 'I shouldn't be here in physical form enjoying the immense tranquility of this spectacular moment.' After staring at our phenomenal galaxy for at least another half hour or hour while reminiscing about my life I crawled back into my tent and went back to sleep. That night the weirdest thing happened. As I slept, I had a longboarding dream. In my dream, I slid to a stop, and I was consciously aware of what I did differently as I was sleeping.

The next few days we had to play catch up and ride out then back in to make up some missed kilometres after getting a ride to basecamp. We got up, packed our bags, then my dad and I headed off for the day. We began to walk to the highway and as I walked through the parking lot, I decided to try the arm and foot positions I did in my dream that caused me to slide to a stop. I ran a few steps, jumped on my board, and took a few big kicks through the parking lot. Once I got enough speed, I put out my arm and turned the board sideways and slid to a stop. It worked exactly like it did in my dream. I was as shocked that it worked like it did in my dream as I was confused on how it happened to come to me in my sleep. But I was excited it finally came to me and incredibly grateful it happened THE DAY we got to some of the craziest hills the country had to offer. I was confused on how I could be sleeping but still consciously awake and aware at the same time. I recalled as a kid when I slept, I still had the conscious awareness of things. For example, while I was sleeping, the sound of the door opening would trigger me to wake up. Not because it was noisy but because it meant someone was there and, while sleeping, I could still be consciously aware of that.

The extent of my abilities of being conscience while sleeping at the same time goes back to my childhood. As a child I remember always having bad dreams and dreams about dying and I would either be drowning or falling to my death. I had them so often that I started to recognize when I was having a bad dream or a nightmare while I was in it. If I even suspected my dream was going somewhere I didn't want it to, I would wake myself up from my sleep while I was still sleeping. I would do this by consciously rolling my eyes to the back of my head and it would immediately break me out of the deep sleep realm. I think the first time it happened it was by accident but over time I began to be able to control it with my own will. That at times got annoying because I would wake myself up from my sleep when I didn't need to, I'd just suspect my dream was going bad and force myself to wake up then I'd have to spend hours trying to fall back asleep again.

Once my father and I got to the Trans-Canada Highway, we turned left and began to push down the never-ending road. After a while we got to a small, blue bridge that crossed a little creek flowing from the woods on the right side of the highway into Lake Superior on our left. After the small, blue bridge, we continued down the highway and came to a left turn. Around the bend, we were now facing a long, monstrous uphill that we spent the next half an hour walking up. Once we got near the top of the hill, there was a small parking lot with a viewing area of the lake on the right side of the road where we stopped to catch our breath. Overlooking the lake to our left we could see the big, beautiful bay, the white sandy beach, and the tree line our basecamp was located at, just a few kilometres away. There was a sign at the viewing area stating that part of the country was the hardest part of the Trans-Canada Highway to construct out of all of Canada, and we would soon see why. The beauty of the view was stunning, so we sat there and had a sip of water enjoying it for a few minutes. Between the views of the Milky Way Galaxy, the astonishing beauty of my country, and all of the stupendous occupants in it, I was mentally being shaped and I was mentally being moulded. The best part of it all, I didn't even have a clue it was happening.

For the first time in my life, I felt like everything I went through and survived to get to this point, was all worth it. I felt like the luckiest person on the planet to still be here, and to witness such phenomenal things across my country. It was a blessing of its own. It was the first time I began to see that everything happens for a reason. My cancer diagnosis, strokes, drug use, mischievous behaviour, petty crimes, fights, and arrests were all what led me to be right here, right now. In that moment I knew if I had to go through it all over again just to be here, I wouldn't have even hesitated. This was it. This was life to me. Not sitting in a classroom or working a dead-end job. Travelling my country, witnessing, experiencing, and being entirely enveloped in everything it had to offer was more like living life to me. I could have died right then and there, and I wouldn't have cared. I would have been incredibly content, happy, and more ready than I've ever been. This inner happiness was what I always wanted. It was the kind of happiness that no amount of money could ever buy, it could only be earned. The profound happiness and inner peace we all think can be had by winning the lottery was found, experienced, and achieved by just pushing across my country and following my heart. I had suddenly found myself the winner of the lottery of life, sure I wasn't rich in material wealth, but I was completely fulfilled and rich with my spiritual and mental self, and that in my opinion is much more rewarding, satisfying, and more beautiful than any amount of dollars and cents could ever be.

We got back on the road continuing to walk to the top of the hill where the road turned right, and we entered a canyon of rock. On both sides of the highway were massive rock faces about twenty- or thirty-feet high. Every few metres you could see the old drill marks coming straight down where they had to drill out the rock for the explosives to blast out the way for the road. All day was spent pushing down the highway in this canyon of rock. Occasionally, the rock would disappear into the ground and the forest would emerge. With so many twists, turns, ups, and downs it boggled my mind how much manpower, money, and equipment it must have taken just to build this one section of road we pushed that day.

After hours of twists, turns, ups and downs through the valley of blasted out rock and forest we made a long, left turn and were now facing the second colossal uphill of the day. We got off our boards and began the hike up the super long hill. After about twenty minutes of hiking up the hill, it took a right turn at the top before the road levelled out. I looked to my left at the top of the hill just before it levelled out and for as far as my eyes could see was the blue water of the massive lake. To keep cars and trucks from going off the huge cliff and plunging to certain death were wooden posts every three metres or so with a single, inch-thick wire that came out of the ground and ran through the sides of them. I couldn't help but think 'yeah that's really going to stop a fully loaded big rig truck' I could see it maybe stopping a small car but if you saw what was on the other side of that wire and straight down, most would need a change of underwear.

After riding for a while on the level ground it was time to turn around and head back to camp, but not before I took off from my dad and bombed the hill that I saw in front of us after a left turn in the rock wall canyon. At the start of the hill, there was a jagged, light-brown wall of rock on both sides. After pushing down the slight hill for a bit to get more speed, the sides of the roads now had wooden posts that had three wires running through them and I laughed thinking, 'the massive cliff had just one wire, not three. Here the three wires protected you from a wall, not a hundred-foot cliff down a rock face into ice-cold water.' I thought it should have been the other way around. As I rode down the hill, I was using my own lane so I had to constantly keep looking behind me to check for traffic but there was none until about halfway down when a dark-grey Toyota car slowly went by me as I now rode in the oncoming lane with a view all the way down the hill. As the rock walls dropped into the ground and disappeared the protective wires on the sides of the road also disappeared. For a short distance there were just walls of trees on both sides of the road. Then the wires came back just as a black Chevy truck pulling a massive white camper trailer drove by me in the oncoming lane. I flew past the truck then noticed a small bridge coming up. I was going at a decent speed from the hill, so I took a quick look for traffic, saw none coming either way, and as I got on the bridge, I put my slide glove down and came screeching to a stop without flipping around and wiping out. It was the first time I was able to go from ripping fast to a dead stop in a very short distance. After I slid to a stop on the small bridge, I got off my board and looked over the edge as I waited for my father.

There was a very small creek that came out of the forest and ran under the bridge towards the freezing-cold, ocean-like lake. The very shallow creek was full of big and small boulders that sprinkled out of the forest and beneath my feet, continuing on under the bridge. As I was checking out the creek, I saw something on the concrete wall of the bridge. I went to check it out and it was a big, gross-looking bug. The big beetle had six long, lanky legs with two huge antennas that came out of its head and towered three times bigger than the beetle itself. It was a really gross-looking bug. Once my dad got there, I pointed out the nasty bugger and he said "neat", and I couldn't have disagreed more. I thought it was disgusting as I'm not a bug person at all. After we looked at the bug for a few seconds, we walked up the hill we just rode down, and began our ride back to base camp where Kathleen made us dinner. After dinner, Kathleen's son, Jay, and I grabbed a couple badminton rackets and smacked a birdy back and forth off to the side of the camp for a bit. With the sun now setting behind the lake and hills, we smacked it back and forth as I started to reminisce about a few of the things that happened on the big hills on the way back to camp.

The first thing I thought about was when we were coming back to the second huge hill we got to that day. As I rode the flat part of the road, I could see in the distance it descended as it turned left. I knew this was the start of the huge hill, so I was full of excitement and started to carve back and forth in the empty, oncoming lane. Only as I kicked more and got more speed, I started carving too hard, and my board slid out on me. It only slid a few inches, but I wasn't expecting it and it scared the bananas out of me. I let out a "whoa fuck" after it unexpectedly startled me. Then the road started to descend more as it made the left turn. I gave a few more kicks as I approached the corner just as a small black car drove by in the oncoming lane. I then gave a few more kicks and lightly carved to get a feel for my board, the road conditions, and how it all felt under my feet. I saw the yellow downhill sign for the trucks on the other side of the meridian and clapped my hard plastic slide pucks together in excitement. The view to the right was an amazing view of Lake Superior. Beyond the cliff that was on the other side of the road, you could only see the ocean of water. Trees stood at the top of the cliff face on the right side where the road was flat prior to the land drastically descending.

As I looked down the hill around the long slow bend, I could see a truck coming my way in the oncoming lane I was riding in, so I moved over to the empty lane on my right until they were gone. As I started to get going faster and faster the dark-blue GMC truck came up to me pulling a small trailer. As he drove by me the older man with a big, grey beard stuck his left arm out his window and gave me a big thumbs up in approval and smiled because he knew I was just starting to head down a monstrosity of a hill. After the guy drove by giving me his approval, I bombed down the hill half bent over with my arms behind my back and body pointing forward in hill bombing position and started to fly down the hill looking for traffic every few seconds, however I got to ride the whole hill without needing to move for traffic. It was nice to see the view at the top of the cliff overlooking the lake, then coming down the hill and getting swallowed by the forest. I was now riding in the outgoing lane and turned around to see a black truck coming up behind me, so I moved back over into the oncoming lane just as the wall of rock on my left came out of the ground towering over me before disappearing back into the ground as fast as it came out. Once at the bottom, I stood on the shoulder listening to music as I waited for my dad. The whole way downhill from top to bottom was only about two or three free minutes of ripping at least sixty-plus-kilometres-per-hour. It made for a nice ride in the stunning beauty around Lake Superior. When my dad came up to me, I told him about the guy that gave me a thumbs up and we had a "you know the hills are big when" moment.

Then I started thinking about the first big hill we climbed up and got to bomb down, just before we got back to camp. We came up to the first hill and, with my adrenaline going, I got super excited as I came around the left corner at the top. The only thing that killed my excitement was listening to the aggressive "beep beep beep beep" of the GoPro dying. Riding in the oncoming lane, I went around the left turn slowing down as I knew the parking lot to the lookout was coming up on my left. Once I got by the look out spot I saw the right turn on the halfway mark of the hill, I ripped it the rest of the way down with no slowing down or needing to move for traffic. That hill was pretty intimidating, even for me. As I was ripping probably eighty-plus-kilometres-an-hour, I couldn't help but think, 'I should really be wearing motorcycle leathers.' If I fell going that fast in my shorts and T-shirt I would be losing the majority of my skin and wouldn't have been able to ride for who knows how long. With the thought of 'you are so fucked if you fall' I religiously kept looking for traffic as I ripped down the hill. I always loved gaining so much speed the laws of physics kicked in and you physically couldn't go any faster, until you tucked down even lower to reduce drag from the wind. I was at the bottom of the hill that took us what seemed like an hour to walk up after just a couple minutes. Now coasting the long, slow right corner, I took a quick look for cars before I put my hand down and came sliding to a halt. I got off my board to wait for my dad and when I turned around to look up the hill, I spotted him, but he wasn't on his board. When I looked up the hill to the halfway turn, I saw him running in the outgoing lane with a dump truck hot on his tail and his board riding solo in the oncoming lane going into the ditch. I couldn't help but think, 'whoa careful, dad.' After a run and a rolling tumble, he popped back up on his feet, got his board back, bombed down the rest of the hill, and caught up to me on the side of the road. We then began to push the flat road back to camp. As Jay and I were passing the birdy in the air, every once in a while, I'd look at the hill my dad wiped out on and had a little chuckle while being glad he didn't get run over by the dump truck, injured more than a bit of road rash on his elbow, or die.

After playing badminton for a while, I sat down on the bench that overlooked the beach and the lake. With the sun now setting lower, I had an incredible view. There was the big, beautiful, white sandy beach that overlooked what seemed to be an ocean with the sun setting way off in the distance on the other side of the water with the sky lit up in a bright-orange colour. To my left was just beachfront that ran along the waterline in the bay. To my right, I could see the same but a few kilometres off in the distance the beach ended were the first big hill we had to climb was. That's where the land rose out of the water turning into a big, rocky, tree-covered hill that took over from there. It was an incredibly relaxing view, and I couldn't help but again feel like I was the luckiest person alive and thought, 'I shouldn't even be here seeing this right now. I should be dead; be grateful for this moment,' as well as, 'I honestly couldn't care if I dropped dead right here, right now.' Not because I wanted to die or because I was upset. But because I was so content, relaxed, and at peace in the purest moment of happiness that I had ever felt. I was so at peace even the thought of death couldn't intervene, and it was immaculate. For the second time of my life, death, my greatest fear of all, didn't leave me paralyzed when I thought about it. It was exactly how I felt after myself induced LSD experiment when I had my life's first epiphany. Only I wasn't high on drugs, I was high on life.

 I reminisced as I sat there relaxing completely at peace with life. I couldn't help but continue to think how lucky I was to be from such a clean, peaceful, and beautiful country. It was in that moment I had my third 'I could care less if I dropped dead right now I am so blessed' moments of that day. How could that be possible? I've only had one of those moments in my life when I was seventeen and here, I had experienced it multiple times that day. As I sat on the bench watching the sunset over the hills and ocean-like lake I had this incredibly overwhelming feeling. One I've never had before. I felt as though my mind, body, and soul were one. Not only that, I felt connected with everything around me for the first time in my life. It was like when you truly become one with yourself, you also become one with the land and all that there is, I don't know how else to explain it. Both the inner peace and the feeling of being one with everything overtook my body, mind, and soul for minutes. It was like every atom in my body was connected to every atom of my surroundings. I was not only one with myself mentally for the first time ever, but I also knew without a reasonable doubt that I was also one and somehow connected with everything there is, was, and ever will be. The feeling was so surreal I felt like I wasn't even a human anymore, but I was billions upon billions of atoms that were there in the moment just existing in space and time with everything else all connected as one. As I sat there in this profoundly euphoric, content state of mind my dad came down the pathway behind the bench and took a great picture of me and my longboard as I pondered on the bench.

 After my dad's close call on the massive hill, we had to have a quick chat about things. With the treacherous terrain drastically increasing the odds of something disastrous happening to one another we made a verbal agreement. That was, no matter what if something ever did happen to one of us, we would finish the trek across the country in the other one's honour. The hills were getting so big and steep that people didn't even like driving down them and here we were standing on pieces of wood maybe two or three inches off the ground with no breaks flying down them at eighty-plus-kilometres-an-hour in plain clothes. With death cliffs on the sides of said hills and being in the middle of nowhere with next to no population and zero cell service—if anything was going to happen to one of us, it was going to be here. This was the most dangerous part of the entire trek and that is why Kathleen gave us the warning back in North Bay at her house, and this is why she decided to put us up for five weeks. This part of the trek was literally a death sentence to some, so I agreed with my dad that no matter what happens (injury or death) to one of us, the other will continue on and finish it in the honour of the other.

Later on, my dad and I would find out the hill he got speed wobbles on that made him have a run and tumble with the dump truck on is tail was called "Montreal Harbour Hill." Once we found out the hill had a name, we then had our second "you know the hills are big when" moments. After supper, I grabbed my computer and plugged in the GoPro camera to see what footage I was able to get. As I was sitting there with my computer on my lap at our campsite, a man came walking by and asked, "How are you getting Wi-Fi out here?" I told him, "I have no connection. I'm just charging and downloading pictures off the camera." He replied, "yeah that's what I thought but I was just checking," and continued on his walk.

After a few days we had to move base camp to Wawa about one-hundred-kilometres away. There, the routine would continue on for a week or two. My dad and I would be on the road trekking through the endless rock and forest all day while Kathleen and her family would be sure we came back to food, fire, coffee, beds, and be able to relax for the rest of our evenings. With their truck so full of people and gear, we began asking other people if they would be able to give us a ride out towards our new basecamp. After a while, one of the girls working said she could give us a ride when she was off work later that afternoon. Instead of waiting around the whole day, we asked Morgan if she could keep an eye out for us on the side of the highway as we were going to get skating and get a head of some kilometres. As Morgan worked all day we pushed through the beautiful hills and the blasted-out rock for a second time. It was a very beautiful and peaceful ride so I couldn't even complain. All morning and into the afternoon we went up and down the twisty hilly terrain witnessing some the most magnificent sights our country had to offer.

Later on in the afternoon, Morgan drove past my father and I and pulled over on the right side of the road. My dad and I jumped into her car, and we drove for maybe two or three minutes before she took a right turn off the highway to where her cabin was. We got out and said hello to the other provincial park workers that were off work and already there for the night. We had a short chat with a few of the young women and had a chance to refill our water supply. At one point I asked the girls, "Are there any hills coming our way?" only to be devastated to get nothing but "I don't know" and "I don't think so" for answers.

We got back on the highway continuing on through the woods, and after we came around the small lake the girls' cabin rested on, the road then made a left turn and on my right in the outgoing lane I saw a yellow downhill sign. I got super excited and clapped my slide gloves together before I took off and pushed for the hill as fast as I could. I came flying by my dad on his left and began to cruise down the hill as it turned right at the top before descending. We pushed past a small lake at the top of the hill, then bombed by another lake on the way down, and past yet another lake at the bottom of the hill, the amount of water in Ontario was astonishing.

Between the lakes, there was nothing but forest and big-brown rock walls on the sides of the road that came and went. We skated through the woods for a little before we came up to a left turn in the road and as we came around the left turn, I was thrilled to see another yellow downhill sign on the other side of the road. I clapped my slide pucks together and started to vigorously kick the road for some more speed. This hill I could see went on for what seemed like a few kilometres, and I could see all the way down once I came around the turn at the very top. It was really long but had a very gradual descent. I kicked and kicked until I was going so fast, I physically couldn't keep up with kicking the road anymore. Then I got down low and coasted down the long hill for about three or four straight minutes.

For how long the hill was, I thought I would have gone faster than I was going but I couldn't complain as it was a free few kilometres of effortless coasting. As I was crouched down on my board I was looking around for traffic and at the beautiful scenery that I was completely entranced by. On both sides of the road was thick, lush, green forest. To my left, you could see the forest went on for a short distance before it vanished, and Lake Superior took over the landscape. To my right, was forest that went on and on as it blanketed the rolling hills. The green hills on the land frequently rose and dropped like ripples in water. The air was so fresh with every breath I could feel it rejuvenating me while simultaneously cooling me off as it rushed over my entire body.

After I looked for traffic and saw none in the oncoming lane, I moved over and got to use the whole lane to myself for probably half the hill before moving over to the other lane to let a few cars go up. Surrounded with nothing but peace, beautiful land, and nature made for an incredibly awesome and peaceful ride. There were no office buildings, no over-populated areas, no trains, no power plants, and no massive line ups of traffic. There was nothing but nature's harmony; silence, and tranquility. It was only disrupted with the odd car passing here and there. I don't think I've ever felt so disconnected from society as I did in those moments, and I absolutely loved it with every atom in my body.

I found there is something about the land in my country that made me really feel grounded, grateful, safe, and at peace with myself. Time and time again, I experienced this incredible feeling, and it was more than magnificent. I felt as if the land and myself were connected. Not by a cord or a string, but connected by an unfathomable spiritual bond that couldn't be seen, heard, or touched. It could only be spiritually felt. It was like mother earth had an invisible umbilical cord connected to my soul, feeding me the nutrients I needed in order to grow into the young man I was becoming. It was unlike anything I've ever felt before.

After riding downhill for a few minutes, I took the momentum of the hill and started spinning doing three-hundred-and-sixty-degree spins on my board for fun on the flat ground. With my arms out like helicopter blades, I stood spinning and spinning, slowly coasting to a stop next to another little bridge on the highway where I took a short break and waited for my dad. There, I looked right to see a small creek come out of the forest and go under the bridge that held the road, then when I looked left, I was stunned. The small creek ran into the huge lake and just off to the left side I could see a monstrosity of a cliff face coming straight out of the water that probably went a hundred feet into the air holding thousands of trees on the top of it. It was quite the view.

As my dad rolled up, I pointed out the cliff before we continued down the road and found a left turn into a parking lot beach area to check it out. There was a nice blond, sandy beach area where we could look out at the water and get a nice view of the massive cliff, so we decided it was a great spot to take a short break. My dad asked a nice young couple there if they could take a picture of us on my dad's phone and we hung out on the beach enjoying the view for a few minutes having a sip of water. Two of the girls that were at the cabin ended up venturing down to the beach as we were there. The two ladies and I walked through the sand for a bit and had a chat. They asked me more about my cancer and stroke experiences, so I told them all about what it was like. I really wanted to tease them about telling me there were no hills around the cabin, but I didn't because I wasn't sure if it was those two that said anything. I was just glad I had my crushed hopes of "no hills" turn into spending the next five kilometres riding mostly all downhill to Old Woman Bay. With no cell service for weeks and completely consumed by the stunning beauty of the Superior landscape, I felt incredibly disconnected from normal society and at times, even reality.

It was probably the most amazing feeling and experience of my life. It was in these sequestered wild places I unexpectedly found my happiness. But most of all, I found myself again, and by again, I mean for the first time in my life. Day after day I was so content and had an unfathomable amount of peace, gratitude, and happiness it would give me those "I honestly don't care if I die right now" moments again and again, daily. It is something I'll never forget and something I still hold onto and feel in my current day-to-day life. I've never felt more grateful and content with life than I have in this part of the country. Though I was incredibly saddened, heartbroken, and angry to realize that our society and the way we are told to and forced to live our lives, has completely robbed us from these incredible, priceless, and truly magnificent experiences. Yet at the same time I felt incredibly blessed that I was able to feel that unfathomable, spiritual, soul-bonding connection to earth in my life. That blank canvas that was my life before this profound journey was now the most intricate, beautiful, colourful, and priceless pieces of art that I had ever seen.

After our short break at Old Woman Bay, we turned left back onto the highway, and I thought to myself 'I hope there are some more hills coming up.' We got maybe a hundred metres away when the road turned right and went straight up at a steep incline. "Careful what you wish for," I remember then saying to myself. All that nice downhill we got to ride to the bay we had to hike up for at least an hour. Right when I thought the massive uphill was over, it went flat for a left turn then went right back uphill. At least this one wasn't as steep of an incline. After an hour of hiking uphill, it finally levelled out and I thought about turning around and ripping down the huge hills, but I didn't feel like spending another hour plus walking back up. On top of that, the hill was so big it intimidated me, plus the left turn at the very bottom of the super-steep hill I don't think would have been physically possible to make. I would have likely been thrown into the woods going one hundred plus kilometres an hour. That was if I didn't get hit by or hit a car on the blind corner.

After trekking through what seemed like an endless number of rocks, trees, and lakes everywhere, we eventually made it to the Tim Hortons where we were to be picked up. I was more than ready for a break, some water, and supper after the long day in the hot sun. Luckily, after Kathleen picked us up, we went over to some locals' Kathleen knew for chats and food. After driving into the woods through a small mining town, she found the massive camper trailer where we relaxed, had chili for dinner, and hung around chatting for an hour or two. One of the guys there was wearing a "come hell or high water" shirt he got to help support Calgary through the devastating flood that happened.

After supper, chats, and a refill of water we got back pushing on the road. After coming around several corners and up and down a few hills we got to a construction zone. Again, they had half of the freshly paved black tarmac closed off as it had no lines painted on it so we had the entire fresh road to ourselves for kilometres to come. I loved that part of the road construction. Fresh, empty, clean roads with pylons I could use as a slalom course to carve around.

Kathleen and her amazing family were such an incredible blessing, not only for their tireless effort and support but also for events unforeseen by everyone in the coming weeks. After a week or so staying at Wawa we moved base camp again. This time we went to White River. Only our stay there was very short as it was too much for everyone to handle. The bugs were very bad and we stayed for a night, maybe two, before we decided to leave. So we packed up and moved base camp to Neys which was yet another beautiful campground just outside Marathon, Ontario.

My father and I pushed through the woods all day to Marathon as Kathleen and her family set up base camp for us again. Our arrival into Marathon was really enjoyable as there was another long gradual hill that was a good two or three minutes of effortless coasting into our destination. The forest was on both sides and the hill looked like it was leading down to Lake Superior off in the distance. At the bottom of the hill, it made a slow left turn. After skating by a small gas station on our left we continued on until my dad found a coffee shop to set up his computer and get a hold of Kathleen. The nice long hill into town had me itching for more hills so I grabbed my board and went to explore Marathon as we waited. Not wanting to get lost and miss my ride, I tried not to go too far, or for too long. When I returned, my father told me he went to the store to get some supplies where the cashier told him that her son Trevor was one of the few local longboarders in town. He also said we still had a while to wait so I decided to go adventure some more.

Shortly after I left the coffee shop, I found a hill and bombed down it passing a school on my right before coming into a community of houses. As I was slowly pushing along the sidewalk, I ran into another longboarder. It was Trevor, the cashier's son, I was literally just told about. I laughed at the small-town coincidence when he introduced himself. I asked him if he could show me some hills and he took me on a little skate through town to show me the few they had. After bombing a small hill down to the bay, we hiked up through a small wooded area and sat on our boards enjoying the views for a few minutes before we continued our skate through town. After a half hour or so I decided to head back to the coffee shop. Only now I had no idea where I was or where I needed to go, so I asked Trevor if he could show me the way to the shopping plaza which he was more than happy to do. We jumped on our boards, skated around, and bombed the hill we went down a few minutes earlier one more time. Then after following the waterline for a few blocks, we made a right, went up a small hill, then down another block or two before he pointed to the strip mall I was looking for. I said, "Thanks a lot, man," gave him a fist bump and skated down the street to the coffee shop where I had everyone waiting for who knows how long.

We all jumped into the truck and headed over to camp at Ney's National park. On the way I saw another incredibly beautiful sight. As we left the small town of Marathon, I looked out the front window of the truck and for as far as I could see on the road were the endless rolling hills. With the setting sun turning the sky a nice bright-orange colour and the endless, green rolling hills while completely surrounded by nature—it made for one incredible sight. I wish I had told them to stop so I could take a picture because it was definitely picture worthy. Once we got to camp, we had dinner around a camp fire, chatted for a bit, then Jay and I smacked a birdy around for entertainment for a while. After that, Kathleen made me a coffee and I sat around the fire drinking it as we chatted into the night.

The next morning, I woke up disgusted and immediately climbed out of my bed and tent then puked in the bushes a few times before I went back to sleep. Right after that, my dad tried to wake me up to get going but I wasn't having any of it. So, my father took off and went to skate the kilometres he missed that morning as I rested. I would get a ride and skate in from Marathon the next day. As I rested, I couldn't help but think of all of the gnarly hills we had been riding around Superior and how freakishly fast I'd get going down them on my longboard. I then had an idea about using Kathleen's Canadian flag as some sort of parachute to help slow me down on the colossal hills. I also recalled from the train tracks just off the highway into the park there was a nice little downhill cruise. I had a few hours of sleep while my dad rode the kilometres he had missed and when I felt a little better and my dad returned, we got in the black Suzuki truck after I tied the top and bottom half of the flag together by the rings on the corners and headed to the top of the hill for a test run to see if it would work. I gave Jay the GoPro to record the test as my dad and I jumped out of their truck. I wrapped the flag around my body like a cape and once Jay shouted, "Go!" we took off.

I gave about a dozen good kicks or so and went around the slight right bend on the road. With my dad right behind me and Jay in the truck behind him, we were off. After getting a bit of speed, with one tied end of the flag in each hand, I lifted my arms into the air and the wind caught the parachute-shaped Canadian flag and it drastically started to slow me down. Jay in the truck saw that it worked and let out a, "Yeah!" I brought the flag back down around my body as we turned a slight right corner then gave a few hard kicks before tucking down low to gain more speed and reduce the drag.

I got more speed as we came around a right bend and the road split left and right which made a little island with a huge piece of driftwood in the middle of it. I turned right as the other way led into trees and would have made me lose the speed I had. After the road went slightly to the right it made a left turn. After that turn we passed a 40kmph speed limit sign on the right side of the road just before another right turn. I started to lose speed on the flat ground, then even more so once it started to go up a slight hill. My dad cruised by me as we got to the top of the small hill, but it went right back down. I gave a few good hard kicks and went by my dad on his right then tucked down to gain more speed down the small hill. We stood on our boards just hanging out coasting for a bit. With my dad behind me coasting a few feet away on my right, we started to gain more speed, so I threw up the flag and it instantaneously slowed me down again. My dad past me and went in front as I tucked down lower to try and get some more speed again. We then came around a left bend when the road dipped down for fifty metres or so before coming back up and continuing on the left bend through the forest. The road went uphill a little bit, then turned right, and went right back down. I was still tucking down and past my dad on the right just as a lady riding her bike went by us on the other side of the road, heading out of the park.

Continuing to tuck, we came up to the camps registration site. I went left in the oncoming lane to avoid the speed bumps and the longer way around the office. The truck had to slow down to the 20kmph speed limit and go over the speed bumps, but my dad and I flew by them in the straighter oncoming lane continuing to effortlessly coast down the road. The truck had to go slow so my dad and I were already gone around the left and right turns before they got through. They had to do a bit of catch up and found us around the second long right corner. That's when an obnoxiously yellow Dodge truck came around the corner and drove by us, leaving the beautiful national park.

I threw up the flag, slowed down, and noticed Jay and the truck right behind me so I quickly put it down and began to kick again. We then came around another left turn now on flat ground, so we started to kick the road. We then rode past a big brown sign that said, "Build fires in fire pits only." I thought that would have been self-explanatory or common sense, but I guess some people needed a reminder to not burn down the massive forest we were all in. We then came around a long, slow right corner that had a sign indicating parking, restrooms, and a picnic area at a place called "Prisoners Cove". Coming around the right turn I gave a few good hard kicks to get me to the left turn up ahead. After the left turn the paved road turned to gravel as we entered the camping grounds. So, I turned into a little gravel area and got off my board to drive back to camp where we relaxed for the afternoon into the evening. As the sun set that night, it turned the sky into fire, so I grabbed the GoPro, and we all took a walk to the beach only a few metres away. I thought I was taking pictures, but the camera was still on video mode, and I caught a short video of the beautiful, bright, fire sky as we walked around chatting and enjoying the beautiful view.

I was excited to skate the hills from Marathon to Neys the next morning, until I got up to the sound of rain hitting the top of my tent, however I was feeling much better that day. I hated the rain with a passion and was very disappointed I would now have to ride the hills in it. Wishing I manned up and skated with my dad puking on the road the day before, I started to help pack up the truck and as we were loading everything up, it got incredibly foggy. The fog that comes off the lake is insane. We couldn't even see ten feet in front of us. This was going to be an interesting day. I expected the fog to stay around the lake and knew the highway was a fair bit away, so I thought I'd be clear of the fog on the roads.

Before I got on the road, we all pulled into the "Prisoners Cove" area to check it out. Only the fog was so thick you could cut it with a knife, and we couldn't see anything but down, and only down. Looking down, I could see we were standing on solid bedrock that had big holes in it filled with water and green algae that grew in the rock bowls' stagnant water before the bedrock went away and the white sandy beach began. We walked around for a few minutes then got back in the truck and headed into Marathon. I thought the fog would lighten up once we got to the highway or at least into town, but I was sadly mistaken. We got into town, and I jumped out by the gas station dropping my headphones without realizing it. I got on my board and pushed a few times to the highway then made a left going down the Trans-Canada heading back to camp. I decided to bring the flag-chute for a few reasons. One being to slow myself down on the huge hills, also so I wasn't wearing out my shoes, and to throw it up in an attempt to help me be more visible to the traffic in the thick fog and rain.

The rain was on and off lightly for a bit as I rode in the oncoming lane. I chose the oncoming lane so I could see the traffic in front of me and didn't have to constantly be checking over my shoulder for cars that might come into my space. It wasn't long before the roads got sketchy as can be, they twisted and turned with cliffs on both sides of the foggy, wet roads. The fog was so thick I couldn't tell where the fog ended, and the sky began. On top of that, I couldn't see around any corners I was coming up to. After a while I went to put my headphones in and play my rainy-day song, only to find out I had no headphones, and I got mad. I stopped and tore my bag apart looking for them and couldn't find them anywhere. I then remembered I had them on my lap as I was untangling them in the truck, and they were probably back at the gas station. I figured they were probably still there but also thought of them as a lost cause, because if they were not run over and broken by now, they were soaking wet and likely ruined. Plus, with the current riding conditions I figured taking away my sense of sound wasn't the best idea, so I continued on knowing I had my main better pair of headphones at camp.

On the left side of the road, the rock wall disappeared and turned into a short ditch with a wall of trees behind it. On the other side of the road the wall of rock came out of the ground lifting the entire forest that grew on top of it. At first, the road was pretty dead with nobody travelling on it. Each corner I came up to was a mystery whether it was going to be a left or right turn, if it was a car or truck that came around it, and if I had any shoulder to ride on. I still wished I had my music, but the eeriness of it all was quite adrenaline pushing. However, at the same time, it was incredibly nerve racking, so my anxiety and paranoia was running wild as I came to a long slow right turn in the road that then straightened out.

With the crazy thick fog that came off the lake and out from the trees and one lonely me on the side of the road in the middle of nowhere, it looked like the beginning of someone about to get slaughtered in a horror movie, I looked so alone and out of place. The ditch to my left dropped lower and lower as the safety posts and wires came up keeping anything from falling into it. At the bottom of the steep cliff, stood trees that came out of the ground, grew above the cliff, and still towered higher than the highway. On the other side of the road, it was still a wall of rock with the forest protruding out of the top like a spiked-up hair style. The road started to straighten out and the rain came back. I decided to take a break and have a sip of water, so I put my longboard down on a big boulder that rested on the side of the highway, popped a squat on my gross wet board, and sat in the rain on the side of the highway resting my legs while I had a few sips of water. As I sat there, I saw everyone in the black Suzuki truck drive by, heading back to camp on the other side of the road but the fog was so thick I was hardly able to see them through it, and not a single one of them saw me. I couldn't help but think, 'Thankfully I'm not laying here dying after being hit by a car.' I couldn't help but think about how screwed I was if anything did happen. Nobody would know for hours, then everybody would struggle to be able to see me when they came looking. The cliffs on each side of the road meant if I had to suddenly hit the ditch, I would have my legs taken out by the wires around my shins and knees before I went summersaulting over them, down a twenty-plus-foot cliff, where I'd lay until I died or I was found. As much as I had recently felt that I was ready to die, that didn't sound like the way I wanted my day to go, so I had to be extra careful.

It then started to rain hard again, and I got soaked. My attempts to hide under the flag I had wrapped around me didn't do much to help either. I was now freezing cold, wet, crabby, and without music, thankfully I was alone though. This was the dumbest shit I had ever put myself in. "Yeah, just go for a leisure longboard across Canada…what a great idea," I sarcastically said to myself as the fog got incredibly thick again. It was like something out of the movie "The Mist." I couldn't see if traffic or whatever was coming, I couldn't tell if the road turned, or if there was a hill until I was maybe fifty feet away from it. I half expected a monster to come out of the woods and drag me away as it made slurping noises. To make things better, the huge ten-foot shoulder I had, went down to maybe two-feet. I couldn't see in the wet and very slippery conditions with semi-trucks now passing me maybe two- or three-feet away on my right. Each one spit up a cloud of mist that surrounded the big transporters and hit me as they drove by. Coming into the afternoon, traffic was really starting to pick up and there was semi after semi after semi. It was almost like they all decided to leave at once. Here I am on a tiny shoulder, sandwiched between a massive rock wall on my left and big rig after big rig on my right within an arm's length away. I could just make out the road started to turn left into the fog. Following the big wall of wet, dark-brown and black rock on my left, I continued on, hoping I made it back to camp in one piece.

The entire time I had the flag up waving it as much as I could slowing me down as I went downhills and around blind corners. The road continued on what seemed like this endless right turn with a massive twenty-foot rock wall on my side in the oncoming lane. The massive ten-foot shoulder I once had came back for maybe a hundred feet before it was gone again. With no music, I took a good listen and look for traffic before flying to the outbound lane to see the shoulder there was non-existent and just went into the ditch with a wall of trees. I had another look and listened, heard nothing, and flew back over to the oncoming lane with the small shoulder. The road went straight for a bit and I thought I could see cars coming my way so I moved over as far left as I could on the tiny shoulder.

That's when the rain came out with a vengeance, and I got pelted with the sideways rain. I jumped off the road and hid in the trees trying to get cover while I had another sip of water. After I had another shower in the trees, I got out of the tree line and back on the road. As I rode on the tiny shoulder, I looked up to see a semi-truck just on their side of the white line and my right wheels were just on the other side, pretty much touching that same white line. I hardly had enough time to jump off my board and into the ditch. With my heart now in my throat, I couldn't help but let out a "Holy fuck!" I was so glad there was room for me to jump off onto a shoulder and it wasn't just a cliff or a rock wall like it had been for most of the way.

As I caught my breath and shook off another near-death experience of a head on collision with a big, white Mack truck, I went into the ditch, got my board, and got back on the move. My little shoulder got even smaller as I came down a long, slow, left turn with the massive wall of rock again on my left. Finally, The fog and rain started to lighten up on me and I was able to see a bit farther, so I started to rip down the hills a bit faster. With my flag-chute in the air I came flying down the long, slow, left downhill turn as big rig after big rig kept popping out from behind the wall of rock on my left. The wooden posts and wire running through them were all that stood between me and the cliff face. As I came around the corner, the fog seemed to have collected in one spot and my hundred feet of visibility turned into maybe fifty. A small silver car came out of the fog and drove past me, by the time I turned my head right to look behind, the car had already been swallowed by the fog and was gone without a trace. Things were getting freakier, and I wanted to get off the road as soon as I could, so I started to kick more and more and at a faster rate of speed. I looked for cars and didn't see or hear any. Then I looked to my left into the ditch and the fog was so thick I couldn't see farther then the third tree into the forest, they were all encapsulated by the heavy fog.

I knew if I couldn't even see the trees right beside me, then traffic likely couldn't see me at all. The fog then got even thicker. It got so thick the semi-truck that drove by me only a few feet away was just an outline and the sounds of a motor with wet road under the tires. Then there was a guy on a motorcycle that went by, and I couldn't even see or hear him coming. The big trucks made plenty of noise, but this guy was super quiet on his bike, and I hardly noticed it go by. I took another look for traffic and saw none, not that my visibility was any good, so I listened and heard nothing but the water running under my wheels. I looked on the other side of the road to see if I had a big shoulder to push on, but I couldn't tell. However, I was able to just see another fait yellow downhill sign. I was super excited but probably even more nervous as the hill-bombing conditions were less than adequate. I took another good look and saw nothing, so I listened hard and also heard nothing before I quickly crossed to the other side of the road. Of course, just as I did, a big rig came around the corner and I hardly made it across to the shoulder on the other side in time.

The ditch on that side dropped away turning into a cliff and the trees at the bottom again rose high above the highway and I could still only see maybe three or four trees deep off the road. Just as I'm thinking about how blind I am, and how I don't like it, I started to go faster and faster as I began to come down the top of a hill that I couldn't see down. Once I got going a bit too fast for the conditions, I started to drag my left foot before I remembered to use the flag. I threw up the flag and started to slow down to a more comfortable speed with it in the air. I then flapped it around a bit so the passing cars would hopefully see me.

I had a white SUV pass me just as the shoulder started to get smaller, and smaller, eventually completely disappearing leaving me on the road in the oncoming lane. I looked and listened before bolting over to the other side of the highway in the outgoing lane which luckily had a small shoulder. It was a good thing I crossed over when I did, because just as I got to the other side in the outgoing lane a semi followed by a few cars went by on the side of the road that had no shoulder and I probably would have been hit, ditched myself off the cliff, or caused an accident of some kind.

I was still going downhill at a steady pace, so I threw up the flag again. The massive twenty-foot rock wall on my right side stood towering above everything around. I still couldn't see very far even with the rain and fog dying down a bit. Everything was still wet, slippery, and grey. I was soaking wet, cold, and had been really sick of this stupid-ass day for hours. I just wanted to be in dry clothes, sitting next to a warm fire, while drinking some hot bean water.

With no death cliff down and a decent shoulder on my side in the outbound lane, I decided to stay put. I looked around and listened for traffic but with all the corners, hills, fog, and rain, things were coming out of nowhere and I couldn't even trust my own senses, which was an uncomfortable feeling to say the least. I was going pretty fast for the wet road, so I used my left foot to slow down a little bit. As I was slowing down, I saw a yellow watch for moose sign on the side of the street. It was still hardly recognizable even with visibility improving.

My nice shoulder ended so I went back over to the other side of the road as fast as I could after looking and listening. As I crossed to the other side, I looked behind to see a big semi-truck coming my way, so I threw up the flag to be more noticeable. The big truck passed me with a car hot on its tail. I was still going downhill and even with the flag up, I was going too fast for my liking so I decided to foot break to avoid hydro plaining around the coming corner. I put my left foot on the ground until I got to a more comfortable speed. I then came to a slight bend in the road, just as the shoulder on my side ended so I looked and listened before I shot over to the other side as quickly as I could. There, I had at least a two-foot shoulder to ride on.

With my longboard a little more than a foot wide, riding on a two-foot shoulder, it didn't leave me with a lot of wiggle room. The shoulder widened to about five or six feet but that was short lived and went right back down to about two. I finally got to a straight, flat part of the road and could now see cars coming a couple hundred feet away. I saw a car coming my way and as it went by, I saw there were two or three more behind it that I couldn't see until they got close. The highway was now starting to get busier as car after car and truck after truck came passing by me. From vehicles passing me every few minutes, it seemed like they were now passing me every few seconds. I really wanted to get off of the sketchy road but didn't really have any other option, so I kicked on.

I started to go downhill again, and the shoulder went back to a nice, big eight- to ten-foot size so I had lots of room. I continued hoping for the best as the fog came back, and I again was unable to see more than one-hundred feet away as car after car passed me. Car after car, truck after truck dashed past me. As they did, I was looking at the drivers and passengers to see if they even noticed me and not a single person did. I was just blindly putting my trust in the drivers that they stayed in their lanes as I stayed on my tiny shoulder.

Again, the paranoia set in, and I couldn't help but think about 'what would happen if I got hit'. No one would know for a few hours, then it would take hour after hour to find me, and if I went into a ditch or off a cliff, I'd be lucky to even be found at all. But above all that, my biggest fear was causing a pile up of cars and big rigs if there was an accident on a foggy corner. With little to no visibility, nobody would have time to react or stop and it would have been a disaster of epic proportions. Plus, with being in the middle of the forest, in the middle of nowhere, with no cell service, and no cell phone, it would have taken a very long time for help to even get there. My mind went racing with the "worst case Ontario" (scenario) on replay.

I came up to another hill that was long and straight, so I ripped down it as fast as I comfortably could with the flag in the air keeping me at a perfect speed just as the fifteen-foot rock wall came up out of the ground on my right and disappeared back into the ground just as fast. After the small embankment that led to it, the pine trees created a tall wall on my left. The fog was back and overtook everything in sight and I could hardly see twenty feet in front of me. The rain had died down to a tolerable sprinkle which was nice, but I had been dripping wet from every limb for hours now, so it really didn't matter much anymore. With the road covered in puddles and every semi-truck kicking up that cloud of mist from the multiple tires, I was running into wall after wall of mist as every big rig went by me. The worst part was when you had your mouth open and you got the mist in your mouth, eyes, or up your nose. I had to close my eyes and hold my breath with every passing truck, so I didn't get the dirty road water in them.

The fog then got so thick I couldn't see a thing and I got off my board, took off the camera, looked at it and said, "I can't see fuck all," in my disorientation while pointing the camera around. I then put the camera back and repositioned the flag in my hands for a better grip. I decided to take a break from my board, so I picked it up and started to walk for a minute or two. After walking for a bit, I saw the road took a long slow right turn as it dropped and disappeared. I put my board down and began to kick for the hill. On the other side of the street was a huge fifty-foot jagged rock wall that soared over everything else. On my side was a small two- or three-foot ditch then another colossal thirty-foot rock wall. By now, we had been travelling through these walls of rock for about four or five straight weeks. It boggled my mind realizing how much energy it took to blast out that much rock and then move it all for one incredibly stunning road from Marathon to Ney's, let alone over the entire Canadian Shield and across Canada.

After the short hill, the road turned left and appeared to be flat, also the fog let up a bit so I could see again for about a hundred feet. The flat road started to sink into the ground just as I passed underneath some powerlines that crossed over the road in the middle of nowhere. I again lost my nice big shoulder just as a white semi-truck came straight for me so I turned my board onto the hard gravel dirt shoulder and bailed off the road to let it pass. As a truck pulling a white mobile home drove by, I went and grabbed my longboard from the side of the road before I took a little walk. Then after looking for traffic, I got back on my board and started to push away. After looking and listening for traffic, I rode over the two lanes to check out the shoulder on the other side, only it was tiny, probably smaller than the oncoming lane, so I looked around then rode back over to the other side. I was not only really unimpressed with the lack of shoulder but more so with all the back-and-forth zigzagging I was doing. I was nearly invisible to traffic going both ways in the dense fog, so I needed to limit my road crossings to a minimum. Traffic still had maybe fifty feet to see me and react accordingly at the best of times.

After coming around another corner, the fog was the lightest it had been all day, I had a good half kilometre of sight and looking down I could see the road descended as it turned right. Once I saw the hill, I started to kick harder and harder going faster and faster, filled with excitement. As

I got closer to it, the road dropped down and was suddenly lost to the fog. The flat part was clear but as soon as the road dropped down, the fog returned. Again, I couldn't tell where the fog ended and where the clouds began. I couldn't see more than fifty feet in any direction; it was just grey everywhere I looked. It was like I was in an airplane high in the sky with the clouds and not on the ground.

Right before the turn on the other side of the road I could see a big blue sign that said I was now entering "Ney's" Provincial Park. The fog wasn't as bad as I thought, and the hill was a long slight incline, so I just stood on my board not needing to push and coasted in the oncoming lane with a good line of sight. Suddenly to my right, I noticed the store which was where I had to turn left to go into the campgrounds. I quickly threw up the flag, only I was going much faster than I originally anticipated and when the wind caught the flag-chute, it stopped me so fast it pulled my arms so hard I could have sworn it dislocated both shoulder joints, it was incredibly painful. But now that I slowed down enough, I was able to make my left turn onto the road and past the dark-green sign that said, "Neys" which was being held up by two old, half cut down trees that stood in an island on the road separating the two driving lanes that went in and out of the park. I looked for traffic and saw none, so I began to push until I got to the 40 kmph sign and coasted around the corner to the train tracks which was the start of the hill into camp. Once at the train tracks, it was the same five-minute cruise I tested the flag on the day before and I cruised right through to the gravel road where I got off my board and walked over to camp still dripping wet, cold, annoyed, and very lucky to still be alive.

Luckily for me once I got back to camp, everything that I wanted was ready and waiting for me. Kathleen, now dubbed "Favourite," had a fire going, and while I finally changed into some dry clothes, she made me a fresh hot coffee. That day was by far the scariest skate day of my entire life. I then sat around the fire reminiscing about how many times I could have and almost just died on that short ride. I honestly think if I didn't have the flag, I would have got going too fast, hydroplaned, and fell off my board on one of the corners that had endless semi-trucks coming around it. I likely would have ended up rolling right under the eighteen wheels of a semi. Shortly followed by another eighteen, eighteen wheelers, cars, trucks, trailers, motorcycles, and knowing my luck, probably an emergency vehicle or two responding to the scene. After I warmed up around the fire, Jay and I grabbed some badminton rackets and smacked a birdy around for a while until we had dinner. At dinner, we sat around the fire and chatted as the sun set in the background behind the lake. As it got darker and day turned into night, our fire burned out and we all went to bed.

The next day, my dad and I were back pushing on the highway through the endless Canadian forest. After a while, we came around a left bend that then went hard to the right, and straight up a massive hill. As my dad and I stood there looking at our next vertical obstacle, a guy in a black truck pulled over to the right at the bottom of the hill and jumped out. He called out to us, "Hey guys! Do you want a ride to the top of the hill?" That wasn't something we were going to pass up and my dad shouted back, "YEAH, MAN! THAT WOULD BE AWESOME!" as he put a thumb up in the air. The guy hanging off the side of his truck said "Yeah? Are you sure?" To which my dad replied, "We would love one, man. That would be great!" The guy offering us a ride then said, "Okay," as he got back in his truck and drove away up the huge hill, leaving us behind.

My dad and I stood there and asked each other, "Did that really just happen?" as we burst out laughing wondering if he didn't hear us right, or if he was just trolling us. After the slow roll, the long walk up the hill began. Step by step, it was like we were walking up a stair stepper at the gym that just never ended. We got about halfway up the hill when we turned around to take in one incredible view.

We saw a big valley of trees off in the distance. The valley was filled with dense fog that looked like a "witch's cauldron" my dad called it, which wasn't far from the truth. The valley of trees on both sides of us ran for miles until the valley on both the left and right sides seemed to connect creating a big bowl for the fog to collect in. As far as you could see behind it, the rolling hills slowly dissipated off in the distance. My dad took a quick picture of the witch's caldron, and we got back to the huge hill we had to hike up.

Once we finally got to the top, the road went flat again, and after catching our breath and having a quick sip of water we got back on our boards and began to push down the highway. The road was flat for about a kilometre, then as we came to a big left turn at the top, it went right back down. Now riding in the oncoming lane, I could see the yellow and black downhill sign on the other side of the road. I got excited and started to push for the hill as I moved over to the outgoing lane while clapping my slide pucks together. I started to fly down the huge hill and carve all over the empty road a bit too excited for the hill. I came around the left turn and the road just dropped. It had a nice big right turn in it that continued to drop before it was lost around the corner. As I'm flying down this huge hill, I wasn't paying attention to traffic, and I was hogging the outgoing lane in the middle of the road like an idiot.

Suddenly this silver car comes ripping past me doing well over the speed limit, probably trying to get as close to me as he could to give me a subtle reminder of how stupid I was being. I not only put the both of us at risk but also anyone in the oncoming lane as he had to slightly move into the oncoming lane to get around me. I wasn't expecting it, and it rightfully scared me enough that I screamed a cuss word or two. I then started to constantly check up and down the hill for traffic, paying attention while ripping down the massive hill, like I should have been. After the scare I ended up taking that hill a bit easier and pulled over to the small blue store that was at the bottom of the hill on the right and waited for my dad before we walked into the store and got some more water. As we looked off toward "Jack Fish Lake" with the rolling, tree-covered hills behind it, we took some sips of our nice cold drinks.

From there, we came around a corner to find the road in the oncoming lane was half closed off. The road was freshly paved with no lines, so they closed half of the new road off to control traffic onto one side. We saw it again and again and I loved it every time as we would get nice fresh smooth roads up and down hills and around corners for kilometres at a time. People lined up in their stopped cars would snarl at us in disgust as we moved through traffic on our boards faster than the actual traffic. Once the construction ended it was back to normal roads and a nice shoulder to ride on for a while until we reached Terrace Bay.

My dad jumped off his board so I could take a picture of him up at the blue and white "Terrace Bay" sign. There, we found a Subway and grabbed a much-needed sub to refuel before we were back on the road to Ross Port where we were going to be picked up. I came flying down this hill and there was traffic stopped with a temporary red light at the bottom for the construction zone. As soon as I knew there was no traffic coming, I ripped down the hill in the oncoming lane. When I got to the bottom, the light was still red and I figured I also had to stop for the heavy machinery so I came squealing to a stop in the empty shoulder on the side of the oncoming lane and waited for my dad before continuing on our way. As my dad and I waited for our ride I sat on my board looking out at Lake Superior.

With all the incredible scenery, stupendous people, and profound experiences I was having over the last few weeks, I had never felt more contentment, peacefulness, and mindfulness than I did when travelling my stupendous country. Each and every day, my fear of 'I wonder if I'm going to die today' turned into 'I could care less if I died right here, right now.' Again, and again death became nothing to me. It was now just a word that described an inevitable part of life. It no longer conveyed the same paralyzing fear into my mind, it no longer made me emotional, and it no longer had me questioning what I should be doing with my possible remaining days. It was now just like any other five letter word. It was like I was once a quadriplegic unable to help myself, but now I was out of a wheelchair running full sprint for the first time, and I had never in my life felt so good, so blessed, and so free. As I sat around the fire that night, I couldn't help but feel it and know it from my blood to my bones that I was the luckiest person alive.

Not because I managed to squeak by three separate twenty-five percent chances to live. Sure, I was lucky and blessed that way too. However, I felt more lucky, blessed, and grateful that in my nineteen years alive, I was able to see, feel, and experience such profound joy, peace, contentment, tranquility, and pure happiness. Most people go through their entire lives as a modern-day, chainless slave. They get up, go to work, come home, and go to bed. Only to wake up and repeat the cycle all over again. This routine eventually becomes all that we know, it becomes our everyday lives, it becomes our entire existence for being here. But most of all, it keeps us distracted from finding our happiness, our purpose, our dreams, societal independence, and even worse, it keeps us distracted from finding ourselves. I felt so blessed to have finally found happiness, gratitude, peace, and myself in this life. I think that alone is more than what most people will experience, accomplish, or achieve in their lives. Therefore, I felt incredibly blessed to have found, accomplished, and experienced all of that before I was twenty and before I died.

The next morning at Ney's, "Favourite" got up and went to brush her teeth in the restrooms. While in the restrooms, she sparked up a conversation with another woman. She began telling Stacy what she was doing, putting my dad and myself up around Superior. Stacy was blown away and wanted to come meet us so she went and got her husband Tyler, their beautiful daughter Reegan then came to our campsite to say hello. Stacy and Tyler happen to live in Thunder Bay which was the next major city we were to reach. They asked us if we needed anything and if there was anything they could do to help. We told them about the usual things like transportation to get around, some new longboarding equipment, and a place to stay while we were passing through. Stacy and Tyler told us to give them a call once we got to the Sleeping Giant National Park parking lot a day or two later and Tyler handed my father a business card to get a hold of him when we arrived.

When we did a few days later, it was the moment I had been regretting since we met Favourite and her family, the day we had to say goodbye. But it was going to end with a bang, and we took a day trip to go drive out to the "Thunder Bay Lookout," "Silver Islet," and "Ouimet Canyon."

We drove down the Sleeping Giant Peninsula for about a half an hour before taking a right turn down a dirt road that seemed to go on forever. After some time, we got to the parking lot of the lookout. At first, I thought we were driving on a paved parking lot, but a look down revealed I was on a sheet of solid bedrock. They parked the car as I went to the washroom in the little outhouse that was there on a small hill to the left. After the restroom break, we all walked around the hill that the outhouse stood on then down a little pathway that led to the lookout. The pathway started as dirt before turning into wood, the wood eventually turned into steel, and once you got further over the edge of the cliff the steel bars had an inch or two gap in them so you could see the hundred-foot cliff you're walking off below you.

The fence that was intended to keep people off the edge of the cliff was tiny, so I easily jumped over it and took a closer look. Later I'd find out how stupid that was because the edges of the cliff were shale and could give way if you're on the wrong spot. As I got closer to the cliff, I was getting nauseous and dizzy from the height over the edge. It was a long way down, so I stopped a few feet from the edge and took a few pictures with the GoPro on the GoPro stick standing among a few trees on the side. I wanted to take a picture down between the metal cracks of the overhang, so I walked back over and took what I thought was a picture, but it ended up being a video of banging metal as people walked around on the platform.

On the overhang when I looked down, we were suspended probably one-hundred feet in the air above the ground that had tall trees on the left and right growing at the base of the cliff that ran for a while in both left and right directions. Looking out, you could see water for miles before you saw the land off in the distance where the city of Thunder Bay was. To the left, the water continued for as far as you could see. Off to the right you could see the water ran into the land of the forest-covered hills a few kilometres down the peninsula. On the rock wall beyond the fence, you could get a good picture of the overhang suspended over the edge of the cliff; so, I went over there as well to take a quick picture.

It was a beautiful spot and I had never seen anything quite like it before, so I was very content, at peace, and happy as I looked around. From there, we went to check out Silver Islet which was a small town that was once the site of the world's richest silver mine located at the very end of the Sleeping Giant Peninsula. Once we drove back down the dirt road we finally got to the paved road where we took a right and continued on to the end of the peninsula. When we got there, there were some cool, old houses that rested along the waterfront with the road that ran along it. After we got through the houses there was a blue building with a sign that said "store" on it, which was once the old community store back in the day but was now boarded up and closed. However, it was still there to keep the historic small town feels. Behind the old, closed store was a big dock that went onto the water but was blocked off by locked fences and big concrete blocks.

To the left of the docs looking out to the distance onto Lake Superior, I could see some huge rocks that popped out of the water which was a manmade seawall made with massive boulders. I found the end of the seawall and walked over to where it met the side of the road before I climbed onto the big rocks and began to walk around it hopping from one huge rock to the next, doing my best not to step on or into bird poop that seemed to be almost everywhere, all the while doing my best not to fall into the cold lake. Once I got about halfway around the seawall, I noticed these little green jelly-like balls that had collected looking like it was growing off a log that rested just below the surface of the water. So, I took the camera off and plunged it into the water to look at them closer when we got back.

I then continued my walk around the seawall till it ended and I had to turn back. After, I took a short walk down the road and sat on a bench that rested on the right side overlooking the water and soaked up the incredible view. As I sat there looking around, I looked at the shoreline where the water met the land on a rocky, sandy beach that was only maybe a foot or so wide. I looked left and right down the beach line and to my right I saw a small beach ball that had washed onto shore. I got up, walked down the steps onto the tiny beach, picked it up, and brought it back to the parking lot area where everyone was hanging around.

From Silver Islet we headed back down the peninsula to Ouimet Canyon. It seemed like it was a bit of a drive away but it was well worth it. However, before we took off, I wanted to bomb down the hill that went onto the Sleeping Giant Peninsula from the #11 highway. We pulled over at the top of the hill and everyone turned around to tail me in the truck. Once they got behind me, I started to kick the road hard and once the start of the hill began, I got down low and started to rip down.

With everyone in the truck behind me, I didn't have to worry about unexpected traffic coming from behind and kept my eyes forward most of the way. Once I got going fast, I still turned around and took a quick look to see they were still right behind me with nobody behind them. Once the road levelled out, I coasted down the road, went by a small house or store with a dog tied outside that was barking at me until I lost most of my speed and did a quick slide to a stop. I then grabbed my board before I got back into the truck and we were off. I was told I was going around seventy-five kilometers an hour on that hill. It was steep and short but it was still a good rush.

Once we got to the parking lot it was a short hike through some trees on a trail that led to the wooden fence and lookout spot. The view was priceless, we were looking around one-hundred-feet straight down over the edge of the massive canyon. On the top of the cliff, we were in the thick, dense Canadian forest that turned into the brown rock of the huge cliff face once you got to the edge. I looked left and the massive tear in mother earth continued for about a kilometre or so. At the bottom, trees grew where they could, but at the base of the cliff faces you could see that fallen rock had piled up over the millennia claiming most of the valuable real estate the trees needed to grow.

Looking right, the massive cliffs went on for another kilometre or two before slowly getting lost to the rolling hills that were covered in trees that went on for as far as one's eyes could see. In the valley of the canyon, once the tear in mother earth ended, you could see a small lake collected and pooled before the rolling hills began. The massive, brown cliff faces rose up into the sky lifting the entire forest bed with it. It was one of the most incredible sights I've seen in my country. I didn't even know places like that existed here, until then.

After our spectacular day of adventure and sightseeing we went over to the Sleeping Giant parking lot where Dad called Stacy and Tyler while I found a restroom. When I came back, I saw my dad packing things into a brand-new white GMC Denali that was in the parking lot. Turns out Tyler and Stacy grabbed it from their dealership, Dominion Motors and drove it out there, hid they keys in a super sneaky spot, and left it for us to get around town with. My dad and I were blown away by this incredible act of kindness from these amazing strangers we met in the middle of the forest. We loaded our stuff into the truck and said our heartfelt goodbyes to Favourite and her wonderful family before we got in the truck and headed into Thunder Bay. After stopping at Dominion Motors to thank the kind team and take a picture we went over to Tyler and Stacy's beautiful home.

We hung out at their house for a bit, and I probably spent too much time checking out Tyler's circular, custom-made, chilled wine cellar. I'm not even a fan of wine, but the cellar was a thing of pure beauty and had me questioning why I didn't. Upstairs was a beautiful walk out patio overlooking the Sleeping Giant that rested in the water a few kilometres off shore. It was an incredibly nice view of the Sleeping Giant Peninsula and Lake Superior from the top balcony.

After, we went over to their restaurant, Lot 66. There, we had a wonderful meal and a drink to celebrate our halfway across Canada mark. In terms of kilometres, Ontario would be our one quarter, one third, and halfway across Canada mark, so the Dolcetti's treated us to a wonderful meal to celebrate. The skillful and kind chef personally came out to talk to us and ask how things were. The meal was outstanding, and we sat there chatting for a while before we headed back to their house for the night. I remember lying on the couch upstairs as everyone went to bed and I started to have a hot flash. I thought I would quietly go sit outside on the walkout patio and cool off for a minute or two. Not even thinking anything other than to be quiet so I didn't disturb anyone. I grabbed the door handle and opened the door.

"BEEP BEEP BEEP WOOOOOP WOOOOP" the alarm went off and I woke up everybody in the house. Tyler comes running out of his room ready to hulk smash the intruder breaking into his beautiful home, only to see me at the door with the look of an idiot on my face, totally like a deer in headlights. Now I was that asshole that woke everyone up in the middle of the night. I didn't even think about someone setting an alarm. I apologized to Tyler and told him I wanted to go sit outside for a minute to cool off, so he turned off the loud screaming alarm and I sat outside for five or ten minutes enjoying the nice summer breeze before going back inside and falling asleep on the couch. I suppose I should have been praying to the house-alarm Gods like I did in Sudbury.

The next day, Stacy and Tyler took us over to the local skate shop called Static to see if they could help us out with some gear that we desperately needed. My dad and I both needed new slide gloves as I worn through mine over the hills around Superior and he had lost his in a marsh we cut across to switch roads quite some time ago. We got to Static and had a chat with the manager and the people working that morning. They were all amazing people and kind enough to hook us up with the new gear we desperately needed. After the guys and gals at Static hooked us up, we got dropped off down the highway to do our skate in.

As we pushed down the "Terry Fox Highway of Courage" on the nice bright sunny day I couldn't help but think of Terry Fox and his tremendous, monumental accomplishment of running across Canada on one leg. Then Linda came back to my mind and her story of meeting him at Middle Cove beach. I couldn't help but again think, 'What are the odds she was able to meet the both of us' and again wondered, 'How many more people on a mission would she meet?' We eventually got to the turn for the Terry Fox monument they had just outside Thunder Bay so we decided to go take a break and check it out, because you can't do a cross-country trek without stopping at the monument of the Godfather of all cross-country treks. We walked up the short hill that turned left leading to the historical site. Now that we came across a washroom, I went inside to go pee and to fill my water bottle before we took a look at the Terry Fox statue, read the information carved on the monument, and took some pictures. As I walked around looking at the statue reminiscing about his story and struggle, I couldn't help but think of the small similarities to our cross-country missions. I remembered being in Chestermere and our schools would shut down for Terry Fox drives. I thought what he did was the coolest, craziest thing ever. Now years later, here I am doing something similar and I'm experiencing the coolest, most incredible, and craziest things ever. I can directly remember being in grade five and my school was doing a Terry Fox run around the parking lot. I did my few laps and was out of breath being the short, chunky kid I was. As I was trying to catch my breath, I thought about running across Canada only to realize you couldn't pay me enough to do something like that, yet many years later, here I was doing something like it for free. Sure, I was trying to give back to the world while desperately trying to find direction in my life, but I couldn't help but laugh at the irony of it all and how I was doing something I once knew I'd never do in my life.

After another 'funny how things change' moments I got on my board and bombed the small hill that went down to the highway. I came ripping up to the stop sign faster than I was expecting to and slid to a quick stop just as a car went flying by on the highway. It was kind of fun, so I walked back up and rode it again and again. My dad finally came down the hill and told me we were waiting for a few people to show up. A few Thunder Bay local kids wanted to ride into the city with us, so we waited for the locals off the highway in the meridian turning spot for a bit before they showed up in a minivan. The three local kids jumped out and began to lead us into the city by starting to longboard the opposite direction, which I was temporarily confused about. But the locals knew a safer way into the city that wasn't on the main highway and so full of traffic. My dad and I with these three youngsters started to longboard into oncoming traffic on the shoulder of the fast lane as it was the biggest lane for us, but we still only had the width of our boards to ride on.

A few minutes later, the shoulder shrunk and turned into rumble strips just as we went to get off the highway and turned right down a side road. After we crossed over some train tracks, the road went down and to the right and rode along the waterfront all the way into town. After an hour or so, we got to a little dam on our right side, of which, about every hundred feet, I could see the concrete slab the water ran down dropped several feet and this continued on until it got to us at the road before the water ran under us into the water of the lake. All the way down, the sloped concrete slabs there were big boulders with a few trees growing on concrete and rocks. After that, we continued our skate into the city and I had asked one of the kids if there were any big hills around so they took my dad and I over to the huge steep hill that was around. Once we got there I was stoked, it looked like a hill from San Francisco with the steep, short incline. I slowly made my way up but once I got halfway, I stopped, put my board down, and jumped on it. I came flying down the hill only to realize there was an intersection with a stop sign at the bottom. I freaked out and turned the board sideways and slid to a stop in the middle of the street just before the stop sign. I almost lost it and fell when the panic of 'Holy I need to stop right now' while ripping faster than expected took over.

Now that I knew there was an intersection at the bottom that I had to stop at, I pushed over to the bottom of the hill and began to walk up. That's when I heard some noise to my right, and I looked up to see an elderly man sitting on his balcony looking at me. He asked, "You sure you can do this one, it's a big hill." I told him, "Yeah, as long as I can stop and not fly blind into the intersection, I'll be just fine." He said, "Okay," as he sat there sipping his beer watching me. I went three quarters of the way to the top this time, put my board down, and jumped on going flying down the hill faster than I was expecting—again. By knowing I had to stop this time, I was more prepared and did a huge slide down the road with my wheels making an awful screeching noise. I kicked back to the bottom of the hill and went back for another round. This time I went all the way up and got on my board. I came flying down the hill and once I got to the bottom where it levelled out, I came up to my slide marks in the street, so I put it sideways to leave one more and stop. But this time, I was going so fast I slid right by the building on my right and into the intersection at the bottom. Luckily for me there was only one car coming on the other side of the street and not in the lane I ended up in, but the lady driving saw me come sliding into the street and shook her head at me as she drove by.

After our hill session, we headed back over to Tyler and Stacy's house. After dinner, we all relaxed, and I looked up some YouTube videos on hills that were in Thunder Bay, and I found a video of a nice run that went into downtown Port Arthur. So, I looked up how to get there, grabbed the GoPro and I was about to take off when Stacy told me she knew where the biggest hill in town was. Stacy and I got in her car with my board and took off to the hill. After a short five-minute drive we arrived, turns out that was the hill my dad and I had been riding with the three locals earlier that day, so we drove back to her house and I went back to my original plan.

I left their house and took off down the street on the rough road that went slightly downhill before coming to a construction zone that had the streets in ruins. I got off my board and walked through the construction zone. With no working city lights, I couldn't see anything till it started to go back up hill and after taking another turn, I was there at the top of the hill. I took a picture of the street sign I had to turn at to get back to Stacy and Tyler's, so I didn't get lost before I looked right and left on the street, and after seeing nobody coming, I got off the sidewalk and walked uphill on the road a bit more before I turned around and started to push down the hill. I saw a car coming from behind me so I went to move over for it but it took a right turn onto a side street and disappeared by the time I looked behind me again. Continuing down the hill, I kept gaining speed and had one or two cars go by me in the oncoming lane, but I had the outgoing lane to myself, freely carving over the entire empty street.

Just as the cars went by, the road had a left turn in it with a fork to the right down a steeper hill that was much shorter. I thought about going right and taking the short, steep hill but the massive crack across the entire road had me hesitate, so I veered to the left down the longer, gradual hill.

I coasted by a small, green space to my right and approached an intersection with lights. I had a green, so I slowly cruised on through the intersection watching for cars that might come from behind me. The road continued to turn slightly right as it leisurely descended through the buildings of downtown Port Arthur, now on my left and right. The hill levelled out as I came to another intersection with a red light. I looked around to see no traffic in any direction, so I took a few kicks, bombed through the red light and on into the empty, small-town streets, slowly-coasting with no idea where I was, or where I was going.

I started to lose my momentum and slow down, so I gave a few good hard kicks to get going as I came up to another set of red lights that turned green just for me. After looking around for traffic and seeing nothing, I kicked some more through the dead quiet ghost town only lit up from the streetlights. A few more kicks and I made it through another green light, then I took a few more kicks and made it through another light that just turned amber as I passed underneath it. Now I was coming up to the waterfront and gaining speed going down the small hill, so I took a look for cars before screeching to a stop, right before the stop sign at the intersection. I picked up my board off the road and walked back to the top to do it again. On this second run, I had wanted to go on the road to the right with the big crack and rip down the steep, short slope, instead of the same run as before. But I forgot to check out the crack on my way back up, so I just did the same run taking long, slow carves all over the road as there was still no traffic out this late at night. Once I got to the bottom, I was starting to get tired and decided not to go for one more as I still had to make my way back to the top to get back to Stacy and Tyler's house for the night.

I made my way all the way back to the top and began to look for my turn to get back to the Dolcetti's house and only found it because of the picture of the street sign I took with Janelle's old iPod. Once I found the left turn, I slowly made my way down the little hill knowing the road disintegrated into rubble at some point, so I got off my board and walked through the dark, unlit construction zone. After I made my way back, I was showing everyone the video I took, and when Tyler saw me coming up to the road where I could have turned right on the short, steep part, he said, "Go that way!" I told him I thought about it but noticed the big crack along the road and paused the video to show him. After showing everyone the little two- or three-minute run downhill, I got ready for bed, and I crashed hard for the night.

The next day we went out to look at Kakabeka Falls just outside Thunder Bay before we pushed back into town. It's the second highest waterfall in the country next to Niagara Falls in southern Ontario. It was a pretty big fall, about one-hundred-and-twenty-feet tall and a hundred feet across. It was definitely something I wouldn't want to fall over or get caught in, that's for sure. The water that poured from the top looked like it was mixed with a dark-brown, liquid syrup, it looked like a waterfall of brown pop. But once it ran over the edge and was aerated, it turned white as it continued to cascade down the edge hitting the wall of rock protruding from behind and underneath the falls.

About a quarter of the way across the falls to the left, a rock face came out enough to separate the water for ten or twenty feet. The big rock emerged from the falls before it dropped and flattened out enough near the bottom to create a small island that was habitable for a few trees and small shrubs. To our right was a big tree that took up the close view I had of the falls. When we were squished over to the right, I saw the dark-black wall of rock come out of the left side of the falls then channel the endless amounts of running water into a river at the bottom. You could tell the rock was as slippery as ice from the years of running water because it glimmered in the daylight, even on the cloudy, overcast day.

At the top of the falls up stream, you could see two bridges crossed over the river that led to the falls. On top of the big wall of rock that came out of the left side of the falls channelling the water downstream stood a thick wall of trees. There was a clearing in the trees on the other side of the falls where it looked like someone had built a cabin of some sort. The small place backed onto the falls and I was incredibly jealous about it. A place like that, even a tiny cabin on that spot would be a dream home for me based on its close proximity to the falls. However, I'm not sure it was even a house, it was likely a small store or information centre.

From the falls we took a right onto the highway and skated for a few minutes before we took a left to ride down another road that would take us to the Port Arthur side of town. On the sides of the highway there was nothing but the same forest that seemed to never end. With two lanes in the oncoming side of the highway and only one on the other, we decided to ride on the shoulder of the outgoing lane, even though the shoulder was hardly a few inches wider than our boards before the small ditch that led into the thick wall of trees.

After skating through the forest for some time, I saw a downhill grade sign on the other side of the highway. It was only a four percent grade, which wasn't much, but I always got excited for some free momentum and began to push to get a bit more speed before the hill began. I came up to my dad, went around him on his right side, and continued to push down the long, gradual hill. The hill descended as it curved to the right into the valley giving me a clear line of sight down the entire hill. Looking at the other side of the valley I could see the massive, dark-green ripples of the tree-covered, rolling hills that came up and down for as far as my vision would let me perceive. I could see some light-green patches of grass in some places but most of the land was dark green from the endless amounts of impenetrable Canadian forest.

As I came down the hill, there was a silver minivan driving up the hill in their right lane, so I moved over to my right lane as I rode down the long, slow hill. When they passed me, the driver, and the passenger both turned their heads, looking at me with a funny look, like a deer in head-lights. I laughed about the funny look they gave me as I got down lower to the road to get going faster. As I came down the long, slow, right bend, I was approaching a bridge. Bridges usually have a decent size gap between the steel plates that connect the road and bridge at both ends. These gaps can be bad for smaller skateboard wheels as I've hit a few of them and went flying into the street once or twice in my days. So, as I came up to it, I cautiously looked to see how big of a gap there was.

It wasn't too big, so I went over it with the full speed of the hill. As I hit the gap with the front and back wheels of my board it made a loud clunking noise and gave me a little jolt forward. After hitting the first gap I was still going at a decent speed, so I had a look for traffic, and I did a one-hundred-and-eighty-degree slide. I stood up now riding backwards, put my arms out, and started to spin in circles on my longboard. I noticed it continued downhill for a little bit, so I took a few big pushes then did another slide and some more spins until I got dizzy. I then got off my board and stood on the side of the oncoming lane and waited for my dad still wobbling and dizzy from all of my excessive spins.

Once my dad got there, we began to walk up the long, slow, gradual hill similar to the one we just rode down. Once we got to the top it levelled out again but there was almost no shoulder for us to ride on. Stuck on a shoulder as wide as our boards, my dad and I pushed down the road on the shoulder of the oncoming lane. After an hour or two, some guy in a truck either wasn't paying attention, or was paying too much attention to us on the side of the road and coasted over the solid white line onto the tiny shoulder we were riding on. We had no time to do anything else but react by jumping off our boards into the ditch. With our hearts now beating in our throats we grabbed our boards from the ditch and got back pushing into town. After our skate that day, I skated down to the marina and went by a small restaurant. Outside, stood big silver teardrop-like figures. I kept pushing and went by a small skate park that had a few kids skating and biking on the ramps and continued on until I got to an embankment with big boulders. There, I got off my board, took a seat on one of the big blue and white rocks just down the embankment, and sat there looking out into the abyss of the massive ocean-like lake. With the overwhelmingly intense vibes of genuine love, compassion, and respect from every single person we met, I continued feeling completely at peace with my mind, body, and soul for the first time of my life. I felt so content, complete, and at peace with everything in my life that it gave me a new profound outlook and understanding on life. To this day, I'm convinced as I sat there and stared out into the distance my mind was opened. Opened to life and its never-ending unlimited potential. Whatever it was, whatever happened there in that moment, it gave me a definitive sense of who I was—a survivor.

I was still alive and able to live life to the fullest, I still had the possibility of having my entire future ahead of me if this AVM in my brain left me alone. I was still here and had access to life's unlimited potential, unlike the millions upon millions of poor souls that never had that second or third chance like I did. I realized not only did everything I go through bring me here to this spectacular moment, but it was also what made me into the person I was becoming. Tragedy after tragedy, battle after battle, fight after fight, these were the events I had to get through and overcome to be the person I was becoming. The further we went along on this remarkable trip, the further my mind was being opened from all the amazing people and phenomenal realizations that came my way. For the first time ever, life was starting to make sense to me.

Off in the distance to my right, I could see grain elevators that filled up the massive, ocean-going vessels when they came in. Directly across the water from me, about seven kilometres offshore rested the sleeping Giant Peninsula. It was there we went to the Thunder Bay lookout with Favourite just a few days before. At the very right end of the Sleeping Giant Peninsula was Silver Islet but the town was so small and hidden I couldn't even tell there was anything there. Off to my right beyond the seawall there was a big "Salty" (huge ocean-going vessel) that was waiting in the bay to pick up or deliver its payload. The big, blueish-white rock that I was sitting on started to hurt my butt, so I got up, got back on my board, and began to skate back over to Stacy and Tyler's for our last night with the phenomenal family.

The next day, we were back on the road heading to Ignace before going through Dryden and finally over to Kenora. It was still nothing but rock and forest the entire way. The peace, quiet, and isolation was incredibly nice. I'm more of the strong, silent type. As much as I enjoy a good jam session with a few guitars and fun people, I also like my isolation, peace, and quiet. This part of the country was nothing but peace and quiet, I absolutely loved it. If it's in nature, even better. I've found every single one of my moments of peace and gratitude have been when I'm surrounded by nature. Not once have I found that soul-touching peace and tranquility in the chaos of a cement jungle or a major over-populated city. So being sequestered in nature in the middle of nowhere was amazing for me. Especially when it was this beautiful. It was my favourite part of the trek thus far. It took a day or two to get to Dryden, then another day or two to get to Vermilion Bay then one long day to get to Kenora. Kenora would be our last stop in the big beautiful O. The five-week, seven-hundred-and-fifty-kilometre detour was coming to an end.

The day we got to Kenora I was hardly able to make it. I could feel I now had a massive blister that formed on my left kicking foot and I couldn't put any weight on it. I went to tell my dad but it was drastically slowing me down and he got way ahead of me. I tried to walk to see if it was better but it was just as bad, if not worse. Push by push, my dad got farther and farther away and I started to lose him when I came around the rock wall corners. It was like when I found a good song that motivated me, I just started to push away then I'd realize a song or two later I had no idea where my dad was. Bit by bit I was getting increasingly frustrated as I wanted to kick faster and harder to catch up to my dad, but the pain I was in physically held me back from doing so. For the last forty-five minutes to hour, I struggled to even touch my foot to the road, let alone skate on the side of the highway. But I had no other option but to continue on.

I came around a right corner that then went left into the forest again. Gratefully, at the bottom of the hill, I could see my dad standing on the side of the road just after the left turn. With him was a white SUV that had its four-way blinkers on. We finally made it to Kenora where some more incredible people put us up via couch surfing. My dad and I got into Kathryn's car, and we drove over to her house where we met her amazing daughter Sam, and her fabulous sister Sue. On the way to her house, we passed a train yard and I looked for graffiti to see it on almost every train car. I even recognized a well-known Calgary writer. Once we got there, I had a nice, much-needed shower and changed out of my gross, sweaty clothes.

While I was in the bathroom, I finally got to see why my foot was so sore. When I took off my sock, I was disgusted. On the palm of my foot was a blister that was bigger than a toonie. That blister then headed up towards my little toe and just under my pinky toe, I had another blister the size of a quarter and the two blisters were connected by a long skinny blister and all of it was bulging off of my foot quite a bit. It was gross but made sense why it was too sore to even walk on. I took a tiny piece of the blister off, drained it as best I could, then sterilized and cleaned it up before getting in the shower.

After my shower we grabbed all our dirty laundry and got to wash the few days' worth of dirty, sweaty, dirt-covered clothes before we sat down and had dinner. After dinner we relaxed and hung out. As we chatted away into the night, Sam was showing us the pictures she took when she went to Burning Man a year or two prior and I got incredibly jealous as I've wanted to go for some time, but I wasn't even old enough to go to America for the event. After a while I was tempted to go ride the hill that was just outside their house, so I grabbed my board and went out the front door. I hardly got to the sidewalk before my foot was hurting so bad, I turned around and went back inside. I told my dad about the two blisters connected with a blister and we decided to tape up my foot so it wasn't rubbing in my shoe and making my problem worse.

The NOT FLAT Prairies

The next morning, we wrapped the end of my foot with gauze then wrapped it with a stupid amount of tape and put on my clean grippy socks from Beau. The combo prevented my blisters from getting worse. The pressure of pushing on them still sucked, although it was much better than not having it taped up at all, that's for sure. July 30th marked another completed part of the trek. We finally got to the Ontario/Manitoba boarder after our massive detour across the incredible, beautiful, peaceful, and stunning O. My dad walked over to the "Welcome to Manitoba" sign as I took off the camera. I put the GoPro on the ground and walked over to my dad as the camera took pictures of us. We raised our boards and arms in excitement before trying some other poses in front of the sign. We raised our arms and did a slow-motion high five for the camera to be sure we got it and after a quick sip of water we continued on. The clouds covered most of the sky that afternoon and it looked like it might rain. We eventually got to a small hill that went down and back up a slight valley in the trees. Fresh out of Ontario and heading into the Prairies it was what I thought would be the last hill we saw for a while. After our skate for the day, we got to a place called West Hawk Lake.

There, we stayed at the local motel for the night. I was excited to see that the road outside the motel was a nice, big hill that went down to the lake, so I got to spend the evening sliding down the hill and bombing it a few dozen times. Each time going faster and sliding farther. After at least a dozen runs I got tired, and my blistered foot was incredibly sore from the skate that day. Walking uphill over and over again wasn't helping so I headed back to the motel room and left my slide marks all over the road. Once I got back, I uploaded the photos we took to Facebook. I posted the high five picture as it turned out to be the best one, as well as the tiny potential last hill we saw on our way to the lake. From West Hawk Lake it was a few days to get to Winnipeg, which would end up being one of the most boring times of my entire life. But the crazy awesomeness of stupendous Canadians would continue to ripple on.

We got about halfway to Winnipeg when the Mercedes-Benz dealership called my dad saying they heard what we were doing and wanted to help. They told my dad to come by and grab a car for the weekend in Winnipeg if we wanted one. My best guess, our new friends from Dominion Motors in Thunder Bay made a call to their friends westbound. Having a form of transportation in a big city was critical for us to get around to gather supplies, and not to mention a huge necessity to organize things for the Winnipeg longboarding fundraiser that weekend. My dad and I couldn't have been more happy and grateful for such a wonderful surprise.

However, heading into Winnipeg was so boring and not scenic at all. We went from one of the most scenic places that I've ever seen in my country to probably the least scenic and most boring scenes I've ever seen anywhere. The road went on for as far as you could see. On both sides of the road was grass, wheat, dirt or whatever the farmers were able to grow and harvest on their land. Lots of the endless land was green, other parts were brown with dirt, and sometimes endless fields of yellow. With the straight road going slightly uphill for as far as your eyes could see, it was incredibly off-putting. We saw the kind of rolling hills like the ones in Ontario, only they were short, tiny, ever so gradual, and this wasn't beautiful. To me it was uninteresting, vast, boring, emptiness. Looking at the road was incredibly daunting because we knew we had to push that road for hours, days, and weeks to come. The endless open land meant there was no hiding from the rain, no shelter to go take a break, but worst of all, absolutely no hiding from the horrendous head winds that whipped across the sloped land straight in our faces, making it a struggle to go a few kilometres without taking a rest.

We spent two or three days pushing on this road that crossed the slightly-sloped land for as far as you could possibly see. Just looking at it all day knowing you have to push all the way down that endless road was intimidating enough, it made me want to quit. Thankfully, I still had music to get me through these horrible, lame, hard, and annoying days. My music was probably the only reason I made it through, although I began cursing and chirping at the wind more than ever before.

Once we got closer to Winnipeg, we took a right onto another road so we could cut up to the other highway that went into town. We skated down this long empty road for a while before we came across a house on our left that had some people outside working on it. They waved at us as we rode by, and we waved back continuing down the road. After a while the sun was lost to thick dark clouds, and it started to pour a waterfall on us. Right when the downpour started, we were going to make our left turn onto the highway that would take us into Winnipeg. Luckily, there was a small store on the corner of the two roads and we ran inside to hide out the storm for a bit. The hard rain then turned into light hail, then the hail quickly got bigger and bigger. You could hear it ferociously striking the roof of the building. It sounded like there was an entire construction crew redoing the roof pounding away with their tools. The store worker and another customer were looking outside as they were talking about the crazy storm that came out of nowhere. After a while, the hail lightened and turned back into rain and looked like it was about to stop. Then as the wind began to pick up and howl like crazy it suddenly started to rain horizontally. We thought it would be best if we got a ride into town and caught up on our few kilometres the next day. So, after an hour with it still raining, we started to ask people if they were heading into Winnipeg. Only everyone we asked was just leaving Winnipeg. So, we sat on the front porch of the store where they had some benches on the deck covered by an overhang and we continued to ask people for a short ride into town.

My dad went inside to talk to the lady working when I saw a man pull up in an older blue and white pickup truck. I asked him if he was heading into Winnipeg, and he said he wasn't, but unlike everybody else he then asked me, "Why?" and "What are you guys doing?" I began to tell this stranger what we were doing and he said that we rode past his house while his family was working outside. He was the guy on the roof that waved hello to us just down the road. After I told the kind man our mission, he decided to take time out of his busy day to help us out and give us a ride into town. But first he asked if we would go to his house and say hello to his family which we happily did. After we said hello to the man's kind wife and kids we got back in his truck and headed into Winnipeg. We turned left off his property, drove down the road for a bit before we turned left at the little store where we met him, and headed into town.

We got dropped off at the Tim Hortons just on the outskirts of town and thankfully it had finally stopped raining. From there, we skated through the soaking-wet roads to go spend the night at Darryl's place. But first we rode past a Subway and, with tummies rumbling, we decided to go grab a bite. After hearing what we were up to, the considerate young woman working happily donated us a couple of subs to keep us going. After our much-needed meal, we went outside and my dad took a picture of the young woman, me, and the Subway sign in the background before we got back on the road to Darryl's. Darryl started the "How We Roll" longboarding community in Winnipeg and organized an event for us as we came through town to show his appreciation.

The timing of our arrival would be really ironic as when we got to Winnipeg going west, we crossed paths with a fellow named James who was also longboarding across Canada that year in honor of his late grandfather, only he was going west to east. The longboarding community put us in touch with each other and he also came over to Darryl's place that night and we got to meet the man. James was a tall guy with a big beard and even bigger back pack that I could hardly lift. How he was able to longboard with it on at all was impressive, let alone going all the way across Canada with the weight of a human on his back. The kind man was a beast with his strength; it blew me away.

We did a bunch of chatting that night as Rayne Longboards sent my father and I brand-new longboarding decks. My first Landyatchz was toast and my custom Sayshun was rapidly falling apart on me. As my dad and I opened up the boxes with our fresh boards, we sat around chatting about the trip, life, our mission, and Darryl's involvement within the longboarding community.

The next morning, we went over to the local skate shops in town with our new decks to see if they could complete the new set-ups to help us complete the second half of our trek. We went to one shop who gripped our boards with grip tape, and I put their obnoxiously huge green sticker on the front of my helmet before we went to "Boarders Anonymous" there they hooked us up big time. I got new wheels, trucks, and bearings and my dad got new ones as well. On top of the hundreds of dollars in gear they donated to us, Darryl was given a new complete longboard to thank him for all his hard work within the longboarding community. Back at Darryl's, we set up our boards and I put the Boarders Anonymous sticker on the only available spot left, which was on the very top of my helmet and added it to the growing collection of stickers given to me by all the skate shops that helped us out along the way. After putting our new boards together, we had some kilometres to catch up on, so we all skated out to "The Mint" just outside Winnipeg where they produce the Canadian coins in circulation and manage Canada's coin supply. When we got there, we each took our turns doing media interviews. As we skated around the empty parking lot, I accidently ran into James as we were both messing around on our boards and dented my new deck. We tried to get a tour of The Mint, but we were of course denied from even entering the secure building. On our way back into the city, we were all skating in the outbound lane and we passed a big, brown sign with white writing that said "This is the geological centre of Canada" with its GPS coordinates. I laughed at the irony of literally running into another man also longboarding across Canada, in the very centre of the country.

Once we got back into the city, we went to the Mercedes-Benz dealership to pick up our sweet ride for the weekend. My dad and I walked into the dealership, told them who we were, and they grabbed the set of keys to a black Mercedes-Bens GLK350 and gave them to my dad. From there we went to the market to meet a couple of locals that had made me a beautiful one-of-a-kind board. We gathered at the marketplace with Ryan who painted the deck and Colton who made the deck.

The board was a beautiful blue colour and it had the outline of Canada that showed the natural colour and design of the wood it was made from. Also, in the wood grain design, it had "St. Johns, Halifax, Ottawa, Winnipeg, Calgary, and Vancouver" listed down the right side with the Long for Life logo beside the outline of Canada before there was a darker blue circle that had a neat double triangle design inside of it. The shape of the deck itself was unique as it got wider by a few inches for your feet and it also had a nice slight concave to it. It was a thing of pure beauty to me, and from the second I saw it I wanted to get it grip-taped and ride it, but I couldn't bring myself to destroy such a collectible, beautiful piece of art. After we hung out and chatted with Ryan and Colton for a bit, we got back over to Darryl's for another night.

The next day, we packed up the Mercedes and got ready for the longboarding event. We all met at a local school, there we waited for the media to arrive, and once they did, they wanted to get footage of me riding around. I jumped on my board and started to skate the giant concrete pad that was in the back of the school for the basketball court. Only problem was the playground was right beside it. The concrete basketball court was covered in tiny rocks and it was very difficult to do even the most basic longboarding things. Just pushing around without having a wheel jam and going flying was an accomplishment of its own. One of the riders even came up to me and said, "Sorry, it's not really a good place to skate for your interview." I told him, "Don't worry buddy, it's all good." Looking back, I probably should have just walked to the front of the school and rode on the nice, smooth street for the interview instead.

After our interviews we all went to the front of the school and gathered together in a group on the street, then took off. With over a dozen of us, we took over the street kicking down the road doing tricks and dancing on our boards for fun. We rode on the road for a few twists and turns until the road paralleled a paved pathway going into the trees. We all cut over the little patch of grass that separated the street and the paved pathway—Darryl went up the curb, leading the way with me following right behind.

The pathway twisted left and right through the trees for a bit which reminded me of Fish Creek Park back home in Calgary. After a short time, the trees vanished, and we came to a small field that had the occasional tree and bush here and there, with a few benches to stop and rest at. We continued on the path through the little park then it began to parallel the road on our left before it took a long, slow right turn that broke off from the road and paralleled the river that cut through town. The path then took a slight left and started to get farther away from the river embankment on my right and looked like it was going back into the community. On the right between the pathway and the river you could see some well-used bike trails that broke off from the path back towards the river. There was a guy and two of his kids just off the paved path on the bike trails. One of the kids asked Darryl what we were doing as he rode by, and he replied with, "Riding for cancer, buddy." The kid then said, "Wow, cool," as he watched the pack of riders continue to keep coming around the corner. Darryl thanked the young boy as we continued on our cruise through the trees after taking a right turn.

The pathway paralleled the road for about a hundred feet before it turned back right into the trees. Darryl then warned the two old people we passed that there's a big group of skaters coming behind us. That's when the pathway turned into the road, and we started to skate down the street again. Up ahead, you could see the pathway continued on the other side of the road, so we pushed down and across the street going back onto the pathway at the next corner where we could ride back onto it at the crosswalk.

The path turned into another small field with some benches and about a half-dozen trees scattered around before it then turned again going down the roadway that led into the parking lot of the small park. We cut back over onto the path again and as Darryl went up the curb and cut over the two or three feet of grass on the right side of the road, he made a "woop" noise. I carved hard to the right and headed for the curb. I had just enough momentum to make it up the curb, over the grass, and onto the pathway. After skating down the path, we entered the parking lot. We rode by a few outhouses on our right that stood on the edges of the parking lot which was under construction and continued back on the path. We could either take the pathway or take the road, but we had lots of people behind us, so we decided to pop a squat and hang out in the grass to wait for everyone else to catch up so we didn't get separated.

We hung around chatting, cracking jokes, laughing, and listening to the music Darryl had on his portable speaker while we waited for the six or seven stragglers that were behind us. Once everyone was there, we continued on the pathway to the "fun little hill" one of the riders mentioned. First, the path went slightly downhill for a few metres then came back up and turned to the left, shortly before it went back downhill. After it turned right, the pathway straightened out for a little bit before it zigzagged left and right a few times through the small forest of trees. After a few more turns in the bushes, it went flat and straight for about fifty metres before taking a long, slow left followed by a sharp right around a group of trees.

There was a wall of trees on our right and a small seating area to our left where there was a family that had a massive barbeque, bigger than their car under one of the two tents. Under the second tent, was the family sitting around in a group hanging out having a meal and enjoying the day. I looked up and the pathway took a right corner and we passed another family birthday or event of some sort before we got back onto the roadway that had car after car after car parked along the right side of the road from the family gatherings. Then we made a right turn to head over to the "duck pond."

We took a turn onto a brick pathway that rumbled our wheels every few inches. Down the rumbly path we came up to a seating area with a big roof over the group of benches where a bunch of people sat eating their lunch. It was our destination to stop. Darryl informed everybody about the tent on the other side set up by the Twelve-Tribe's community that served us all free, delicious hot and cold tea. I probably had half a dozen cups of the amazing cold tea. As I was riding with the group, my dad took off in the Mercedes-Benz to Subway where they hooked us up with a box of free subs and a box of drinks for everyone at the end of the charity ride. As the people under the hut left, we slowly began to sit down and eventually took over the whole seating area as we waited for my father to return.

Meanwhile, Mother Nature had once again turned on us, the scattered clouds turned into one big, ugly storm cloud, then the temperature dropped about ten degrees, and it started to storm down on us. We had arrived just in the nick of time as the heavy raindrops pelted the roof of the hut we sat under. The wind came howling through the hut as it was just a roof that had one wall for the bathrooms. However, the wind wasn't coming from the direction that had the bathroom wall, it was coming from the other way, and tore through the little hut we tried to take refuge under.

With my dad back from Subway handing out subs and napkins, they flew everywhere when the wind viciously tore through the area. The sub wrappers and napkins were picked up and thrown across the hut and everyone scrambled to clean up the current mess, as well as the mess left behind by the other people that were there before us and took off without cleaning up. As we cleaned up the messes, the rain continued to pound the roof of the hut and the ground. Once the rain finally stopped, we all gathered on the big concrete pad outside the hut and my dad took a picture of all the riders and myself with my new custom-made deck in my hands.

After the cruise my dad, James, Darryl, and I got into the Mercedes and started to drive over to the restaurant the Twelve Tribes guys and gals had in town. On the way there, I looked to my right out the front passenger-side window of the car as we sat at a red light and this lady looked at me and then suddenly busted out laughing for some reason. Wondering if I was really that fugly-looking, I realized that all four of us were still wearing our helmets in the car. Just four guys driving around in a brand-new safe Mercedes GLK 350 all wearing helmets like my dad's never driven a car before. I pointed it out to my dad and the boys, and we all had a good laugh at how funny we must have looked.

Once we got to the restaurant (still wearing our helmets for the laughs of the general public) we took them off and put them all on the coat hanger just outside our booth and took a picture of them all. After a delicious healthy meal, they asked if we wanted to go on a tour of the place. I thought it was a small restaurant and there wouldn't be much to see but we decided to take a tour anyway. The kind man took us around back and down a hall then he opened a door that led to a fully equipped and operational, metal workshop. We took a walk around and checked it out before we went back inside the building and he took us down the hall and opened another door that led to a complete operational woodworking shop. I was baffled, from the outside it just looked like a small restaurant. Then to top off the tour we went upstairs to the second floor. Up there was industrial-sized equipment for packaging the delicious in-house tea that they made. It was a very impressive set up. I never would have guessed they had two full workshops, an industrial tea-packaging system, and a restaurant all in the small building, it was very impressive and reminded me how deceiving looks can be. After our tour we went back over to Darryl's for one more night there with the rad young men.

The next day, we were on the road heading west and I continued to realize I was lied to my entire life by everyone that ever told me "the Prairies are flat." They look pretty flat and there's lots of flat, sure, but going east to west from Winnipeg to Calgary is literally all slightly up hill. There is over an eight-hundred-metre elevation difference between the two cities, and to make things even better it was also against the gnarly trade winds. I remember James saying he was pushing one-hundred and forty kilometres a day across the Prairies with ease, but he was going with wind, downhill. So we would push once and go maybe four or five feet instead of the usual fifty, it took us twice as long to cover half of the distance and I was incredibly frustrated, hollering, and cursing at Mother Nature as we rode. This is where I tried to unleash all the bottled-up anger I had for my old probation officer, the useless court system, and useless governments. Day after day, I pounded the ground thinking of the shitty uselessness they all provide and, day by day, I slowly shed the overwhelming disgust and anger I had like a snake sheds its skin.

For the next few nights leaving Winnipeg, we stayed with Ryan and his wife. I got to see where the magic of the beautiful board he painted for me happened in his personal studio. There, we also used some sort of sealant to coat every inch of the edges of the wood on our boards to protect it from getting wet and waterlogged like my first board that you could now see through sideways. We also cut a few inches off the back ends of our board because when we walked dragging the board by the front end, the back was scraping the ground, so we cut off a few inches and sealed the ends as well. I cringed at the sight of the jig saw going through the fresh new boards, it just didn't seem right even though it needed to be done. Ryan poured me this amazing drink that had diced watermelon, ginger ale and vodka in it before he told me his recipe for its summer day deliciousness. He lived on the back of a big greenspace with paved pathways, so I went for a little ride to check it out. But there was nothing worth checking out, it was just a big, flat field with houses all around it and the flat paved path wasn't very exhilarating so after I got to the end of the field I just turned back.

The way out of Winnipeg was just like the way into Winnipeg; incredibly boring and probably the least exciting part of my entire existence. With no rock walls, water, rock, or groups of trees, it was just vast empty land that had the tiniest of hills. We would walk up the slanted ground and with the head wind being so strong we would have to kick down the other side of the slope. I thought getting lower to the ground would help so at the next tiny downhill slope I kicked as hard as I could, then I lay down on my board and started to street luge it down the hill but I was still just slowing down. I started to cuss and curse at the wind now using my hands to paddle myself down the hill. I was again the product of a trucker and sailor who had a baby; my late papa and great-grandmother along with my grandmother's and mother and father would have been ashamed of my mouth. I knew Tony was there cussing with me while having a laugh at my five-year-old tantrums. Luckily, everyone still with me in physical form was too far away to hear any of it.

With no twists, turns, or sights to see, it was like a dog turd covered in glitter; pretty shit. It was like going from one extreme of incredibly full and beautiful land to another extreme of the barest, most boring land you ever saw. It was about as much fun and excitement as coming home from the Dominican Republic (or any tropic place) to a minus fifty-degree Celsius Canadian winter. But seeing how much open and empty land we had was absolutely mind boggling. The best part about the Prairies was definitely passing a cow or a herd of them. I noticed as you rolled by a cow, one by one they would look at you, and as you're riding by, all their heads would turn collectively as one staring at you with a half-turned head wondering what this thing floating by on the road was. The entire herd of cows would all move at the same slow pace while looking at you like you're the most alienated thing they ever saw. They looked very confused, and they wouldn't take their eyes off of you until you were gone, it was quite comical. The next funny part was realizing that cows, fucking "moo" cows were the greatest part of the bare landscape in the Prairies. Not bears, mountain lions, coyotes, cougars, wolves, foxes, or a beautiful landscape, but big I'm-just-going-to-stand-here-and-eat-grass-all-day-while-I-moo COWS. If that doesn't tell you how boring the NOT FLAT Prairies were, then I don't know what will.

As my dad and I were pushing down the Trans-Canada leaving town, I noticed this small, black Scion sports car rip by us and the occupants (particularly the passenger) gave me a serious look. I thought nothing of it at first and figured they were just checking us out, wondering what we were doing. So, I continued down the road listening to my music and pushing away.

Once we got to our hotel for the night, I checked my Facebook quickly to see I had a message from an old co-worker of mine. He said he saw me longboarding down the highway outside Winnipeg (he was the one in the black Scion going to visit family and friends). He also told me that he was impressed that I was actually longboarding across Canada. When I was working with him, writing **a book** and longboarding across the country was just all talk and ridiculously absurd things that I would never do. At that time, I was very busy going to court, probation, and in and out of jail. God only knows how many times he had to cover me as I dealt with my legal issues, so I could definitely see where people had their doubts. I told him how stoked I was to finally be on the road and how much epic fun it's been, and couldn't wait till I was back home.

Over the next day or two we pushed our way to Brandon, Manitoba. Right before we got there, I took a big push into the wind and next thing I know it got a little breezy in my private square. I looked down to see a huge tear in my jeans from my groin area down to my right knee. I then had to push the rest of the way into town with a huge hole in my pants. Luckily it wasn't very long until we got to the Super 8 Motel that was on the left side of the highway and nobody was exposed to my junk.

Super chapped that I ripped my jeans and had to skate in them I grabbed a donation request letter from my dad, took a second to remember the way to the local mall, got on my board, went outside and took a left onto the road and kicked down it until my left turn. I made my left turn and was coming down into a small valley where I was half-tempted to get off the sidewalk and bomb the hill down the middle of the street but there was lots of traffic at the bottom of the hill at an intersection, so I stayed on the sidewalk hitting the cracks every three feet, vibrating my whole body. As I gained speed, the vibrations increased to the point when I let out an "a-h-h-h-h-h" as I rode down the hill. It sounded like I was hitting my throat. After I did it, I had a mild laugh at the funny sounds that came out of my mouth as I rode down the hill with the hole in my pants flapping around in the wind. I was actually surprised that this was the first time I tore a pair of jeans on the trip as I used to tear a pair or two a week every summer when I was longboarding around.

As I came down the hill, I looked to my left to see a little shopping area and thought I should stop at the Walmart on the way back and get a cheap pair of sunglasses to keep the sun, dust, and dirt out of my eyes when traffic past us on the road. The big semi-trucks kicked up quite the amount of dust and blinded us as our eyes watered like crazy trying to flush out the contaminates. Being on the side of a road with speeding cars and trucks was not an adequate time to be even more blind than I am, so I told myself to run in there on my way back.

When the big semi-trucks past us on the highway, the gusts of wind they created as they drove by would actually give you a nice push if they were travelling in the same direction. However, if you were not paying attention that same gust of wind would catch you off guard, and either scare you from the random push or cause you to lose your balance and wobble all over the shoulder on the road. I did notice the big trucks that had the angled flat pieces under their trailers wouldn't give you that little boost, as they were too aerodynamic. Sometimes there would be a line of semi-trucks passing us and if they didn't have the angled flat things under their load, every truck was a boost, and it was nice when we got boost after boost just from the passing trucks. It's like when you follow one really closely while you're driving and you get your car in the wind tunnel the truck generates, it will just pull your car along and you hardly have to use the gas. Only it's incredibly dangerous to do so, so I wouldn't recommend it. The only downside to having trucks pass us so close was the cattle trucks. Sometimes a truck with a full load of cattle would come flying by us. With some of the animals backed right up against the sides when they pooped, it would come right out of the holes in the trailer and onto the road. I didn't even know they pooped out the holes like that till a truck came flying by me and some freshly produced poop came flying out of a butthole and nearly hit me. Luckily, I was a foot or two to the right and missed it. But when it hit the road and exploded everywhere in front of me, I nearly crashed into the ditch trying to swerve around it.

The trucks had their pros and cons like anything in life, and when we were riding in the oncoming lanes, we would be battling the outrageous headwinds and then when a semi passed us, it would give us that same push but only the wrong way. It was like running into a wall of wind for a second and you lost lots of momentum. That wind also kicked up dirt and dust and threw it in your face. After a while when I saw a truck coming in the oncoming lane, I would crouch down low to try and bust through that short burst of headwind, and it worked decently well. You still felt the wall of wind but it wasn't as forceful when you're a little ball, so on top of pushing, I was now doing squats on my board with every passing big rig.

Once I got to the bottom of the hill in the shopping area, I got off my board and began to walk up the other side on the sidewalk. With all my clothes disgustingly dirty, I was still in my crotch-less jeans walking up the hill heading to the mall. I got to the top of the hill, crossed right at the lights to the other side of the street using my board to try and cover the huge hole in my pants as it was rather embarrassing. However, it was something I was also used to as every summer I tore out the crotch of four or five pairs of jeans a month, and if I was on the other side of the city, I'd have to take the bus and train home with my boxers hanging out of my pants.

Once I got to the right side of the street, I got back on my board and pushed up to the mall that was coming up on my right. I turned off the sidewalk, rode through the parking lot to one of the doors, and entered the mall. I began to aimlessly walk around looking for the West 49 with the hole from my groin to my right knee. After ten minutes or so, I came walking around a left corner in the mall and spotted the store on the right side and walked over.

I walked into the store where the nice lady said, "Hello," and greeted me with a big friendly smile. I said, "Hello," back and started to tell her my story about trekking across Canada and my issue with the lack of fashionable and functional pants. I asked the lady if there was any way they could help me out with a pair of pants. She wasn't entirely sure, so she called the owner of the store and started to talk to him as I walked around the store stopping at the shoe selection to see what they had for Vans. After checking out the shoes quickly I walked back over to the counter where the lady was working and I saw her check me out top to bottom once or twice and I was thinking to myself, 'Did she really just blatantly check me out like that?' As I got to the counter she says to the man over the phone, "Yeah, he looks like a professional." I had my slide gloves, helmet, and GoPro on, the only unprofessional thing about me was the huge hole from my crotch to my knee.

She then asked if I could speak with him and answer some questions, which I was more than happy to do so. I grabbed the phone and started speaking to this man who was asking me all sorts of questions just trying to verify I'm not some random guy coming in trying to con myself some free jeans. I told him all about my battle with cancer as a child, having strokes in my teens, and the longboarding trek across Canada. He then said, "Well, we don't usually just give things away to anyone that walks into the store. There's a process to donating goods," he told me.

Feeling like an idiot, I suddenly remembered about the donation request letter in my bag and told him about it. He said that was exactly what he needed. I told the man I would leave it with the lady at the counter as I pulled it out for us to fill out. I thanked the man over the phone for his support and gave the woman the phone back. After a few more words she hung up the phone and told me to go grab whatever jeans I would like. I went over to the jeans section on the far wall of the store across from the till and started to look for my size.

Once I found a pair in my size and tried them on to be sure they fit, I popped the tags off of them, walked over to the lady at the counter, and gave her the tags with my old jeans. She put the tags with the request letter, and she threw out my old breezy, crotch-exposing jeans for me. I then asked if she would be okay if we took a picture outside of the store for Facebook, which she was happy to do. She ran to the back of the store and grabbed one of the guys in the back to take the picture for us. We went out front of the store and got a picture of me, the West 49 crew, and the West 49 sign before I thanked them all very much and I started to walk around the mall looking for some cheap sunglasses. I couldn't find any there but I found the door I came into the mall and left wearing my new jeans. I jumped on my board, gave a few pushes to get out of the parking lot and onto the sidewalk then pushed down the sidewalk for a bit until I got to the lights on the corner of the property and crossed over to the right side of the street. I got on the sidewalk and gave a few light kicks to get me going down the hill hoping these jeans wouldn't rip on me in a day of riding or before I got back to the Super 8.

I got to the bottom of the hill and remembered I needed to go to Walmart to get some glasses, so I made a right into the shopping area and pushed over to Walmart. I got off my board, walked inside and found the sunglasses selection. I've always hated how I look in glasses in general, so I tried on a dozen pairs before I just said whatever and grabbed the cheap four-dollar NASCAR ones. I paid for them and left before I skated straight to the end of the parking lot, got off my board, and turned right heading up the hill. I got to the top of the hill and made a right onto the road and headed back to the Super 8 for the night.

Once I got there, I changed into my swim shorts and went for my first swim of the trip. I had every opportunity to go into countless lakes or swim in Lake Superior for the five weeks we were there, but the water in the lake was so cold I couldn't bring myself to go in past my knees, let alone swim in it. I wanted to see how well the GoPro worked underwater so I brought it with me to the pool hoping nobody was there thinking I'm a pervert with a camera at the swimming pool. Taking pictures every few seconds I tossed the camera from one end of the pool to the other and swam back and forth diving down to get it at the bottom. The place was completely empty, so I had the pool and hot tub to myself. After swimming for an hour or so I sat in the hot tub for a while when another man and his wife came in to relax in the hot tub as well. The couple who was also from Calgary, started to chat with me. He and his wife asked me where I was from, what I was doing, and where I was headed so I told them what my dad and I were up to, and it blew their minds. Once I got back to the hotel room, I had a nice cold shower to cool down and wash the chlorine off of me then just relaxed chatting with friends online before I headed to bed.

The next morning the instant I woke up, I was absolutely disgusted. Wanting to puke all over the room I started to roll and make noises as I was waking up. I got some clean clothes and jumped in the shower hoping I would feel a bit better afterwards, but I didn't. I slowly got myself ready for another day on the road wishing I could turn my brain off, and we left.

From Brandon we were heading west to Regina. It was the same boring, dry, long, empty, slightly up hill, against wind push we had been skating for a few weeks now. We skated west to the Virden area, where we were picked up by friends of Kathryn's (from Kenora) and taken to their place just south in Reston, Manitoba. We had a delicious meal with Lori and Fred then we got to take a tour of their farm and land in the area before we chatted into the evening and went to bed.

The next morning, we did an interview for the local paper called the Reston Recorder, took a picture with the amazing family that put us up, and got dropped back on the road continuing to head west. We were about halfway to Regina when my dad got a call from the Regina Mercedes dealership saying they loved what we were doing and asked if we would like to grab a car for the weekend while we regrouped and reorganized in town. Again, we got an offer we couldn't pass up, and the tsunami of generosity continued on.

After hours of pushing, we got to a rest stop and on the right side of the road there stood the big green Saskatchewan sign where we stopped to take a break. The top of the sign was wide and flat so I thought it would be funny to take a picture of me longboarding on the sign. I took off the GoPro, put it on the ground taking pictures every few seconds, and walked over to the sign. Then I realized it was too high for my abilities to jump up it. So, I leaned my longboard against it and I used the trucks on my board like steps to get to the top. I then pulled my board up, put it down, and stood on it for a second before I got down into hill-bombing tuck position. I thought it would be funny as everyone thinks Saskatchewan is flat, so for the irony of it I got into hill-bombing position.

From the boarder, we pushed on down to Moosomin, then from there it was over to Whitewood. All this time still going uphill against the wind. Now more than ever, I really wanted to punch every person that ever told me the Prairies were flat as we were going uphill for a good three or four weeks now. From Whitewood it was off to Indianhead, and after another long day in the wind uphill, we crashed as soon as we got to our motel.

The next day it was the same routine. We got up, packed our bags, filled our waters, and left for the highway. I got on the highway super excited for some reason and I ran about five steps then jumped on my board and I gave three huge kicks as hard as I could. However, I had made one drastic mistake and by the time I kicked the road for the third time, I pulled my hamstring. I forgot the number one rule in Zombieland; limber up. I didn't stretch that morning, and pulling a muscle at the start of the day really makes the rest of that day pushing not so pleasurable. Every time I kicked the road, I felt the pulled muscle aching with a sharp, knife-like pain. It made the few thousand pushes into Regina incredibly terrible, and it seemed like it took four times longer than it should have. When we saw the Regina sign on the right side of the highway, I went over to it for my dad to take a quick picture of me and the sign before we got back on the move into the city.

Once we got closer to the city, I saw the road was covered in what I thought were rocks, but as I got closer and closer, I saw that these rocks were moving around. I continued on ,and once I got to what I thought were rocks were most definitely not—they were grasshoppers. Millions upon millions of them took over the highway. There were so many of them, it was like a blanket that covered the entire road. With so many of them it was impossible to not hit them. Every time

I kicked the road, I could hear them crunch under my kicking foot. As we rode on, we could hear them crunching under our wheels. It literally sounded like we were skating over dry crackers, and if we got kicking fast enough, like riding in water, the four wheels of our longboards began to spray grasshopper guts and limbs off them and into the air, it was absolutely disgusting. This continued on for a good half kilometre or so. At one point, I turned back and could see the wet tracks my wheels made from the grasshopper guts. Trying to avoid them would be like trying not to step on blades of grass as you walked across your local school's soccer field, it just wasn't going to happen.

After we got to Regina, we entered this mall area, and across the street was a skate shop that we went to check out and to say hello. We open the doors, and it led down a set of stairs. We went down the stairs like were heading into a dungeon then took a left at the bottom and walked down this little hallway that led into the shop. The shop itself wasn't very big, but I was impressed by the time we left. They had the usual skateboards, accessories, shoes, even a small selection of glass. The guy working started to tell us how they teach kids to skateboard there. I thought he meant in the tiny shop and made a joke about it. Then the guy took us down the hall we had entered through and opened up a big sliding door. The door led into a massive underground warehouse that had been converted into an underground skatepark. They had a huge half pipe, some quarter pipes, ramps, and rails everywhere. It was quite the skatepark and it was all underground, available year-round. It reminded me of the old Source indoor skatepark they had in Calgary years before. I was pretty impressed with the set up to the point I wanted to get on a skateboard and go skate, but I hadn't touched an actual skateboard in years, so I never did.

In junior high, I ended up in the hospital urinating blood with internal bleeding from a mountain biking accident, which was when I quit mountain biking and started longboarding. The last time I rode an actual skateboard was before I got into mountain biking, so I figured I better not attempt to get back on one and end up in the hospital, again. Instead, I took a quick walk through and looked around. After our chat we got back on our boards and headed over to the Mercedes dealership where we got another sweet ride for the weekend.

When we were at the dealership, I was talking to my dad about how we need to go to a car wash to clean the bug guts off of our boards and wheels. The guys and gals at Mercedes told us we could go around to the side of the dealership and use their pressure washers in the wash bay. As my father and I waited for them to bring the car out front we walked around the building to use the pressure washer. When I was spraying one of my wheels with the pressure washer, I got my wheel spinning incredibly fast and because of all my sliding, my wheel was slightly cone shaped. So, when my wheel got spinning really fast it shook the board like an uncontrollable jackhammer, even if I put all my weight on the board, it would still vibrate to the point my dad and the worker could feel it shaking the concrete pad beneath their feet. We laughed and I had some fun spraying my wheels and shaking the building for a minute or two.

It wasn't till after we left that I realized we were lucky the wheel didn't just explode. I've heard and seen longboard wheels exploding when they're mis-shaped or lose the outer layer of polyurethane that kept it all together. If you got through that outer layer or coned your wheels from sliding and got going really fast, the wheel would sometimes explode into hundreds if not thousands of tiny pieces of rubber scattering everywhere, as you went flying headfirst onto the road you were on, it's a pretty terrible experience to have. However, at the time, I forgot exploding longboard wheels were a thing, and it was just too much fun doing it because, you know, cow watching had been my greatest form of physical entertainment for the last month, so, by comparison, it was kind of fun. They pulled the car around for us and my dad said something about being careful putting our boards into it. The worker just laughed, popped the back of the SUV, and threw our nice clean boards in the back for us before closing it up and handing my dad the keys.

The next day we drove over to another skate shop in town to say hello. We parked the car and went inside to have a chat. This shop wasn't anything like the underground one we saw, but it was a nice big shop that was nuzzled in a shopping plaza area across from a Tim's. There, we sat around and talked to the workers as we waited for a lady to come do an interview with us. I saw these sweet sunglasses they had on the counter, and I tried them on, actually liking the way they looked on me. I told the guy I liked them, and he told me the price tag. There was no way I was going to be paying that crazy amount, so I put them down and continued to walk around the store.

He must have saw my heartbreak when he told me the price tag. Because he then told me there was a small defect to them and they were going to get tossed in the garbage, so he told me I could just have them if I wanted them. After we chatted and waited around for an hour or two, we went outside and met the lady who was there to interview us and take our picture for the article. We went out in the parking lot and had a chat before she took pictures of us riding around trying to get a good shot of the both of us, but it wasn't going well. So, we got off our boards and kneeled down on the ground side by side with our boards and she took the so called "money shot" for the article she put together.

As we waited in the skate shop, my father and I met a rad local guy named Brandon. He told us about the Regina beach festival that was going on that weekend and told us we should come if we could make it. Brandon was a good guitar player who was going up there to hang out and jam. My dad got the location from him and the next afternoon we drove over to spend it at the festival.

There was a big outdoor market area where my dad set up a table with some t-shirts, the map of Canada showing how far we've gone, and hung out there telling people what we were up to. Brandon stood jamming away on his guitar and DJ-ing at the turn tables to our right under a white tent that protected the equipment and him from the outdoor elements. After a while, I got bored and took a quick walk through the market to look at what was there before I remembered there was a nice hill that we parked on. After I got the keys from my dad, I got my board from the car and walked to the top of the hill. I turned around, gave a few kicks, and started to rip down the hill. It was very busy because of the festival, and I had to be very careful and turn the board sideways to slow down a few times every run. At the very bottom of the hill was a nice sandy beach at the boat launch area. As I ran out of road, I turned sideways and slid to a stop just before I ran into the water. My dad wanted to stretch his legs, so he got in the car and picked me up from the bottom and drove me to the top for the first few runs.

The hill was big enough and steep enough I could do four or five huge, long slides as I went down. One of the times I went down, I had to dodge a car as it came up the hill and I swerved to the right just making it around it, then cut hard left around a family crossing the street. I decided I should slow it down a bit, so I did a big slide and almost slid into the back end of the Mercedes my dad now had parked on the side of the hill. Luckily, I was able to kick my left foot out just enough that I avoided sliding into the rear end of the SUV. Once I got back to the bottom, I walked back to the top to do it again. Traffic was clearing out as the day was starting to wind down, so I asked my dad if he could move the car off the main street and onto a side one that was just beside us. I then walked back to the top of the hill and bombed it again.

When I did my first slide, I slid to a stop at the end of a camper-trailer parked on the right side of the street. Just as I screeched to a halt, some guy popped his head out the side window and asked me what I was doing. I told him I was just having some fun ripping down the hill. He then invited me to come in and have a beer with him and his buddy. I walked around the small RV and the kind man opened the door for me as he gave me a fresh ice-cold beer. He and his buddy cracked one open as I opened mine and we sat around drinking our beers talking when one of them asked me, "How'd you walk up the hill five times so fast?" I told him, "My dad was picking me up at the bottom and driving me to the top the first few runs." I then told them my cancer and stroke stories and all about what my father and I were doing that summer. One of the gentlemen had a soft spot for what we were doing and began to tell me about his wife's cancer diagnosis that tragically took her life only a few years prior. As a few tears trickled down his face he told me the heart-breaking story of his wife having an inoperable brain tumor that wouldn't stop growing. Everything the doctors did was not helping her, and two months after the diagnosis the pain got too much for her, so she ended her life on her own terms. It was a heartbreaking story and as he described how fast it all happened, from the diagnosis to finding her lifeless body in eight short weeks, I myself almost broke down in tears as I listened. The three of us sat around chatting and finished our beers. As I was getting ready to go slide down the hill again one of the guys reached into his pocket, pulled out five bucks, and gave it to me. I thanked them for the beer and the five bucks before they wished us luck on our journey, and I went back to ripping down the hill like a maniac for a bit.

Once I got tired, I walked back up the hill and over to the table my dad was at in the market area where he stood talking to a young lady about what we were doing. I walked over and gave him the five bucks from the man in the RV and he introduced me to the young girl who was probably already drunk and asked if I wanted something to drink. I said, "Sure." She then told me to open my mouth, and I foolishly did. She started to pour vodka mixed with Red Bull out of her water bottle into my mouth and I had a few good chugs of it, before she did it again. Perhaps for a third time. By now, my dad was telling me to relax and (a few minutes later) warned me about taking random drinks from strangers, but the drink was really good, and I couldn't help it on our day off. She then asked us if we were going to stay for the bands at the bar and my dad thought about it for a second before he asked her where and when. She gave my dad the complex directions of walking fifty feet down the alley and around the corner before she gave me a hug and said, "I'm proud of you, and everything you've overcome." Then she said goodbye, wished us luck, and walked away down the alley. As she walked off, it hit me. That was the first time that I've ever heard those words come from a stranger's mouth. "I'm proud of you." Her words felt as good as they were to hear, and I got some random warm and fuzzy feelings.

I had no idea why for a moment, but it felt good, no it felt absolutely incredible. It was the feeling of finally being on the correct path in life after years of being lost driving life into the ground and having complete strangers respect you for it when they had no idea what you had to do to get there physically, but even more so mentally. All the love, respect, and positive vibes we got from every single person we met was incredibly overwhelming for me. I was the one being told I'd never amount to shit EVERY SINGLE WEEK for the last year and a half. I was always the one being told I would go nowhere, achieve nothing, and end up a worthless piece of shit, either dead or in jail. So this new abundance of endless love and respect I was getting from everyone was completely strange to me and beyond my abilities to digest. Who knew all I needed to do to get respect and love from people was to stop hating life and wanting to watch it burn, to start loving life, and wanting to watch it flourish. For far too long, my anger, depression, and the drugs had all blinded me from, and pushed the idea of a flourishing life so far beyond my grasp, I never really considered it. But holy shit did that idea ever sound nice. The idea of having a future, the idea of building a legacy, and the idea of a life that flourished sure sounded better than being dead by twenty. But could I do it before I died was the real question.

With some liquid courage, and good feels in my belly, mind, and soul I took back off down the hill for another run. By now, there was hardly any foot or vehicle traffic as the day was coming to an end and I had the whole road to myself, so I carved left and right all over it as I went down the short, steep hill. Once I gained enough speed I would do a slide, each time going faster and faster. As I got to the bottom, I got a little too close to the boat launch and the beach area. I ended up sliding on some sand and almost had a good wipeout but recovered just in the nick of time before I made my way back to the top of the hill with the sun on my right setting in the west. When I got to the top, my dad was packing up the table of stuff so I, put my board down, and helped him load the car before we went over to the bar.

The bar happened to be just down the alley, conveniently right where my dad moved the car earlier. We walked down the alley, out to the front of the buildings, and into the bar. The place was already packed with people, front to back, so we walked around for a bit and finally found a table where we sat down. I enjoyed a burger with a beer accompanied by my dad chowing down on some hot wings with an ice water. After dinner, we watched the bands play for a while however, we still had a long drive back down south to Regina so we couldn't stay very long. While my dad paid the bill, I grabbed the keys for the car, walked down to the alley, and again ran into Jessica (vodka-Red Bull lady) still going hard and she asked if I wanted another drink. I said, "Yes please," assuming it was still vodka and Red Bull. She handed me her water bottle that still looked like the yellowish Red Bull colour, so I took a huge swig and swallowed to find out it was now straight tequila. As my throat burned, I said, "Whoa, maybe a little warning next time, eh." She had a good laugh at me as I couldn't help but remember my dad's warning an hour or two before about taking drinks from strangers. I told her I was going back to the car to head back south and continue my journey, so she kindly walked me back to the car, gave me a huge hug, and wished me the best of luck as I got into the car and waited for my dad who was just popping out of the alley. He got in the driver's seat of the Mercedes and over the next hour or so in the darkness of night we drove back south to Regina.

The next morning, we got up, drove around, gathered the last bit of stuff we needed, and then went to drop the car back off at the dealership. When we got to the dealership the back of the Mercedes was still full of the stuff from the festival like a fold-up table, chairs, bins with t-shirts, a map, and sign that my dad had made for the first Long for Life event. We were going to see if we could leave it all with them until we had someone come get it or have it shipped. The manager, Jason, asked my dad, "Well where do you want it to go?" And my dad replied, "Back to Calgary, Alberta." Jason then said, "Well, I'm going there next week. Just leave it in the back and I'll bring this car to Calgary, and drop it off for you, I just need an address."

Wait, what the fuck?

Let's take a second to have a little recap here. Meeting Josh in the middle of the woods led to Kathleen putting us up in North Bay and five weeks around Lake Superior. Which led to meeting Stacy, Tyler, and the Dominion Motors crew, Which in turn led to the Mercedes we got in Winnipeg for the event, which led to the car in Regina for the weekend, and finally to Jason bringing our stuff back to Calgary. It was a ripple effect that went well over three-thousand-kilometres long, just by being in the right place at the right time. I think it was more like a tsunami than a ripple effect, but I was astounded by the convenience and incredible support we were getting from everywhere by everyone. But to actually see the tectonic plates collide, shift and then watch the tsunami of positivity wash over nearly half the country right before our eyes was on a whole other level of stupendously crazy. Again and again, I was coming across the most amazing people who were slowly painting the majestic picture that was my life and I wouldn't even have sold it for billions. For the first time in my life within my mind, heart, and soul I had the kind of happiness, joy, and life fulfillment that no amount of money could ever possibly buy. I became the richest I've ever been and ever will be, just from that alone.

Each time, I couldn't help but think how this never happened to me. I was so used to being the person people put down all the time, I was the angry, misunderstood rebel that lashed out at the world and got help from nobody, ever. But now, everyone was going well out of their way not to bash me or put me down, but to help me achieve my goal, lift me up, and fill me with an unmeasurable abundance of love, positivity, and respect. It was something I wasn't accustomed to and I was still trying to figure out how to take it all in. The generosity from every single person we met along the way was incomprehensible to me. My faith in humanity was not only being restored, but I started to see, believe, and know without a reasonable doubt that everything I battled through, fought for, lived, and survived, was for a reason. Again, I knew it within my soul that it was all what was going to make me, *me*. For the first time ever, the canvas of my life was a priceless incredibly intricate and beautiful piece of art. It was so beautiful, just looking at it could blind you from the overpowering awesomeness that it possessed.

After we dropped off the car, we were on the road going westbound on the Trans-Canada. That day we pushed to Moose Jaw on the usual lame, boring, dry ride through the Prairies going slightly uphill against wind. I was getting increasingly frustrated with that situation as it was our life for almost two months now and I was over it. No, I was fucking sick of it. From Moose Jaw it was off to Swift Current. After Swift Current we got on the road and pushed all day uphill against wind while I continued to curse at Mother Nature like never before. I don't think I've ever swore so much in my life as I did in the Prairies from the wind. It wasn't even a close rival to the three weeks of rain in the east. I was on the highway kicking along the right side of the road pushing with traffic while my dad was a ways ahead of me when I heard the sounds of a car behind me so I turned around to see this big white diesel truck creeping slowly behind me on the shoulder. As soon as I turned around the loser in the big white truck punched the gas and blasted me with a big cloud of black smoke that came out of his exhaust on my side of the road. After drowning me in a cloud of black diesel pollution, I gave him a big middle finger and continued on. Why someone feels the need to be an asshole like that bugged me until I realized, I was that same asshole when I was in my early to mid-teens going through life just pissing people off, it was just a minuscule taste of my own medicine I suppose.

We spent another day pushing into the wind and after hours we turned left off the highway to where Google Maps told us our motel would be for the night. Only when we got to this town, it was a ghost town and there was nearly no one or hardly anything there. We stood in the middle of the dirt road looking around to see any signs of life and where to go. After standing around for five or ten minutes looking around, we saw a man exit from a small store and my dad asked him if he knew of a motel nearby and he said, "Nope, there's nothing around here." All of our hopes and dreams were shattered and my dad got obviously frustrated as the sun was setting and we had maybe a half hour of daylight left. It wasn't nearly enough sunlight to get to the next town or go back to where we came from. We ended up walking over to the post office and sitting at the side of it so my dad could use the power outlet to charge his dead phone and try to figure out a game plan. As we sat there, I could hear some people having a backyard party off in the distance. I thought of going over to see if they could help us out, however after seeing how everyone wanted to show us a good time and liquor us up everywhere we went, I figured it wouldn't be a good idea to be hungover in the wind uphill the next day, and I had flash backs to how badly I wanted to quit on our first day after getting screeched in on the East Coast. As I thought about our nights with Alby and Vanessa, it seemed like it was an entire lifetime ago. I was so angry then, I still hated life when we met, sure I hated my life in the Prairies too, but that was a different kind of hate.

After the flashbacks of our night with Alby and Vanessa, it was then followed by Jessica and her vodka, Red Bull, and tequila. I couldn't help but think of how terrible I always felt the day after I drank. The last-minute straight tequila really did a number on me that night and I felt horrible leaving Regina. I figured the possibility of ruining another very long hard day wasn't worth it; we were just going to have to find a place that was sheltered.

With the sun fading, it quickly got dark. We remembered passing what looked like an abandoned house just off of the highway, so we walked back over to see if it was at all habitable. We got there and it was definitely not the place to stay as it was covered with mice droppings and what appeared to be years of dust and dirt from end to end. So we said no to the empty, dirty house and started to walk around outside. My dad saw a C-can in the back of the house, so we went to investigate. It was closed but it had no pad lock on it so we opened it up and took a look inside. The C-can turned out to be much cleaner than the house, and with no other option and no sunlight we decided to stay there for the night. We found some folded up boxes that rested against the inside of the C-can that was being used for a toolshed and laid them down for our mattresses, my dad took out the tinfoil-like emergency blankets and we laid on our cardboard beds until we fell asleep. I woke up from the noise the space-blankets made every time I moved but they worked really well and kept me warm all throughout the night. The next morning, we got up, put the boxes back up on the side where we found them, packed our bags, and got back on the highway. We made sure to get up and out really early to avoid getting stumbled upon by workers, so as soon as the sun rose, we were up and out of there.

With hardly any sleep, sore and tired from sleeping in a tin can, we got pushing uphill against the wind. I'm sure the headwind the whole way across the prairies made it seem much worse than it actually was, but it was still terrible. As we pushed, I couldn't help but think how my dad and I had been on the road for about three months now and that was the first night we got stuck not sleeping somewhere comfortable. For two guys that flew to the other side of their country with no suitable shelter, that's not bad if you ask me.

After pushing all morning, we came up to an old gas station. There was an old gas nozzle out back and I put it in the back of my board like I was filling it with gas and took a quick picture. After getting back on the road I saw a hill coming up, the first one I've seen for what seemed like a month. As soon as I saw the road go down and take the long slow left turn, I started to kick to see how fast I could make it down the hill. Only it was one of those days and hills where the wind was so bad and the hill was so gradual, I had to push down the entire hill. Once I got to the bottom, it straightened out and went flat. As I rode the shoulder on the oncoming lane, a big rig truck passed me and blasted me with dust, so I went to put my sunglasses on to cover my eyes only to find they were no longer attached to my backpack. I was disappointed and almost went back to look for them, but I could have lost them at any point that day and wasn't about to skate all the way back for some glasses when I still had the four-dollar pair from Walmart in my bag.

Up ahead to my right I noticed a rest stop and as I got closer, I could see the big brown "Welcome to Alberta wild rose country" sign. After going to the restroom, I went over to the sign, put the camera down set to picture mode and I climbed on the right side of the sign while my dad climbed onto the left side. We took a picture and celebrated another province completed under our belts before we got right back on the highway. I put the camera back on my helmet and we got back to pushing on into Medicine Hat where another amazing Super 8 put us up for a night. After the long day of pushing, we were starving so we ordered a few pizzas and each of us probably ate the whole thing before we crashed for the night. Feeling so glutinously full of my favourite food, I felt like I was going to pop. But after that long night and day, the calories were needed and so worth it.

The next day we pushed over to Brooks where again Super 8 put us up in a warm comfortable bed. I was wondering when we were going to start to see the mountains and expected to see them by now but looking west there was still no sign of them which I was kind of surprised by. We got to our motel in Brooks and crashed for the night. The following day, my mom drove out to Brooks from Calgary to be our support driver. We pushed over and met her at the gas station just down the road from our motel. We threw our backpacks in the back of her red Toyota Rav 4, put the Long for Life sign on the back of her car, and got to pushing on the highway. The highway was still relatively flat which I was not overly impressed about, however I knew of the monstrosities that were coming in the Rocky Mountains, so I focused on that.

It was a long push to get to the small city of Chestermere from Brooks. The push wasn't exciting at all; it was relatively flat with long slow turns most of the way. Once we got to Chestermere, we pushed over to the small skate park off the highway at the side of the lake to wait for some local skaters that wanted to push into Calgary with us. We hung out at the small skate park and waited for the other riders as I had memories of skateboarding and rollerblading at the park many years before.

Once the five or six riders arrived, we got on our boards and began to push west down the highway into Calgary, our plan was to push over to Atlas Pizza and have a bite to eat after our skate in. Once we all were on the road we pushed until we arrived at the "Welcome to Calgary" sign that was off to the right of the highway, down a small ditch. We got off our boards and someone stole my idea of climbing onto the sign for the picture. With the one guy on top of the sign hanging out up there, I stood with the trees on the side of the small hill and everyone else huddled around for a quick picture before we got back on the highway and headed over to the pizza place.

Once we arrived, we walked in and I, like most of the others, didn't know it was also a bar and we needed to bring our identification, which most of us didn't have. So, we all got kicked out and stood around outside wondering what we were going to do now. We figured we would pile everyone in the two cars that were there, drive back to Chestermere, and eat at the Boston Pizza instead. So, the dozen of us managed to cram in and do just that. When we got to the Boston Pizza, we took over a whole row of tables and benches where we sat around, chatted, and had a drink or two before having a delicious meal. I guess two of the riders thought the meal was free and left without paying, leaving my mom to pay for their fifty-dollar tab. After dinner my mom and I drove over to her house for the evening.

We took that weekend off to rest and regroup in Calgary, so my friends threw a party in Spring Bank for my ride through. That evening, a few friends picked me up and we took off to the party house where a few of my other friends were living. There was the usual crazy DJ set up in the basement with our buddy DJ'ing at the setup of speakers that went from floor to roof on each side of the DJ equipment. In between Speaker Mountain was a fog machine and TVs that played colourful hologram images with green lasers and a black light that shined out into the fog blowing from behind the set up.

My friend's boyfriend at the time was talking with me about my story as we had a drink and as I was telling him all about my trek, he broke down crying after I struck a chord with him. I had no idea what to do, so I just gave the guy a hug and he began to tell me about how cancer took his mother's life a few years before. My story had brought back the tsunami of overwhelming emotions of losing her to the devastating disease. I realized that's what I hated most about my story. I hated how many people could relate to it, and how it either broke people down and brought back the worst memories of their lives or inspired them. I loved that it inspired people, but the gamble whether or not it was going to inspire them or bring back their life's worst memories was painful to see again and again. It seemed like there were more people who could relate to the pain that cancer brought, than not. That was an incredibly heartbreaking realization to see.

The party got a bit out of hand that night and some guy had forgotten that you never pass out first at a party, especially in the living room with my assholey friends around. Someone busted out a black sharpie marker and what started with a little smiley face and penis on his arm turned into being covered head to toe with the marker. It was pretty bad. I saw him getting covered in permanent marker and tried to wake him up, but he was out cold and wasn't waking up. I was telling him he was getting drawn on and shaking him like crazy and he still wasn't even moving. At one point, I checked his pulse and airway to make sure the guy was still alive and breathing before I went into the kitchen and poured myself another drink.

I couldn't help but think of the time I went to my buddy's house for the night. The next morning, I got up, grabbed my things, and left. On my way home, I stopped at the store to grab a drink and couldn't tell why the guy at the counter gave me the weirdest look ever. After I purchased my drink, I went home and went to the bathroom to see my friend had drawn a huge penis in black marker across my bleach-white chubby face as I slept. I just realized I walked from one end of the community to the other, stopped at the store, and then walked home before I even noticed. I was so mad, I immediately called him up. Expecting my call, he answered the phone hysterically laughing at me. The asshole got me good, but I told him I'd get him back for his prank one day.

Outside at the party one of our buddies had taken plastic shrink wrap, wrapped the swing set in it, and used the plastic walls to paint some graffiti. It was a cool technique. One of my other friends and myself would go to Fish Creek and he would wrap two poles with plastic shrink wrap and then paint some graffiti as I longboarded around. Random strangers would come up to him as he painted, and both complemented his art, and how he made his own makeshift walls to paint so nothing was destroyed. Everyone would ask the same question at some point; What do you do with it when you're done? He would reply, "I take a picture of it, cut it down, and throw it out," as he points to the garbage bins 20 feet away. Not a single person ever called the police, which was a nice change for once. Sure, it's wasteful with all the paint covered plastic but if you try to paint anywhere else, you'll get a nice $1,000-$5,000 fine and or up to a month in jail depending on if it was your first offence or not. The $1,000 ticket was for your first offence then I heard it's a $5,000 fine or a month in jail for your second offence, then it's just jail time after that. All for people expressing themselves, trying to find themselves, or, like me, trying to escape from their reality using paint.

Excited for the Mountains

The day after the stop through party I rested at home as we were back on the road the next day pushing west to the mountains. My mom continued to be our support driver for the next few days until we got farther out of town. So, after we packed up her car, we hit the road. We were maybe five or ten minutes into the push leaving Calgary when a car in the right lane moved over to the left without signalling or looking and cut off a motorcycle. The poor guy on his motorbike tried to stop and his back tire locked, squealing against the ground. However, it was of little use, he slammed into the back of the small car, went flying over the bike and over the car, before he rolled to a stop in the middle of the highway. My mother being an ER nurse for a few decades, immediately pulled over and began to assist the guy until medical services arrived.

She made sure he didn't move, stayed lying on his back, calming him and assuring him everything was going to be okay. A short time later the ambulance arrived, picked him up, and it was back on the road for us. We got a few kilometres down the highway when another motorcycle pulled over and stopped. It was Dave, my dad's friend, who had attached two tow ropes to the back of his motorcycle and asked if we wanted him to pull us up the small hill we were currently at the bottom of. As tempting as it was, we had to decline his offer as there was already an accident that happened a few miles back, and there was likely to be a higher police and RCMP presence in the area so we avoided the possible stunting tickets and walked up the hill as he drove off enjoying the highway ride on the bright and sunny day.

After an hour or so of pushing, we got to one of the big hills that was leaving the city going into the mountains. As soon as I got to the top and recognized the hill I started to kick hard and took off. Meanwhile my dad was kicking behind me at the top of the hill when his wheel got jammed by a small rock and he flew onto the pavement. With my mom right behind him in her car, she couldn't help but burst out laughing as she sat in the car and watched him get back up and on his board.

I came ripping down the right shoulder of the road heading west and as I came down the hill it had a long left turn as it descended. When I came turning around the corner, it faced me towards the colossal mountains protruding from the ground, reaching for the sky. On the clear sunny afternoon, it looked like the mountains were within an arm's reach. On both the left and right sides of the road were walls of trees that eventually disappeared to the rolling hills. On the right side of the road, as the land started to flatten out, it had a turn off and a merge coming up on the right side of it.

I took a look to see no cars coming down the hill so I went into the middle of the road about halfway down. While I ripped, I kept looking back wondering why my dad was taking so long. Once the road flattened out at the bottom it went straight for a few kilometres heading into the mountains. I could see the huge Rocky Mountains coming out of the ground directly in front of me, and as I went on, they rose on the right side of the highway off in the distance as well. I waited for my dad at the bottom of the hill before we continued to kick down the road until we got halfway to Banff. Once halfway there, we turned off in a rest stop area on the right of the highway, got into my mom's car, and took a short drive to Kananaskis (K Country) so I could take a nice run down the hill that was there. I got out of the car and held my helmet in my left arm as I looked off into the distance at the beautiful mountains with my longboard under my right leg. As I stood there reminiscing about life and everything else, my mom took a wicked picture of the moment before I took off down the short, semi-steep hill for a quick sixty-kilometre-an-hour rip before we went back to Calgary for another night.

The next day, we drove back to the rest stop and got back to pushing down the road. From the rest stop we continued down the side of the highway with my mom behind us and her 4-ways flashing. We went under an overpass, then a bit down the road to our left was a big casino with helicopter tours beside it where a helicopter rested, turned off on a helipad. After we pushed by the casino the road took a long right turn at the base of a mountain. Now, as we pushed down the road, there were massive Rocky Mountains on both of our sides. The ones on our right were mostly covered in trees and rock, on the left side, even though it was nearing the end of summer, you could see that halfway up to the top of the mountain still had plenty of snow. The trees on the left started a few metres on the other side of the highway and went to the base of the mountains. The trees went about halfway up the sides of the immense tectonic plates before the snow took over all the way to the top. We rode past the brown and white Canmore sign as we got to the beautiful small town that was sandwiched between the bases of the colossal mountains on both sides of the highway.

We rode under another overpass and continued down the highway in the stunning valley of mountains and came to a construction zone as the road turned right. We were then suddenly forced from having a two-lane road and huge shoulder to ride on, to being moved over onto the oncoming two lanes of the highway. Just as we hit construction, we came up to a sign on the right that said,

"Banff eleven kilometres" and "Lake Louise seventy kilometres." The oncoming road we moved over onto was freshly paved, nice and smooth, but only had one lane as opposed to the usual two lanes going each way, so we had to be extra careful. My mom sat back until we crossed around the corner of the construction zone then zipped around the corner and waited for us when she had the next opportunity to safely pull over.

After the construction zone, there was a long, slow left turn that had a small dip in the middle of it halfway around the corner. My dad past me on my right side as I adjusted my headphones and changed songs on the iPod. I continued behind him as we came around the long, left turn that quickly turned right. With huge mountains all around us and a nice warm day with the perfect mix of sun and cloud it was incredibly peaceful and a beautiful sight, as well as an amazing experience to have in one's life. I had another one of those "I am so content I could care less if I dropped dead right now" moments. I was in a state of overwhelming peace, in every possible way. For the first time ever, I felt like I was at peace mentally, physically, and spiritually. Again, for whatever reason the land had spoken to me, it connected to me in a way I can't find the words to describe. I felt like not only was I one with the land we were riding on, but all seven billion atoms in my body in that moment were connected to every atom in the universe. It was another profound connection between the land and the deepest part of my soul, and it was absolutely amazing.

After we came around the right turn you could see the road go on for a few kilometres. It had a slight right and left curve before disappearing left into the forest. As we came around the slight left, straight ahead I could see another mountain that rose from the ground and high into the atmosphere with the forest on both sides of the highway still going on as far as one could see.

We continued down the highway with the trees on the left and right sides of the road and the mountains in the background. It was a very nice, quiet, and peaceful part of the Trans-Canada Highway. The huge shoulder we had to ride on from Calgary all the way to Banff was still going strong which we loved. I continued to pound the ground with my grey Vans heading toward more gigantic colliding tectonic plates protruding from the ground, all the while completely enveloped by the forest. The isolation of being in the middle of nowhere, in a place that was so majestic, so peaceful, and, even more, so beautiful, was amazing. I wasn't stressed or worried about anything, I wasn't angry and pissed off at the world. But even better, I was at peace with dying daily for the first time in four, agonizing, long years. 'This was the greatest decision of your life' I thought to myself in another moment of complete euphoria. How one can feel the most euphoria they've ever felt without drugs and just by travelling the land and pursuing their dreams, continued to astonish me.

We came around another long right corner that turned left into what looked to be the base of one of the mountains. Once we got to the base of the mountain, we arrived at a sign on the right side of the road that said "Banff." I got off my board and I climbed into the top of the sign continuing my routine of climbing on signs that I apparently gained at the Manitoba/Saskatchewan border. After the quick picture we piled back into my mom's car and spent another night in Calgary.

The next day, we drove all the way back to Banff to get back on the move. After I said goodbye to my mom and gave her a hug and a kiss she took off as we began to skate down the pathway that we thought went all the way to Lake Louise. Only, after a short time of pushing on the pathway, it spit us out back onto the highway. So, we changed plans. Instead of taking the #1 Trans-Canada Highway, we decided to take the secondary 1A so there was less traffic to dodge, and with my mom off back to Calgary after dropping us off, we had no support behind us that kept us safe.

Just off the highway, we could see the paved path continued on so we got back on the path in a small parking lot. As we rode down the path, there was a small lake that sat off to the left beyond some small bushes and trees. You could see a huge rocky mountain come up out of the ground a kilometre or so beyond it. Shortly after that we popped out of some trees and got forced back onto the highway. The tree-covered mountains on our left ran back into the Rocky Mountains a few kilometres behind it. It made for one incredible view. We had another beautiful day with a bright, blue sky and only a little bit of tiny clouds scattered. When you inhaled, you got a lung full of the purest, freshest, most crisp, and cleanest air you ever had. It was quite literally, a breath of fresh air. I never realized how polluted the air we breathe in our cities were until being out here in the vast open wilderness of my country. When you go from one to the other, the difference is like night and day. The air here felt, tasted, smelt, and rejuvenated better than any city I've ever been to. The feeling it gave you was like having a big cup of ice water after being in the hot sun dehydrating for hours: practically orgasmic.

Going down the road surrounded by the mountains and trees with no sign of society was the best feeling. It was just us, nature, and our boards which was incredibly blissful to me. On our left there was maybe one-hundred feet of grass and small brush that quickly turned into a thick dense wall of trees. They ran all the way to the mountains a few kilometres away, then covered them as much as they could. However, on the side of the mountains were cliff faces that would tower some skyscrapers, so the blanket of trees stopped at the bases.

We continued down the empty roadway that had nearly zero traffic on it. We then had a right turn that led into the forest and the only few scattered clouds seemed to all gather to block out the nice sun we were having, just as the first small car came driving past us turning right into the dense forest being swallowed by the trees and disappearing. We came up to the right turn following the car and we were also swallowed by the thick brush. It then spit us out onto the highway where we had to cross over a bridge that took us to the 1A highway. Once we got on the secondary highway, we took a few twists and turns through the woods until we saw the flat oncoming lane go around a right turn. The outgoing lane went uphill to the right before going up even more and to the left. We began to climb the hill and once we got to the top, it went flat for about a kilometre before we came to a yellow downhill sign on the right side of the road. I pointed to it with my right hand and started to kick the road with a vengeance. The clouds broke, the sun came back down on us, and the day was again bright and warm. Just as I started to approach the left turn that was before the hill, I noticed a car coming from behind me, so I moved over to the oncoming lane to let them pass before I started to kick the road again at the crest of the hill.

I could see the hill was a bit shy of a kilometre long and took a hard right into the trees at the bottom. It was a long hill but very gradual, so I started to kick and kick until I was unable to physically keep up with the kicking. I tucked down as tiny as I could into a little ball and ripped down the hill in my own empty lane as a car and motorcycle rider came by me heading up hill. I went down the hill and made the right turn to see a car coming at me, so I turned around to check my six and saw another car coming up behind me as well. The road I was on only had one lane in both directions so with the speed of riding out the last hill I was forced over to the right side of the road that of course had no shoulder. My front and back right wheels were only inches away from taking me into the ditch going a little slower than the speed limit. Both the cars passed me and each other at the same time, so we were as wide as we possibly could have been on the tiny, secluded back road. I could see my dad was up a bit on the right side of the road waiting for me. I looked forward and back for cars to see none so I decided I would slide and slow down. I got down low, way too close to the left side of the street in the oncoming lane and going faster than I thought. I did a slide that ended up with me going right into the small grass ditch. "Ahhh!" I let out a little girly scream as I fell into the small hill. I got back on my feet, grabbed my board, and got back onto the road reminding myself how lucky I was for that to happen on such a tiny hill and not a massive cliff face like around Lake Superior. I pushed over to my dad in embarrassment, and we continued on until we got to the next left corner.

A little way down the road, it looked like we were about to go downhill again so I took off kicking away. I passed my dad on his right side as we rode in the oncoming lane. A few cars came up around the corner, so we moved into the outgoing lane on the right side. I was still kicking like crazy for this hill. It started to go down and to the right and I was thinking, 'heck yeah.' But once I got there it went down for maybe a hundred feet before going back up. In disappointment, I let out an "ugh, weak." I wasn't so upset about the lack of hill, but more about how much energy I just exerted for nothing. We went back up the small slope and turned right into the abyss of the forest. After a few more kilometres in the twisty windy forest roads, it spit us out onto a T-intersection. To the right it went uphill, so naturally I started to walk uphill as my dad went left towards the Trans-Canada. After walking uphill, a bit I turned around, put my board down, and started to kick the ground to hopefully go flying by my dad and across the highway. I started to come down the hill and went cruising around my dad on his right as I headed for the overpass with more than enough momentum to make it.

Suddenly, I see that there's one obstacle in the way, an obstacle that would probably mean a trip to the hospital; a cattle/Texas gate went across the entire road. For some reason my first thought was, 'maybe I can jump it with my speed,' but between the landing and the possibility of losing my board to the unknown depths of the gate, I wasn't going to risk it. I put my hand down and slid to a stop barely a foot or two before the gate that wasn't even deep. I grabbed my board, stepped on the few medal bars that went across the road, then ran a few steps and went to jump on my board. Only when I threw my board down and went to jump on, one of my fat feet clipped the side of my board and it flipped as I was mid-air in the process of jumping on it. So instead of running and jumping on my board in style. I ran, threw my board down as I went to jump on it, flipped the deck, landed on it wheels up still expecting it to move, only to go flying forward into the street when my feet landed on the board. With almost two falls within fifty feet, I thought to myself, 'man, what is wrong with you right now.' I peeled myself off the ground, dusted myself off, flipped my board over, and ever so carefully got on like it was my first time riding and I was afraid of it. Questioning my abilities to ride at the moment, I took a few dozen kicks to get to our destination that day, the beautiful Lake Louise Village.

Once we got there, we got off our boards, walked over to the coffee shop, and grabbed a seat to wait for my dad's colleague and friend to come get us. Once Catherine arrived, we all walked around the back of the village along a small creek and enjoyed the peace and quiet of the nature for a moment as we took some pictures. After we looked around and took a few pictures, we drove over to her house in the north end of Calgary where Jason dropped off the Mercedes full of gear for us. We were up early driving north to Red Deer the next day for our second Heart and Stroke longboarding fundraiser event. This is where my life would again be grossly mis-shaped and altered beyond comprehension forever.

Second Long for Life Fundraiser

The next day, September 7th 2013, is a day of my life I will never be able to forget. My father and I got up at his co-worker's house, packed my dad's car with all the stuff Jason drove over from the Regina Mercedes dealership, and headed north to Red Deer, Alberta. The whole time we loaded my dad's car we got poured on by the rain and I was hoping once we got to Red Deer it would be nice and sunny. However, it didn't stop raining the whole way, the storm almost stretched from Calgary all the way to Red Deer. Once we got there, we began to set up, still in the cold rain.

We stood around in the rain waiting for other riders, however only a handful of the dedicated and loyal ones came with it raining hard all morning and getting worse into the afternoon. So with only a few family members, a few friends, and our few committed riders we took off in the rain and started to skate over to a place the locals call "South Bank Hill." When we got there, I came around the corner and did the run that I knew just went straight down and then back up the other side of the hill, like a giant half pipe. With the rain getting worse I had the usual four reverse gravity waterfalls cascading off my wheels. They came up covering my comfortable grey Vans and the lower legs of my West 49 jeans that were still somehow holding solid. Once I was going down the hill fast enough, the water spray off my wheels came up to my waist. With the water seeping into my shoes, it gave me a very uncomfortable squishy feet noise. I rode down the hill and back up the other side then once my momentum was about to take me back downhill backwards, I did a little one-eighty spin on my board listening to the squish squish noise my feet made as I did it before I rode my board back down the hill. The water in my shoes had my feet feeling like I had just went swimming with them on, it was very uncomfortable and reminded me of the eighteen days of rain the trek started with in the East Coast.

The water really came into my right shoe on the way back down the hill and now it felt like it was so full, it physically couldn't hold any more water in it. Once I lost my speed, I popped off my board, went to grab it by the loop on the front, but it was the back end we chopped off, so I kicked it up with my left leg and dragged it up the hill to the top for another run. This time, instead of going straight I was going to try sliding a left turn which was something I still had to learn. I put my board down, kicked one time really hard, and put my feet in position and did the first right slide with no problems. However, I thought I would get enough speed coasting to get to the left turn, but I was hardly moving so I gave one good kick as I came up to the left turn, but I still didn't have enough speed for it. I overcompensated the lack of speed by leaning way too far out, pulling on my board with my right arm way too hard, and I pulled the board right out from under my feet, lightly skimming my knee and tearing my pants in the process. I was genuinely disappointed I ripped another pair of jeans, but I was glad it wasn't the crotch like the last six pairs. So, with a tiny raspberry patch on my left knee, I took a few steps straight onto the other side of the pathway to pick up my board and go back up the hill for another run.

I got to my board and bent down to pick it up with my left arm but as I went to grab it with my left arm, my left arm just didn't work. Confused, I stood up and went to kick it up with my left leg, however when I went to move my left leg, it also didn't work. I knew something was off and even being a stubborn Harrison I went to call out to my dad. I looked to my left to see my dad was talking to the photographer, Sheldon. I called out for my dad, but he was mid-conversation and didn't hear me. I called out for him again and still he didn't hear me over the sound of the merciless howling winds, the downpour of rain, as well as his conversation.

Suddenly, I felt like I had just longboarded across Canada, without stopping. I got the most exhausted I've ever felt in my life, it was like I ran back-to-back to back-to-back to back marathons and within a second, I felt the wear, exhaustion, and fatigue of them all. Only it was an exhaustion like no other, one that I knew was going to put me to the ground. At this point I knew I had one last chance to get my dad's, or anyone's attention. So, I took one big breath and inhaled, then with the last bit of energy I had in me, I screamed as loud as I could. "DAD!" I then saw him turn his head to the right and look at me. In my peripheral vision I saw a few other people turn and look at me as well so I knew I was now being watched. As soon as I made eye contact with my dad my body uncontrollably started to collapse to the ground. I remember the moment so vividly I can even recall my last conscious thought as I sat on my longboard in the grass, which was, 'Fuck sakes. Now my ass is wet.' Then I completely blacked out.

I have no recollection of the events that transpired after I blacked out (obviously) but I was told I sat down on my board and told my buddy I just needed to sit in the grass then started vomiting for a while. After my good ol' puke session was thought to be over everyone tried to stand me, but I couldn't manage that and kept puking while help was called. After a short time, some sort of side-by-side ATV came ripping around the corner of the half pipe-like hill and they put me on the foam padding in the back then ripped up the other hill going into the community and took me straight to the hospital that was miraculously just a block or two away. I can only assume once the medical team there saw my unresponsive pupils, my medical history of strokes, topped with an extremely high blood pressure they would have then put me in a medically educed coma and taken me for a quick MRI scan which revealed another brain aneurism. A massive stroke took out one third of the right hemisphere in my brain. I was told the stars helicopter was called to bring me back to Calgary, however when it hit the storm that was happening, they had to turn around.

This stock (like any other) wasn't worth the multi-million-dollar machine or the lives of the crew members on board. By now, the doctors at the nearby hospital had put a "stent" (a small tube) between my skull and brain to help release the intracranial pressure in my head from the colossal swelling, as well to drain the large amount of blood that was accumulating. They then strapped me to a gurney, threw me in the back of an ambulance, and took off back to Calgary. I had my stroke, collapsed to the ground, I was picked up, taken to the hospital, scanned, had a stent put in, and driven back to Calgary to the Foothills Medical Centre all within the time it took us to drive to Red Deer earlier that morning, the response team and medical personnel were unbelievably fast and meticulous, which I am forever grateful for. Within an hour my mom was at the hospital waiting for my arrival where they immediately put me into ICU connecting me to a room full of machines like a ventilator, blood pressure/ heartrate monitor, an I.V pumping God-knows-what into me, a catheter, a feeding tube, and an EKG machine before they told my mom they didn't know if I'll even make it through the night as I had seizure after seizure flopping around in my bed from the sudden colossal brain damage.

The Hospital Stay

With no idea if I'll make it through the night, my mom sat by my side nervously watching as I uncontrollably flopped around my hospital bed from seizures and involuntary muscle spasms caused by the massive amount of brain damage from the fist-sized amount of blood in my right hemisphere. There I would lay in my vegetative state for the next seventy-two hours. With the sounds of the machines breathing for me, feeding me, and monitoring me, my mom, grandmother, aunties, and uncles huddled around my bed praying and hoping for the best. With the doctors not knowing if I'd ever come out of my coma, or be a vegetable forever, they all couldn't help but worry hour after hour, day after day.

On the second day of my coma my incredibly high blood pressure started to drop. It was still very high, but it was lowering to a more manageable level. The ventilator that was breathing for me was switched to a setting where it allows the host it's breathing for, to begin to override it and take over. Luckily bit by bit I started to override the ventilator. With my blood pressure lowering and myself starting to override the ventilator, they began to talk about taking me out of my medically induced coma. They had no idea what the effects of my massive stroke would be. They didn't know if I would have any cognitive abilities, if I would be able to communicate, or if I would even have control over my bowels, they had absolutely no idea what the scope of the damage may be. I could have been a vegetable forever and the only way for anyone to find out was by waking me up.

When I collapsed and blacked out in Red Deer, to me it felt like just seconds after that, I can remember the faint voice of my mother saying, "Happy birthday, Brandon. I'm so proud of you, I love you." Immediately after that, I noticed I was in an excruciating amount of pain. The entire left side of my body felt as if it were being crushed. From my left foot all the way up to my eyes on my face was numb with an intense crushing pain. When it wasn't an intense crushing pain, it was the feeling of the left half of my body being on fire, burning from the inside out. It was like the left half of my body went into spontaneous combustion. The deepest depths of my limbs felt like they were set on fire. I remember for some reason my rib cage on the left side hurt more than anything. It felt as if I had been beaten till every rib was black, blue, yellow, and green. I also had an incredible amount of uncontrollable muscle spasms. I could not feel (except pain) or move anything on the left side of my body; I woke up half paralyzed.

At first, I wasn't even upset about the pain or paralysis, I was more pissed off that my cross-Canada trek was now unfinished, and over for good. I thought, 'I'll never be able to finish my trek in this condition,' and, 'I won't even be able to walk again' (according to the doctors). That beautiful priceless canvas of my life that had been painted over the last five months was suddenly sucked into a shredder in the bottom part of the frame like I bought the priceless artwork from Banksy. It was suddenly torn to shit while I could do nothing but helplessly watch. Not only was my dream and life's first greatest ambition shattered, so was my entire life, and it all happened faster than I could call out for help or bitch about my ass being wet. Poof, just like that my life was again, shattered beyond recognition.

To deal with the suicidal pain, I had morphing dripping into my I.V and I was taking little Dixie cups full of opiates. Half the time, I didn't even care to go through the list of pills in the cup with the nurse, I just took them as fast as I could, screaming in agonizing pain. Then the gut rot began. My nurse would bring the drugs to me with water, and I'd slam the twelve pills back like a drunk with their favourite liquor. The pain was so unbearable and the high was so intense it was so hard for me to even grasp the concept of my new profound reality. When I was coming out of my coma at some point my left leg thought I was still on the road longboarding because as I lay there drugged up, hardly conscious, and fresh out of a coma, my left leg was slamming against the bed as if it were still longboarding on the highway. BAM, BAM, BAM, my leg struck the bed with the force of one that just pushed a 160-pound human on a longboard over 5,000 kilometres across Canada. My leg was so strong it took several people to grab it and hold it down so it could be tied, but that only kept it from physically moving and knocking someone out. My leg was tied down, but the muscles were still going into spasms. My thigh was flexing like a body builder showing off their muscles at a competition, only they were not puffed up and expanding for show. The muscles would uncontrollably tighten up till it could not constrict any further, then it would keep constricting. With every spasm I felt my muscles in my leg being torn. It felt like a mini butcher took a steak knife and was physically in my leg slicing up some fresh meet to cook. I screamed bloody murder in this agonizing pain as my mom sat by my bed and massaged my leg and rib muscles to help calm them down. Hour after hour, I would be screaming bloody murder higher than I've ever been and she would massage till the muscles calmed down.

As far as my family, friends, nurses, and doctors could tell my cognitive abilities were still intact and my bratty, silly, brotherly, dickish attitude continued. My little brother walked into ICU and as he came up to my bed to say hello, I just gave him the middle finger. My nurse was doing simple tests asking me questions like where I was, who I was, and then she asked me to raise my right arm, which I did. She then asked if I could raise my left arm. I said "yup" as I used my right arm to pick up my left paralyzed arm holding it high and proud saying "see" as my mom and nurse just had a quick giggle.

The physical nerve pain and muscle spasms where not my only issue. Unknown to everyone even me, when I saw my girlfriend, I knew who she was, I knew the road to hell and back we took over the years, and I knew that I should be madly in love with her. I could vividly remember how that intense inferno of love felt. But for some reason that deep, profound, emotional connection to her was gone. The fist size amount of blood in my brain had extinguished that emotion along with every other good positive emotion I had. All the good, happy, positive, and joyful feelings I once had where suddenly replaced with a tsunami of pain, frustration, anger, and every negative emotion you could ever think of, including the feeling of complete emptiness. I first attributed this blank emptiness to all the heroin-like, opioid products I was taking and thought it would come back in time once I was off the hard drugs, but it didn't. How it was even able to happen I have no idea, but it made me sick on multiple occasions. I'd think about everything, her, us, our past, our future, and end up puking from the overwhelming fuckery it caused in my head. Day by day, I was slowly breaking down more and more over the whole situation. The physical pain was one thing, but the mental pain was not only a whole other ball game, it was in an entirely different league.

After my stroke in Red Deer, the Long for Life team stayed there while I fought for my life in ICU on life support in Calgary. Apparently when they did finally make it down to the hospital they took a picture for the newspaper, and left. They didn't bother to come see me, they literally just wanted to use me. That caused a tremendous argument between my mother and the Long for Life team. When one of them came in ICU she apparently said, "Wow there's a lot of equipment in here." My mom replied with, "No shit, he just had a massive stroke."

After a few days in ICU, I was lying in my hospital bed, high out of my sane mind watching the roof tiles melt. Super bored of lying there literally doing nothing but attempting to shit in a bed pan, have a catheter put in and out, taking copious amounts of drugs, and wishing I was dead from the unimaginable pain for days. I guess it was time to mess with the nurses, so I grabbed the hospital bed remote and hit the nurse call button. My nurse responds within a second, "Yes, Brandon, what do you need?" I respond to her with, "Can I get some hookers, blow, and Tim Hortons coffee please; it should be covered by my health care, right?" I then hear at least two or three nurses in the nursing station uncontrollably burst out laughing for a bit. After she caught her breath, she kindly responds, "No, I'm sorry, Brandon, unfortunately I can't do that for you but I'm sure someone in your family can grab you a coffee." I then spent the rest of the day in my hospital bed saying how hookers, blow, and Tim Horton's coffee is the "trifecta", whatever that even means. To this day it's something I joke about from time to time.

About a week into my ICU stay, my dad came by with the Royal and Coast Longboarding families. Some super rad people I looked up to and admired in the longboarding community came to bless me with their good vibes and show their support while they were in town. I was given a really sweet Rayne longboard deck that was signed by everyone, a Royal Board shop hat, and a Royal hoodie from Ryan who had been a phenomenal support of my mission from day one. Although I was incredibly high out of my mind I remember when Striker (the president of Coast Longboarding) came up to my hospital bed and gave me a Bronze, Silver, and Gold Coast Longboarding metal. When he put the gold metal around my neck for some odd reason the awesomeness of the situation snapped me out of my intense drug like state and put me there, back in reality, in the moment with him, which I was and am forever grateful and happy about. However, my nurse was not so impressed with the crew of twenty people cramming into the small, tight ICU. Maybe it was because she had no room to work or maybe she feared the trifecta was now in full swing, who knows…

I still had an I.V in my arm pumping me full of drugs, a catheter up my urethra draining my bladder, a feeding tube up my nose pumping an oatmeal-looking paste into my stomach, and the stent in my head. I wasn't bothered much by most of it, but the feeding tube was driving me crazy now that I wasn't in a coma. So, every chance I got, I'd pull it out of my face. I'd pull it out as soon as the nurse was turned around. After she realized what I did and had a meltdown she would come back and ram it back up my nose and down my throat. Right after she did, I went to pull it out again but my uncle grabbed my hand trying to stop me saying, "Don't do it dude. They're just going to put it back up there." However, I was fresh out of fucks to give and as soon as he let my hand go, I pulled the sucker out again. Sure enough, it was about to go right back in when my nurse saw. My mother started fighting for me saying "He's obviously bothered by it, so leave it out." The nurse said, "Well, it's going to be three days for a swallow test." My mother just laughed and let her know how she felt about that before she grabbed a cup of small hospital ice chips (which she knows I always love to munch on when I'm in the hospital) she came over to my bed and asked, "Hey B, do you want some ice chips?" Without saying a word, I nodded yes, grabbed the cup, got a small mouthful of ice, chomp, chomp, chomp, swallow. I show that there is nothing in my mouth to my nurse and my mom's like, "Well, there's you're fucking swallow test," and finally the nurse left the feeding tube out. If you've never had a feeding tube, when they put it up your nose it feels similar to getting the biggest nose full of water in your life only multiplied by the hundreds. Then when it goes down your throat, it feels like you got a piece of food stuck in it, only there is no being able to cough it up and spit it out, that feeling of lightly suffocating with something caught in your throat just remains, it's not pleasant at all.

The feeding tube and the stent were the only things really bothering me on top of the ridiculous amount of nerve pain, the colossal high, outrageous muscle spasms, mental distortion, and lack of any good emotions. The stent in my head was very itchy and incredibly irritating. It was like someone drilled a hole in my skull (which they did, in Red Deer) then started to irritate my brain (which was caused by the foreign object now put in there) creating an incredible itching sensation. No matter how hard I scratched around the stent it would not be satisfying because the itch came from deep within, under the skull. I was trying to satisfy an itch on my brain, and it wasn't going to well.

At one point I got so fed up with the un-satisfying itch that I decided to take matters into my only hand, and I pulled the stent right out of my skull. My nurse of course had a meltdown (as she should) before she put it back in and gave me trouble before she told me not to do it again. Once she got it back in my skull into position draining again, I grabbed it as soon as she turned around and ripped it out. This time I was feeling the plastic parts of it, kind of playing with the pieces, I suppose. As I'm playing with the pieces in my right hand, I feel the brain fluid its draining start to drip down my head. It started at my forehead, then ran down my nose, and dripped directly onto my upper lip. I felt the bloody, brain fluid start to come closer to my mouth and I knew I'll be puking if it got in there. So, I took a deep breath in through my nose, closed my lips closer together, and I blew out as hard as I could to get the liquid off my lips and away from my mouth.

It was a good idea in theory I suppose, but I was way too high to think the whole thing through. I just wanted it anywhere but in my mouth. When I exhaled blowing out of my mouth, I watched my bloody, clear brain fluid fly across my body, bed, and the machines. My nurse came back to see the stent is now in two or three pieces and my brain fluid is everywhere and all over everything within one-hundred-and-eighty degrees of my mouth. After she cleaned me and everything up, she gave me a stern talking to and put the stent back in. This time, she wasn't taking any chances and she tied my right arm to the hospital bed. Surely, I couldn't use my one working arm to pull it out with my other arm completely paralyzed, right? Well, unfortunately the poor woman had no idea what a stubborn, resilient, twat I can be. After she left the room again, I shimmied, wiggled, and flopped around in my hospital bed till I got sideways. I then leaned my head to my tied-down right hand and as soon as I felt the stent in my hand, I lifted my body back up and pulled it out, again.

My nurse came back a moment later to see me now all cockeyed in my bed and rushed over, probably wondering if I was having another seizure or something only to find me with the stent in my tied-down hand while sitting there with the biggest shit-grin on my face like, "Yeah, you can't stop me lady." Now she's infuriated wondering what she's going to do with this kid that just won't piss off with the personal stent removal. After the steam and urge to strangle me back into a coma left her head, she decided to weave the stent a few times through my scalp and then burrow it into my skull. She shaved my head in a few places then weaved it through the bald spots like she was crocheting. Then she took a metal tool and started to use it to dig a hole in the top of my skull just above my forehead. As she scratched the tool against my skull it made an awful metal-on-bone grinding sound, but luckily for me, I was deemed uncooperative and put back to sleep. She put me to sleep after I pulled it out for the third time so I would finally piss off and give her a moment to take a breath, think, and work. Once she was done crocheting this thing through my scalp and burrowing it into my skull I was awoken again. However, the stent was now itchier than ever, and I felt as though this stupid piece of plastic with tubes, and I were not finished just yet. I grabbed it again and tugged on it. This time it didn't just come out, this time I felt the entire top of my scalp lift up with it. Literally feeling my scalp detach from my skull made me want to vomit more than it hurt. That was an incredibly painful and disgusting feeling, so I immediately let it go, she had finally won. That day she became one of the very few people who have been able to beat me, and that alone is an accomplishment she should be very proud of.

I lay there in defeat going back to the useless scratching and I'm left in my bed looking like I got into a fight with a pair of hair clippers and lost. I had chunks of hair gone here, and a chunk gone there. With my missing chunks of hair, I looked quite ridiculous, so my mom decided to cut it all off to even it out. A picture of me in that condition (pre-buzz cut) I got to see for the first time in the newspaper and wow did I ever look funny with my brown hair shaved in spots. The hair on the back of my head had been dyed bleach blond from the sun as it protruded out the back of my helmet all summer. I had two different hair colours, missing patches of hair, tubes coming out of me everywhere, and two colours of skin from the worst farmers tan you ever saw, I think it's safe you could say I was a mess.

One night, I was having a very hard time sleeping. I was tossing, turning, and waking up what seemed like every few minutes and I was getting super irritated and frustrated as sleep in the ICU is a very precious commodity. BEEP BEEP BEEP BEEP the noises from the machines everywhere were keeping me up. There was some sort of commotion going on, I can vaguely remember a moment waking up and getting genuinely mad about all the noise as every time I woke up, it meant the suicidal amounts of pain and the very uncomfortable high would be back. I was waking up more and more infuriated by the minute, until I wasn't. Next thing I noticed, it was morning time. I stretched my right arm and leg then I noticed the woman that was on the right side of me in ICU was gone. I asked my mother, who was still by my side day and night where they went. She told me the person had died in the middle of the night. Now I find out the reason I got pissed off throughout the night when I woke up to the commotion was because this young person had been fighting for their life, and lost.

I couldn't help but instantly feel like the world's biggest piece of trash. My gut and my heart sank so low I literally wanted to vomit. My stomach turned in knots as I thought to myself, 'that should have been you, dude. You're the one that should be dead right now.' In the moment, I remember being mad that it wasn't me. Not because I was suicidal or anything, but because since that day when I was seventeen, followed by the trek I made my peace with death on numerous occasions. Since those moments I did not only become okay with dying, I outright expected it and it did not bother me the slightest bit. It's just an inevitable part of life we cannot and should not escape, we must accept it. From my self-administered LSD experiment and the intentionality of doing it leading to finding my peace with death for the first time compiled with the countless moments just like that across the country, I was more than ready to die. Hell, when I was fifteen I told my mom to pull the plug if my life ever came to this. I was mentally preparing for my death for years now and I felt like that should have been my time to go. People always say things like, "oh God isn't done with you," or "God has bigger plans for you," and things of that nature but it drives me absolutely mad. It drives me crazy that this so called 'God' would have the chance to take the life of someone who's ready and prepared to die but takes the one raising a family instead. It made me again question if there even was a "God" and it was an incredible test to my spirituality.

As I was in the hospital dealing with my new profoundly painful reality, my dad came by with a few riders to say goodbye as he continued to the West Coast to finish the trek as per our verbal agreement in Ontario. When we made that agreement thousands of kilometres ago and got through the dangerous part of the country without any problems, I was confident that we were going to make it all the way without any issues. But life has its ways of putting you in your place, and here I was half-paralyzed after getting to the doorstep of the last province. Being so close to the finish, only to have everything in your life ripped away in a few seconds was more mentally devastating than it was physically. Sure, either way (mentally or physically) it's absolutely distressing but the mental "what if's" immediately began to torture me. What if I didn't go on the trek till I was stroke free? What if I cared and took better care of my health? What if my goldfish probation officer didn't delay the trek two weeks and I finished the trek then had this stroke? What if I didn't have so much anger and hate in my world and didn't unleash it on people's faces with my fists. These questions tortured me for days and weeks until it finally became clear.

Later on, I would yawn, and for the first time in over a week I saw my left, paralyzed leg move and lift off the bed. I was wondering if I was so high, I just imagined it so I called out to my mother and asked her to look as I yawned again. She confirmed that my leg had lifted off the bed a little bit. This little bit of movement was enough to make me realize I still had a slim chance, this wasn't the end of my life's journey. Sure, the chance was slim, nonetheless it was still very much a chance.

Once the Long for Life president and team finally decided to show up and see me in ICU, I immediately started to question their intentions. I remember being so high on medications, in so much pain, and they would come in and start asking me about business decisions. The president asked me something and I remember just thinking to myself, 'I don't give a flying fuck, dude, look at me right now. Do I look like someone that wants to talk business?' Then they would ask me something and I'd just say "yup" or "sure" so they would go away. I was higher than a space shuttle but it still wasn't enough to blind me from what they would say and do. They came into ICU one day and told me, "They had to make a judgment call on if I wanted to be less or more famous." I honestly could not have cared for fame one bit, I had more real-life issues to attend to. Even in my current, drugged-up condition I still knew it was never about fame to me, like I never saw a single person that got "famous" for longboarding across Canada.

For me, it was all about changing my life for the better, finally doing some good in my life before I died. It was about growing spiritually, physically, and mentally as an individual. It was about finding oneself and one's sense of direction in life. As well to give a little back to the world for being such a little disrespectful mischievous shithead my entire youth. Doing this thing for fame was not only the dumbest thing someone could do, but the furthest thing from my mind. But of course, they chose "more famous" for me and I just nodded in agreement hoping I'd be left alone.

Even the thought of being famous and having random people up in my face all the time nonstop pisses me off. I learned that in my early teens from Eminem's music, and watching what happens to literally every celebrity I've ever seen. 'Fuck fame. To be able to walk would be nice,' I thought to myself right after thinking about the ridiculous question. It absolutely boggled my mind but more so broke my heart that they could have their mind on fame right now, but what was even more preposterous to me was them thinking I've got my mind on fame when I almost just died, lost 100% of my independence, couldn't even stand, and was higher than a damn kite. Fame was (and always will be) the furthest thing from my mind. I just spent the last week trying to shit in a bed pan, but they wouldn't know because their heads had gone so far up their arrogant asses that the mission now was apparently all about fame. It absolutely boggled my mind and made me feel like they only ever wanted fame out of this, which (to me) is the absolute worst form of inspiration and intentions one could ever have. If I had the ability to stand, I would have stood up and bitch-slapped them as hard as I possibly could. My stroke was no longer the cause of my high blood pressure, it was now from the people that solely wanted to use me, my story, my struggle, my pain, and my resiliency for their benefit. When they've literally never been around in my life for any of it.

The nurses and doctors wanted to get me up, standing, and into therapy right away but my mom wouldn't let them put me on my feet just yet. She suggested they try and just sit me up first. So, as I lay flat on my back, they used the hospital bed remote to sit the bed up. As they lifted the bed, the entire left paralyzed side of my body went into spasms, and I started to shake uncontrollably like I was having another seizure. Everything from my face to my leg on the left was vibrating the bed uncontrollably. After they saw I couldn't even be sat up without huge problems they held off for a little bit and transferred me out of ICU over to unit 112.

One day in U112 while I was in my hospital bed, I saw my backpack on a shelf and asked my mom to grab it for me so I could find my headphones. My mom went over to the high shelf and struggled to reach it with her being so short. I started to make fun of her for being short and made a joke about it then laughed. I looked at my little brother on my right and we started to crack short people jokes. Meanwhile unknown to me my mom came up on my left side and lifted my paralyzed arm and tucked it behind my head while I talked to my brother. When I was done making fun of my short mother with my brother, I turned back straight in my hospital bed to see my arm that *had been* on my lap was now suddenly gone and no longer there. As soon as I saw my arm disappeared, I freaked out and screamed, "OH MY GOD! Where the hell is my arm!?" Knowing my arm is normally attached to the shoulder, I grabbed my shoulder and found my arm was tucked behind my head. My mother, brothers, and myself all burst out laughing at my stupidity. Because I have no sensation or feeling on my left side, I couldn't feel that she moved it, nor could I tell where it was. After that, my mom asked me how that karma tasted, and I felt like a complete idiot.

Unit 112 was on the eleventh floor in the Foothills main building. It was about two or three days into my stay in that unit when my nurse got me out of my hospital bed and put me in a cardiac arrest chair so I could eat my lunch. I got in the chair, and he pushed me into the hallway for "a change of scenery." I forced down my lunch as I wasn't hungry at all before I called out for my nurse to bring me back to my room as I wanted to lay down in my bed. He came over to me and pushed the chair into my room, then left. Now I'm just inside the door on the other side of the room looking at my hospital bed. It looked very comfortable and being the stubborn Harrison that I am, I said, "Screw it. I can stand and do chair transfers so how hard could it be to walk a few steps across the room?" I'm now convincing myself I can make it and that I can walk for the first time unsupervised to my bed, just like a stubborn twat. I stood up out of the cardiac arrest chair standing mostly on my right, strong leg. I was very hesitant to step on my left, so as I stood I slowly transferred my weight onto my left leg and it was holding strong. "I got this," I told myself words of encouragement to get going and I took my first step with my left paralyzed leg.

There were likely so many things wrong with my step but to me it went off without a hitch. I then asked myself, "What the heck are you doing in bed and being pushed around in wheelchairs for, when you can still walk you, lazy bastard?" I then took a step with my right leg, and I was getting closer; my mission is a third of the way done. I then go to take another step with my left leg. I slowly move it forward into position. "I got this, just like last time," I told myself some more words of encouragement. I then stepped onto my left foot and as I'm mid-stride with all my weight on my left leg, it gave out and I fell to the ground hard. SPLAT. I hit the floor hard, mostly on my right side. "Ouch!" I yelled out in pain. My nurse instantly came busting into my room and started freaking out, "Oh my gosh, what are you doing, you could have hurt yourself, are you okay?" he asked me. I told him I'm fine, but I just wanted to go back into my bed. He then helped me get back up onto my feet, over to my bed, and then encourages me to wait or call for help before I try things on my own as I just had a massive paralyzing stroke. But I'm too stubborn and impatient for that. I always learn best the hard way apparently.

Shortly after that incident, they got me into some physiotherapy sessions which was the longboarding across Canada equivalent of going from an eight-hundred-kilometre detour across the big, beautiful province of Ontario and into the boring moo-cow Prairies. I went from loving and living life to the fullest. To hating life, not living at all, and hardly able to stand at a table moving a plastic ring from the left to the right. This disgusting reality of going from one life extreme to the polar opposite was how my recovery began. I only spent a week or two doing therapy in unit 112 before I would experience the most mind-boggling, brain-breaking experience of my life.

It was a shower day and I was being washed by a small group of strangers in the shower room. They washed my back for me as I washed my pits and chest. One of them gave me a small cloth to wash my kibbles and bits while they physically held me up to keep me from falling over because for some reason now when I'm under water or in the dark I lose all sense of direction. I started washing my hair and as I was rinsing out the shampoo with my eyes closed, I got an enormous amount of nerve pain in my left hand. The pain felt as if I put my hand in a blender and blended it off from my fingertips all the way down to my wrist, and that's not even the worst part. This pain, the most horrific pain I've ever felt in my hand wasn't where my hand currently was. This agonizing, nauseating, so-painful-it's-just-numb pain I was feeling in my hand, was a few inches in front of my face.

I started freaking out using my only working arm in an attempt to smack the pain away like it's a fly. However, when I opened my eyes expecting to see my left hand in front of my face where I'm feeling this pain, it wasn't there. To my astonishment and incredible disbelief, my arm was lying across my lap where I left it. As soon as I started screaming in pain and flailing around like a fish out of water, they shut down the shower, dried me up, and got me back into my bed before they got my nurse to get me some pain meds. By now the pain inches in front of my face was gone but I was still very sore and tremendously confused on what the hell just happened. My nurse came in with medications and my Heprin needle (blood thinner to prevent blood clots I got twice a day for months). I took my pills, my nurse administered my needle and asked if I needed or wanted anything else. I told her I was fine other than the normal pain and thanked her before she went to do her rounds.

She walked out of the room and as I lay in my bed trying to process what had happened in the shower, it happened again. My left hand went completely numb with pain as if it had been beaten with a hammer until it hurt so bad, I couldn't feel it. I immediately started screaming in pain again as I tried to simultaneously process what's happening. Again, the craziest part about this experience, was the astronomical pain I felt in my hand, was over in the corner of the room by the bathroom door. Having another out-of-body pain experience like this caused me to freak out and scream even more. This time there was no swatting at anything because the physical pain in my hand was on the other side of the room by the washroom door about fifteen feet away. My mind went blank with how it's even possible to be feeling this insurmountable amount of pain in my body, but in a different physical location. It was at this point, I broke down and started crying because I realized how messed up I really was. My nurse came running back in to see me break down in probably the biggest mental breakdown of my life. I asked her what the heck was going on and I explained how the pain in my hand was felt over by the door and she gave me the weirdest, most confused look. It was like it broke her brain as much as it did mine. The only thing she's heard of similar to that was called "phantom pain." She explained that it usually occurs in amputees who have a limb cut off only to feel pain in the leg or arm that no longer exists. I am dumbfound and completely flabbergasted that it was even possible to feel pain in a physical location that was not in my body. I don't think I'll ever be able to forget that. To this day, it remains the craziest most peculiar thing I've ever experienced in my life. After pondering this situation for years, I think it was another event in my life that proved to me that we are all connected to everything that there is. The same way I felt connected to my homeland and felt like I was one with everything there was, was the same feeling I got out of this. It was like I was over by the door. Sure, I wasn't standing there physically, but I hypothesize, I must have been there in super position because nothing about that experience makes any sense to me, and continues to break my brain when I think about it.

My nurse gave me even more pain killers in an attempt to keep the pain away and I waited for them to kick in so I wasn't so sore and could go to therapy. It was about fifteen minutes before therapy when the drugs the nurse gave me finally kicked in and I was suddenly back to being high as a kite. Not only was I incredibly high but after a month of this nonstop daily pill popping routine, I literally felt my insides rotting day by day and on this day, it was particularly bad. So bad to the point I bailed on therapy that afternoon. I had the worst gut rot of my life. My insides felt like someone had been cutting them into pieces and the sharp aching pain was only getting worse day by day. It was an absolutely terrifying experience being in the hospital waking up every day feeling worse, not better. I knew I didn't even know the half of it as I started to think about all the people over in the Tom Baker Cancer Centre next door and how bad terminally ill cancer patients would feel waking up feeling worse every day.

About a month into my stay at the hospital, I was allowed to leave Unit 58 (traumatic brain and spine unit) with my family on a day pass. Unknown to me, Bobby, a local teacher at the Calgary Arts Academy gathered his students and put together a ride for me to help me finish the last thousand kilometres of my trip. So, my mom picked me up in my wheel chair and we drove down to Eau Claire market downtown Calgary. There, Bobby and his students rode up and down the Bow River for the afternoon. While they rode my mom pushed me over to the pathway in my chair. My little brother had our niece sitting on the front of his board as he pushed and rode on the back. Once there I did an interview with Global News and upon watching the interview later, I realized how badly the drugs were affecting my abilities to think, process information, and speak. Of course, this was on TV for everyone to see, but what they couldn't see was that this inability to think and talk was not from the massive stroke, but from the copious amounts of drugs I was taking to deal with the effects of said stroke. It was a beautiful heartwarming event and moment that (to me) was ruined by the interview. Right after I watched my tragic Global interview in my hospital bed, I opened my computer and the first thing I saw when I opened my Facebook feed was an article a mutual friend shared of my old friend going to jail for killing someone. I couldn't help but think 'that could have and probably would have been me if I didn't make the choice to change paths.' For over a month I was being tormented by the 'what ifs' and upon seeing that I realized, that was where I was heading if I didn't change. After seeing that, despite recently being paralyzed, I was incredibly relieved and happy that I did make a change, however my drugged-up zombie mind I just witnessed on TV was incredibly worrisome to me.

It was at this point I started sharing my concerns with a few close friends and family about taking so many drugs to try and manage my suicidal amounts of nerve pain only to get incredibly high, still be in pain, and feel my insides rotting worse day by day. It was near the end of October when I had someone come by for a visit. They heard my concerns from a close friend that I told, and he told me it's a nice day out before he asked if I wanted to go for a roll outside. I had nothing to do so I agreed, and he wheeled me outside in my wheelchair. We went across the street and over to the smoking area where he pops a marijuana cigarette in his mouth and lights it. He takes a few puffs then looked at me in my wheel chair in obvious pain and he asked if I ever tried medical marijuana for my pain.

I said, "No," and he asked if I wanted to give it a try. I thought to myself, 'Why not, I've been taking pharmaceutical heroin daily for two months straight.' I grabbed the joint and took a few puffs off it. Instantly, the pain I had in my left hand, arm, leg, foot, face, ribs, back, and chest were gone, along with the massive headache I had for the last two months. I kicked out the legs to my wheelchair, stood up without pain for the first time, and asked him, "What the fuck is this?" He then started talking another language saying, "It's a forty percent Indica, sixty percent Sativa dominant hybrid." I thought I had an abundance of cannabis knowledge, but I had no idea what that even meant at the time, all I knew is I finally found a worthy medication, now I just had to get legalized. As we stood there having a quick puff, I told him about the puff of marijuana I took after my first stroke that immediately took away my pain. I was in awe of this apparent wonder drug and thought, 'I should really get myself into a post-stroke marijuana study, if it works this well for me then maybe it could help others.' I thought about being a test subject again, but I had no idea where to go or how to go about it, plus I couldn't legally take the drug. But I didn't give a damn about laws in my current condition. It worked and if the cops, lawyers, and judges had a problem with that, then they were going to spend astronomical amounts of money housing me and paying for my recovery from jail. So I dove head first into the rabbit hole that is medical cannabis and hoped for the best.

Once I was finally able to transfer chairs by myself, I was able to go shower without a crew of people. One day I was having a shower, it was one of my first ones alone in Unit 58. I showered without remembering when my head gets fully submerged under water, I lose all sense of direction. If it wasn't for the metal bars on the walls everywhere I would have fallen out of the shower chair. After I finished up my shower without falling, I dried off, changed, got back in my wheelchair, opened the sliding bathroom door, and immediately noticed the disgusting smell of poop. I rolled out of the washroom and noticed a new patient now in my room. He was an older gentleman who was pacing back and forth around the room. As he's walking around the room, I noticed this small stream of fluids coming from one of his pant legs as he walked around.

I looked at the floor beside me and realized I just rolled through a stream of his diarrhea. I was instantly disgusted and called out for the nurse. Apparently, I was in the bathroom too long and the gentleman didn't think to go use the bathroom next door or in the hall, or other unit. My nurse came in, sees the mess, and immediately got a cleaning crew in to deal with it as I went straight back into the shower this time still in my wheelchair to wash off the poop. I couldn't help but feel as it was all my fault as I was the one occupying the bathroom at the time. Then I had to stop and remind myself, 'I'm in a traumatic brain and spine recovery unit,' and, 'Not all the people here have full or any control over their bladder and colon. You could have and should have been the one without self-control, so be grateful you're not,' which I was incredibly happy and grateful I wasn't.

Also, around October, my dad's mother came into Unit 58. That particular day I was in a crazy amount of pain, having a really terrible time mentally, and contemplating if I should just give up and find a way to end my life so I'd no longer have to deal with any of this pain, frustration, and hellish time of my life. It was another day I was cursing at the heavens for not taking me. My grandmother said a quick hello, checked on how I was doing, and dropped off this brown envelope before she took off for a meeting. She came by right before I headed to speech therapy. I opened the envelope and I start pulling out hand-drawn cards from school kids in Reston, Manitoba. I was pulling out these get-well cards and each one was preaching my message back to me saying, "Don't stop believing, you're awesome, you're so strong, **believe in yourself and never give up,**" along with all sorts of positive uplifting messages. It was another moment where I broke down and cried like a baby since my stroke. But this wasn't a cry from pain, it was the first time in my life I was crying from pure uplifting positive emotions. It was the first wave of pure genuine emotion I had felt since I woke up paralyzed and it was incredibly overwhelming.

I was so overwhelmed with my lost emotions coming back I could no longer hold it together. It was in that moment I realized that I couldn't quit, I couldn't give up, and there was definitely no way I could end it all. Not for me, or because my reputation was on the line, or how I wouldn't be able to live with myself if I preached a message all across Canada, then didn't live by it. But I couldn't give up for everyone we preached that message to and met across the country. I had to stay strong for every one of these kids to show them anything is possible. I had to persevere for every cancer and stroke victim that wasn't given another chance like I was, I was also carrying a lot of guilt from getting upset about the woman dying beside me in ICU and I needed to stay strong for the child she left behind. This was my moment of truth. I had this realization just as my porter came to pick me up for therapy. That day, my regular therapist wasn't in, and I had a temp. She could tell I had recently been crying like a baby and asked me what was wrong. So, I told her my story, from cancer diagnosis to the get well cards I just received. She was so overtaken by her emotions that she broke down and started crying, which in turn made me start crying again. After that, we just talked for the session and looked at cute puppies online for a few minutes to try and cheer us cry-babies up.

One of my least favourite parts about being in the hospital was having to deal with "the vampires." "The vampires" are what I call the lab technicians that wake you up at three or four in the morning to take your blood. They would come in and try to quietly wake you or another patient up, but usually woke up the entire room when they turned on the lights and started talking. So, if one of the three of us had to get poked we almost were all waking up. One morning, I remember the vampire came in, woke me up, and asked, "Are you Brandon?" still half asleep I nod and said yes to him. He began to do his vampirey things and tied off my arm, stabbed me with a needle, and gathered his few vials of blood for the lab. Once he finished taking my blood, he looks at his chart and asked, "Your last name is Bailey, right?" I responded with, "No, its Harrison, that's probably something you should have asked me first, don't you think?" By now the older guy in my room woke up and realized the guy messed up big time and he shouted out, "HEY, YOU JUST TOOK THE WRONG GUYS BLOOD, YOU FUCKING IDIOT!" I didn't even have to say it again because the lab tech realized he screwed the pooch. Flustered and probably embarrassed he took off without saying anything. Then about five or ten minutes later a different lab tech came and took the right Brandon's blood before they left.

I got a new roommate one day who had a stroke as well. This guy was much older and a heavy drinker and heavy smoker. One night, his nurse came in and caught him while he was quite drunk and smelled like booze. When his nurse confronted him about it, he denied it left, right, and centre. His nurse then realized he was sneaking out for cigarettes and once he came back in from his next one, she confronted him and took his smokes out of his front flannel pocket as they poked out. This poor guy lost his mind once that happened, he was now yelling, screaming, and swearing at this poor woman just doing her job. He was being such a jerk I almost got out of my bed and hobbled over to him to say something but the nurse was doing her best to deal with him and tried to calm him down with no prevail. The alcohol was making him quite the loud, rude, belligerent drunk. After listening to this guy lose his mind for about fifteen minutes, the nurse finally had enough and called security to come deal with him. Security came in, took him away, and I never heard him or saw him again. So don't mess with and respect your nurses, they know how to make people disappear.

With being in the hospital able to do literally nothing all day, everyday, it got incredibly boring. So, I tried to keep myself entertained. One day I was outside on a nice, warm, sunny day with my mom, and I saw a bunny on the pathway. For some reason I decided to see if I could catch it and I went chasing after it in my wheelchair. The bunny ran right down the pathway with me just behind it cruising as fast as I could in my chair. The bunny then ran off the pathway onto the grass. I thought I would be fine, so I rode into the grass after it. Only as soon as the two front wheels of the wheelchair hit the grass they dug deep into the ground and immediately stopped. The momentum from my speed shot me forward and the back two wheels of the wheelchair came off the ground and I was tilting on the verge of doing a face plant on the front two wheels. Luckily, I leaned backwards, and the chair fell back down on all four wheels. My mom, watching the whole thing, burst out laughing at me and said, "You know what that's called?" I said, "Yes, mom, it's karma," as she continued to giggle away.

The Long for Life president came into Unit 58 after I was there for a month or so. He came to show me "the difference between a signature and an autograph." They got me to do my signature again and again and again on this blank white piece of paper and being so drugged up I thought nothing of it at the time. My porter then came to take me to speech therapy, and They decided to tag along. In speech therapy that day, my therapist told them what she and I were working on; a small, one-page pamphlet about Long for Life. It was just a small test we were doing of my cognitive abilities. It was something that simply stated what my story was, what the mission was, and a little information about it. When my therapist told the president what we were working on they said to her, "I don't want him to think he can take over when he gets out of here." I pretended like I didn't hear them and stared off into space. But really, I was there thinking in my head, 'yeah because making a one-page pamphlet to see if my cognitive abilities and thinking skills were still intact gives me a Master's in business and makes me ready or makes me want to handle a non-profit organization when I can't even dress myself.' I just laughed it off and put it on the list of odd things I was starting to realize about them.

In November, I was allowed to leave the hospital on a day pass to go to my grandmother's house for Thanksgiving dinner. My mom picked me up and we drove to the small city of Chestermere where my grandmother still lived right beside the Lloyd family's old house. We pulled in, my mom took out the wheelchair and I transferred into the chair from the passenger seat. She then wheeled me through the white gates, and over to the front deck where I was now facing about half a dozen stairs. It was my first time being disabled and not having a wheelchair ramp at my destination. Being me, I said, "Screw it. I'll walk from here." I locked the wheels on my wheelchair, moved the armrest and leg rests, then stood up. One step at a time at the speed of an arthritic-riddled grandma moving in slow motion I began to climb up the stairs. Each step probably took a good dozen seconds. It took a while but I made it up the stairs with people all around me ready to catch me if I fell. I got to the top without falling and had a small celebratory moment as it was my first big, obvious progression since my stroke.

Back in the hospital, with the lack of entertainment, I found myself wandering around for hours on end daily. Every building, every level, every unit, and all the tunnels I rolled through, just for a change of scenery. I was heading back to my room one day and the elevator opened so I got off and went left to my unit. As I'm wheeling myself down the hall, I hear a nurse say, "Yeah, I don't think you want to go that way, buddy." I then hear the ear-piercing screams of another woman just down the hall and the nurse said, "There's someone having a baby down there." I suddenly realized I got off at the wrong floor. Every floor was designed and laid out the same way, so it all looks the same and it's apparently easy to get confused and roll into the wrong unit.

The lack of kinesthetic awareness (feeling) on my left side was really tripping me out and to this day I haven't gotten used to it. In the hospital, probably about halfway through my stay, I found myself so bored. I remembered the scene in Ricky Bobby Talladega Nights where he thinks he's paralyzed from the waist down and to prove it to his friends he stabs himself in the leg with a knife, only to realize he wasn't paralyzed, and he could still very much feel it.

I looked at the hospital table beside me and there was a pin sitting on the table. I couldn't help but wonder if I would feel it if I stabbed myself like in the movie. I grabbed the pin and disinfected it with a sterile wipe before I put it on my left thigh and slowly began to put pressure on it until it broke through the denim jeans I was wearing, making a little 'tick' noise when it went through. I then slowly began to put more pressure on it now that it was on my bare leg and I felt nothing. Slowly putting more and more pressure on it I felt it slide into my thigh. But I didn't feel it in my thigh, I felt the needle pierce my flesh in my hand that was holding the needle. Feeling a foreign object going into your body by the tension of the skin around the object has got to be one of the most unpleasant things I have ever felt.

Yet immediately after I stabbed myself with the needle without feeling a thing, I thought about upgrading to a steak knife, because how often does one get the chance to stab themselves and not feel it? I'm sure it was just a stupid boy thing, or more likely a stupid me thing. However, in the hospital the only knives you have access to were plastic. Plus, I figured my nurses would be very unimpressed when I called them for stitches because I drove a steak knife into my own leg. Also, I didn't exactly know where the big arteries in the thigh were and didn't want to run the risk of hitting one and bleeding out so I never could upgrade to the steak knife.

After the feeling of the needle going into my skin, it's probably a good thing I couldn't upgrade to the knife because I probably would have vomited feeling the tension of my skin around the blade of the knife in my hand and not the pain of the knife penetrating my skin. I thought back to when my dad and I were in Montreal when I skated past the guy sticking a needle in his arm, just the thought alone had me quiver and sent shivers down my spine. I can take needles others administer to me all day, between my Botox injections and acupuncture, I've taken forty-five needles in a day and have been fine enough to go skate after but giving myself a needle (to me) is completely different.

At one point in the hospital, it was decided to give me Botox injections to help with my crazy muscle tone and spasms. I was taken to get these injections in my left hand, forearm, arm, calf, ankle, and foot. I got to my appointment and the doctor had an ultrasound machine on my arm looking at the individual muscle groups to inject. He then brought the needle up to my arm as I was watching and asked, "Are you ready?" I said, "Yup," as I looked away, so I didn't have to see the needle going into my arm. I sat there looking off into the corner of the room waiting and waiting wondering what was taking the doctor so long, so I looked back. When I looked back, he was sticking this needle in and out, in and out, and back in different places at different angles like my arm was a pin cushion. Watching this, I instantly wanted to vomit, but I was equally intrigued that I couldn't feel a single thing. It was surreal; I could see my arm there in physical form, but it felt as though it wasn't even a part of me anymore. It was as though my doctor was sitting there stabbing a dummy's arm (I guess he was, if you think about it) nothing he did I felt the tiniest bit and it felt like my arm was no longer my arm, but a twenty-pound foreign object that was connected to my body. I looked away and I stared off into the corner again trying to feel him give me the needles, but I didn't feel a single one. I looked back every now and then to see him still stabbing my arm, wrist, or hand everywhere with this needle and couldn't bear to watch it as it made me nauseous. But at the same time, I couldn't look away because it was a very weird experience to have.

It wasn't long into my hospital stay when I couldn't help but relate the similarities between my stay in jail and my stay in the hospital. In jail, I was physically held there behind steel bars, locked doors, and concrete walls. Then in the hospital I was also physically held there. Not by bars and concrete walls but by my body and the fabric curtains that surrounded my bed. Of course, I could get up and leave at any time unlike jail, but I physically couldn't leave as my body wasn't able to get back out into the world. In each place I was there held against my will, I couldn't leave, I ate terrible nutrient-less food all day, and I was in a building that had a bunch of crazies. I could only adapt to the situation I was in and do my time until I was able to go. It literally felt like a one-hundred-and-five-day jail sentence. The food quality was about the same too, and not in a good way as making twelve-hundred meals three times a day is a monumental task and nearly impossible to make them all look, taste, or feel good. Which was why I was missing breakfast and lunch just so I could force down the rubber textured dinner with no nutrients.

Once I had gotten on my feet and I was hobbling a bit better I was told by my therapist I was able to go home on a night pass to grab some personal effects. After work, my auntie picked me up to bring me home for the evening. As we were leaving my unit one of the nurses came up to us and asked where I was going. I told her my therapist approved me to go home on a night pass to get some things. The nurse however had a different opinion and said, "No," and, "You aren't ready to go anywhere." I again told her my therapist said it was okay, but she didn't believe me. She tried to say I couldn't go anywhere, and my auntie got right in her face and said, "What? Are you calling him a liar? He said his therapist gave the okay, so I'm taking him home for the night." Once my auntie got in her face, the nurse quickly backed off and we left.

On the way home, we stopped by the mall to bring my ring in for repairs. I had no wheelchair, no cane, no braces, and no walker. It was just me on my own walking at my new normal, slower than a turtle walking speed. As I'm hobbling to the store out of nowhere a group of three young teenage boys came walking by me on my left side. As they walked by one of them said out loud to his friends, "Ugh, I hate when people walk so slow." When I was a young impatient teen, I wouldn't have been able to agree with the kid more. However, I've been out of my teens for a staggering-few months and was just recently half paralyzed, I felt that that was another story completely. I said, "Hey, buddy!" All three of the young guys turned around and looked at me and I told them to come over for a minute.

They walked over to me in my big baggy hoodie and jeans then I proceeded to tell them about the last seven months of my life from my longboarding trek to waking from my coma. When the one kid heard the words, "I woke up half paralyzed on my twentieth birthday about a month ago," he suddenly realized the magnitude of his arrogance and I literally watched his face sink lower than the droopy paralyzed left side of mine and I said, "You can't tell what someone has gone through just by a quick glance, boys. Try not to judge a book by its cover." All of them just stood there frozen as I continued on my slow hobble down the tile floors to the jewellery shop.

Back at the hospital a few days later, my mom came to see me one afternoon. Just as she walked in, my nurse came in with my medications. My nurse told me what each pill in the cup was and what it was for. My mom noticed one of the pills she was about to give me I wasn't allowed to take as it was a blood thinner, and my neurosurgeon didn't want me on them (other than my Heprin needle) because they make the risk of stroke higher. My mom told the nurse, "He's not to be taking that medication." The nurse had the audacity to look my mom in the face and say to her, "You can't tell me what to do." I swear my mom almost punched her through the roof. Instead, she got right in the nurse's face and told her that she was my mother and I'm not to be taking that medication and if she's got a problem with it go check my chart or with my neurosurgeon. The nurse walked away and didn't bother to come back, which was probably a good thing.

After my last stroke I've had a very hard time getting to sleep, staying asleep, and feeling like I even got any sleep. If or when I got to sleep it was a horrible, terrible, unrestful sleep and I'd wake up more tired than I was before I went to bed. After a month or two with no sleep, I thought I would try some sleeping pills. I don't remember what I was given but I took this sleeping pill one night and fell asleep. Then I started dreaming. I dreamt that I was back home at my moms with my younger brother. I was cooking something to eat when my brother came into the kitchen and started bugging me. So, I took the kitchen knife I was using and told him "bugger off or else." He stayed mocking me, so I gave him a little cut. He then got a knife and cut me back, so I stabbed him, then he stabbed me, so I stabbed him back, and he stabbed me again. Next thing I know I'm there playing "stab for stab" for some time when my mother came downstairs and sees blood everywhere, both of us covered in blood with multiple stab wounds and she got right pissed. Her being a nurse, she stitched us up on the spot and told us to, "Knock it off" as she starts walking away. But my brother stabbed me one more time as he mocked her. My mother comes charging back, takes the knife out of my abdomen, and starts stabbing the crap out of my little brother. She went full on psychopath-crazy stabbing my little brother until he was dead. I then woke up from my horrifying dream like, "What the heck just happened?" I was then up for the rest of the night unable to sleep because I just watched my mother kill my little brother with a kitchen knife in the most real-feeling, vivid, messed-up dream I've ever had. I haven't taken a sleeping pill since, nor do I ever plan to.

I had quite a few roommates come and go as I was the one in that room in Unit 58 the longest. One night there was this one young kid that came in around nine or ten. My roommate and I were already trying to sleep as the post-stroke life is utterly exhausting. This kid comes in and gets placed beside me as the other Brandon was now gone from the room. Immediately I noticed he was talking to himself and after some short back and forth conversation he decides to turn on country music. He turns on his tunes so everyone could listen as well. The kid then starts saying to himself, "Oh my God yes, yes omg yes." He did this for what felt like ten or fifteen minutes straight. I looked across the room at Dean and he looks back at me as he rolls his eyes obviously as annoyed as I was. He called the nurse, and she came in, turned off his music, and calmed him down enough that I ended up falling asleep.

Next thing I realize it's morning time and the first thing I noticed when I woke was the stench of human excrement, again. I looked to my left where the new kid was supposed to be and there was a crew in there cleaning poop off the walls, floor, bed, roof, and the curtain that separated us. It turns out the kid had a fun time playing with his poop and flinging it around earlier that morning. Again, I was absolutely disgusted but I had to remind myself that some of the people here can't help it nor do they know any better because of their colossal injuries. To this day, I am so grateful that I was not one of those who lost full control over their bladder and bowels.

I didn't have any other place to go but back to my mom's when I was released from the hospital, only my mom just down-sized houses and my older brother moved back in as well. Therefore, the only place for me to sleep was on the pull-out couch in the living room. The absolute worst spot as I would be woken up any time someone came or went and every morning when my brother would use the blender for his protein shakes. It was incredibly frustrating and annoying. But at the end of the day, I'm the one that didn't pay rent for a crack den of an apartment till I left so I guess you could say I deserved it. I finally received the check for that housing charity while I was in the hospital but after purposely skipping breakfast and lunch just so I could be hungry enough to eat the rubber textured meat in the dinners for a few months, the check was mostly spent on food from the café and nearby restaurants and never made it to them like it should have. Then after my 3am incident in ICU and the time in the mall with the young teens, I used the little remaining money to get a tattoo that says "Only God can judge me" on my right forearm as a constant daily reminder to myself that you can't tell what someone has been through by their looks so stop judging them by their cover. Seeing as we live in a world where we are bred and raised to do exactly that, I figured I could use the daily reminder. Plus, after seeing how terrible the one kid felt after I told him I woke up paralyzed, and how bad I felt about getting upset because someone was in the process of dying, I didn't want to experience that same situation. So, I got the tattoo with the little bit of remaining money instead of spending it all at the café in the hospital or local restaurants, which I figured was for the better. Every night I'd wake up two, three, four, five plus times a night in pain, then a few more times in the morning, then I'd have to get up to do therapy as I had ESD (Early Supported Discharge) coming to mom's house doing therapy at home with me several times a day.

Only a few days after being home, I got hungry around dinner, so I went to the kitchen and began looking for food. Of course, I was sold on the box of pizza in the freezer, so I turned the oven on and waited for it to heat up. A short time later the timer went off to tell me the pizza was done so I walked into the kitchen, grabbed the oven-mitt out of the drawer, and then opened the oven to grab the pizza. I leaned down and as soon as the oven-mitt touched the pizza stone, I heard it sizzle like it was wet. I thought 'well that's weird, the oven-mitt shouldn't be wet.' As I'm in the thought process of wondering why it would be wet and sizzling, I caught a whiff of the worst smell I've ever smelt in my life. This disgusting stench immediately brought my attention straight down. When I looked down, I saw my left arm and hand just sitting on the inside of the four-hundred-and-twenty-degree oven door, cooking. I literally screamed like a girl, "Ahh!" as I grab lefty off the oven door with my right arm. I put the pizza on top of the stove then ran upstairs to show my mom my arm and she put cream on my new third-degree burns to help sooth them. I didn't even feel the burns until about a half an hour later which I thought was really weird, but I was glad that I could feel pain that wasn't my normal nerve pain for the first time in four-plus months.

Not being able to walk or function well meant I was unable to work and with not having a doctor willing to prescribe me medical marijuana due to the conservative government changing the laws every four weeks around it, it made it nearly impossible for me to get legalized. It took me ten months half paralyzed in a wheelchair to be able to legally smoke medical cannabis. Not that the being illegal was stopping me from doing so. Because when you are in so much pain you want to cut off your limbs or put a bullet in your head you don't care what's legal, illegal, right, wrong, moral or immoral. All you care about is not being in that state of torturous pain wanting to kill yourself. Luckily for me I had several medical patients help me out and give me some free bags of marijuana until I got my things figured out.

For supplement income, I was on "Alberta works" getting a huge $535 a month to live. My medical marijuana alone at that time was around $600. So, I made a mistake and called the government and said, "You guys don't even pay me enough to cover my medications." The lady responded with, "We send you a health benefits card every month to pay for your medications." This card is only valid in Alberta. I then told her that my medication came from either Ontario or British Columbia at the time, so it was not covered by their benefits. The lady asked what my medication was, and I told her it was "marijuana." She just laughed at me and hung up the phone. The amount of rage and anger that built from that lady still lingers on to this day. I remember saying to myself, "Are you kidding me, you bitch!" and threw the house phone clear across the living room in a fit of rage. Here's a medication that has literally kept me from killing myself, kept me from overdosing, and kept me from losing my life to the opiate pandemic, again and she blew it off, probably because of her negative bias opinion on the subject. I realized the government would rather support big pharma creating drug addicts with the heroin products they push rather than help people. I guess that's to be expected when your healthcare system is based solely on profit, government insurance-based pharmaceutical contracts, and not the health or wellbeing of the people.

I was back to square one, I had next to no income with minimal pain medications, I was unable to work, or even do any of my hobbies. I then realized what my life had come to. Get up, take pills, do ESD therapy for hours on end, then try to go to bed. Only to wake up three hours later and repeat it all over again. After months of fighting, I finally got on AISH (Assured Income for the Severely Handicapped). It was much better pay but still my medications took up half the monthly check and after the Alberta Works incident, I wasn't even going to attempt to call AISH and ask them the same question. My mental health was declining at an alarming rate. With the lack of sleeping, crazy amounts of pain, daily frustrations, and my new dead-end nine to five therapy life, I was getting more depressed and increasingly ready to give up. The thought of death again started to sound to me like something much greater and better than life. Life was once again a heaping pile of rubbish that I just wanted to end.

My first case worker out of the hospital was another joke. The first day I met her, I told her about this therapy device that was recommended by a therapist to help get my left, paralyzed hand working again. I told her about the device and asked if they would be able to fund it. She told me they would and if not them, another organization they work closely with would. I just needed to do a few things first. The first thing was I needed to get my body physically ready for the device as I wasn't even close to being able to use it. I then had to get a prescription, a doctor's letter of medical necessity, get sized and fitted, then have a trial run with the device.

After months of therapy, I had a trial run with the device that went very well. I got the prescription, and everything required for them to fund it, then I brought it all in and submitted it. I then waited for a month, then two months, then three months trying to be patient. After no return phone calls, I went to her superior six months after submitting the work. That day, I got a call back from her that said, "It's too expensive we don't want to fund it." I was so angry. I could have been fundraising or saving to help them the entire time, but I trusted the system would help me out. The most frustrating part was by now I had pretty much adapted to life with one arm and hand and had lost the sense of importance to get the device. It was a comforting yet frightening realization to see that we are adaptive creatures and that it was easier to adapt to life with one arm, than it was to get the paralyzed hand working.

By now, I was on my feet walking and longboarding a bit and the summer went by, then another went by, and the fact I was on my feet but still had not made any progress on finishing my trek was eating at me. So New Year's 2016, I made my life's first New Year's resolution to get back on the highway and finish it anyway I physically could, hopefully without dying. The lifestyle I was currently in was disgustingly boring and incredibly painful. It wasn't long before I realized there were two sides of recovery: the first is the physical side, the second is the mental. I found when you're so enveloped with negativity and pain twenty-four hours a day, you have to find things to focus your mind on. For me, I assumed the "Long for Life" organization would have been that mental escape I needed to recover, but people had other plans.

Once I started asking questions about the organization, I was given the run around. Again and again, I would ask them a question and they would go on for hours talking about something else I didn't ask about, trying to deflect my questions. The more I asked about it, the more run around I got. I clearly wasn't going to be a part of it as it was now not my dream or my vision, but theirs. I was told I could see the books but I was not allowed to go get a second or professional opinion about them, and that was the last straw for me. I was not okay with being the face of an organization and not being allowed to see the details in the background. I then remembered when the president came to the hospital to show me "the difference between a signature and autograph" and had me do my signature again and again. Suddenly I got incredibly uncomfortable with that and became more and more suspicious to the point where I felt I had to quit the organization and did August 22nd 2014.

I abruptly felt I couldn't trust or respect the people who felt the need to take charge of my life story and dream, so I decided to distance myself from all of them. The stress drove my mental health right into the ground and amplified my depression, frustration, anger, and pain. At one point, I was forcing myself to eat breakfast (around suppertime) and while I was putting peanut butter on my toast, I felt like I was about to pass out. I suddenly realized I wasn't breathing. I was so stressed I literally subconsciously forgot how to breathe. Even my beard and the hair on my head started to go grey because of the overwhelming amount of stress. When you are surrounded by nothing but pain and negativity every second of every day, you need that mental release. The only one I had was music, and for some reason after my third stroke music really started to resonate with me. There are many artists that are incredibly good at having you picture life in their shoes or the situations they depict and talk about. I put myself in my half-paralyzed position, in their shoes, imagining living in the world they describe and what they had to do to persevere. It made my brain break from the unfathomable obstacles they had to overcome. The music was an incredible reminder of how good I still had it, and how blessed I am to be from a place that has healthcare and at least some disability programs, but it wasn't quite enough to get my head out of the endless anxiety-filled frustration I was in.

What was I going to do for work now that I physically couldn't work? Screw a dead-end job, what was I going to do for a career? I had spent all this time, energy, and focus on finding myself, making my peace with death, and trying to accomplish something before I died that I completely tuned out what everyone else focuses on, like an education, a career, and a family. I hardly had any independence let alone a job or career path.

I had no clue what my mental escape was going to be from. Besides my music providing a minuscule escape I had to then figure out what to focus my mind on. I started to recall the get-well cards I got from Reston, Manitoba and as much as I wanted to give Lori a call and thank her, I knew a phone call wasn't enough for the amount of hope, courage, love, and inspiration they had given me. I also remembered how much my story impacted a few people at a MADD victims conference I went to in Toronto. I thought I would put together a presentation, go to Manitoba, and give a presentation to the school to personally thank them all. There were only two problems with that. For one, I was absolutely terrified of public speaking, so I knew I would have to start to overcome that, and secondly, I still had to finish my cross-country trek.

As for public speaking, I had no idea what or how to do it so I looked up online a good way to face public speaking and came across Toastmasters. I had been to a few of their meetings before and thought it would be a good place to start. I looked up the closest clubs in my vicinity and went to a meeting to check it out again. The first meeting I went to was filled with amazing people who each had their own amazing character and a profound positive outlook on life as speakers, and as leaders. After the first meeting I knew I had to join this amazing group of individuals. I signed up for six months to test it out and I ordered my books online.

At the same time, I was thinking about finishing my trek in my wheelchair, so I took it out one day, got in, and rolled over to the gym less than one kilometre away. That less than one kilometre took me almost an hour and by the time I rolled there on the mostly flat ground I was utterly exhausted. So, I took my longboard to Fish Creek Park and began to record my longboarding speed which was at a regular person's walking pace around four or five kilometres per hour. I had asked my dad in the hospital if we could take an entire summer to finish the trek. He said it would cost too much, which he was right. To physically and financially finish it, I would have to do as much as I physically could in the shortest amount of time. So, I started to look into other physical modes of transportation. Rollerblades maybe? A scooter perhaps? Both were unappealing and a death sentence with my inability to move fast enough to safely cruise on them down mountain roads. Someone had asked if I could still bike, and I made the terrible assumption that I could. So I took a look online, found a bike, and had a friend take me to pick it up.

While I waited for my Toastmasters books to come in the mail, I continued to go to the meetings every Thursday and every time I went, the confidence of these speakers and how they delivered their speeches was amazing. I realized I was at the "bottom of the totem pole", and I had much to learn from these outstanding individuals. Once my books came in, I began my "ice breaker" speech, which was a basic five-to-seven-minute speech introducing myself to the group. I started to put together a short speech about my life, then I set a date with the chapter to deliver it.

I was really nervous as I headed to the meeting in the taxi. I was the first one there, so I signed into the building and waited for the others to arrive. The meeting started and we did our round of introductions around the long table before I was called up to do my first speech. I have always hated this moment and was a little unsettled and honestly wanted to throw up with anxiety. But between the lack of contents in my stomach and not wanting to be that guy that spewed at his first speech, I held it down and began delivering my first talk. I started to tell them my life story about my brush with cancer and my dances with strokes before moving onto my trek across the country up until I had my last stroke. Before I knew it, the lights at the end of the table started to switch colours indicating the length of time it's been. I wrapped up my speech before everyone took a minute to fill in an evaluation form.

After my speech, there was another speech before we moved onto "table topics" then we were read a single evaluation from the designated person for the meeting and after an hour we closed the session. After the meeting as I waited for my taxi, one of the members came up to me and told me how he was blown away to the point he had a few tears running down his face. As I headed home, I had everyone's evaluations in my notebook but I was too scared to read them because I wasn't at all confident in myself as a speaker, and figured they would all be bashing my abilities. Once I got home, I sat down and made myself go through them one by one. At first, I thought I may have gotten the other person's forms but after looking and finding my name, I was shocked at what everyone had to say. Every single person was moved by my short speech and had nothing but good things to say. I had a little bit of feedback on how I could improve with simple things like eye contact, and body language, but it seemed to go really well.

I was really surprised at how well I did at doing the thing I feared the most in the world. I started to look at my next speech project and got to work, and then the third. At one point, I even won first place in a humorous speech contest at my chapter. Speech by speech my nervousness and anxiety was getting lower and lower. With the kids' get-well cards from Manitoba and their enveloping love still plastered all over my room as a constant, positive daily reminder I started to put together a speech that was just for them and contacted Lori in Manitoba to see if she was interested in having me come out. She talked with the school and gave me a date to come deliver my speech. But I was going to go from doing a five-to-seven-minute speech in front of eight to twelve people to doing an hour-long speech in front of an entire school and faculty, and I was nervous. But first I had to finish my trek, so we planned for me to come a short time after I planned to finish it. It was incredibly weird for me to go from the shy, strong, silent type that never told my story or hardships to anyone, to now sharing it with anyone and everyone. The best part about it all to me was every single time I gave a speech, it had a profound, positive impact on at least one person in the audience. An impact that would forever change the way they think about their own struggles, an impact that helped them persevere and overcome their own physical and mental hardships, which was beautiful to see.

Post-stroke Shenanigans

When you're affected by tragedy, you must keep your sense of humor, I find laughing and having fun is absolutely critical in order for both one's mind and one's body to heal, which is partly why I am **a shithead for life**. Shortly after I was released from the hospital, I was at the store with my mom and two brothers. As we walked down one of the isles, I was kicking my older brother's foot when he was mid-stride walking, like I did to the guy when I was in grade two just being a little shit. I did it once, then twice, then another for fun. My older brother obviously got annoyed and told me to screw off. So I kicked the bottom of his foot one more time. When I did that, he turned around and punched me just as an older lady turned the corner. The lady walked around the corner only to see my brother hit me. I turned to him and said, "You know it's not nice to hit a cripple." My brother said, "I don't care." The lady who turned the corner to see the big buff man punch a hobble head with multiple braces and a cane looked at my brother and said, "Well, that was just rude," and kept her eyes on him as she continued shopping not knowing I definitely deserved and instigated the whole thing.

I was heading home from an awesome Bridging the Gap meeting downtown Calgary one afternoon when my left leg started going into spasms making it very hard for me to walk. So, I stopped, opened my backpack, took out a marijuana cigarette, lit it, and kept walking towards the train station. Within a few minutes my leg calmed down and I continued walking, smoking my medication. I was crossing McLeod Trail towards the train station when I saw two police officers in uniform on the corner arresting someone. Still smoking my marijuana, I walked past the officers and the person they were arresting and kept on walking. Right as I was about to go up the spiral ramp to the bridge at the station I heard "WOOP WOOP" I took out my headphones and turned to my right and there were the two officers now in their van pulled up to me. The officer driving said, "What's in your hand?" Still walking slowly, I said, "It's just some of Canada's finest weed officer, I voted for legalization, so its legal for me, right?" He looks at me and said, "Yeah, not so much." I dropped my jaw and open my eyes wide like I'm in shock and scared to get in trouble. I take another look at the officer driving, and I said, "Okay, well, bye bye then," and as fast as I could, I hobbled to the back of the cop van like I'm trying to run away from them. Once I got to the back of the police van, I stopped and took out my wallet to show them my licence to prove that I'm federally legal. The passenger officer came running around the van with his hand on his baton looking like he's ready to kick my ass. The officer that was driving then came around the van and I gave him my marijuana licence and ID before the officer went to run my name and the other officer and I had a quick chat. When he found out I was legal, he told me his thought process as I walked by them smoking my joint. He said he thought to himself, 'Man, the balls on that kid.' I laughed and started to tell him my story and explained how you have to find little ways to have fun with life after a tragedy, and that includes pretending to run away from the cops to get them going. The one officer driving thought it was pretty funny, but the other officer looked really pissed off at me. After the officer ran my name, he handed me my ID back and (still smoking my joint) I walked away. As I'm walking away, I heard people talking and I turned around to see a group of homeless people at the shelter witnessed everything. Keep in mind this was well before Canada legalized cannabis.

There was also the time I was at a hockey game with one of my friends and we decided to pre-drink at his house instead of paying eight bucks for a crappy beer at the game. I went and got a bottle of rum and, at his house, I ended up drinking most of it myself. Then we got on the train and headed to the Flames game. Once at the Saddledome, we got to our seats and my buddy bought us a tall can of beer for the first period. Once the period was over, I headed to the bathroom. When I left the bathroom, I was walking down the stairs heading back over to my seat. As I was walking back, all of the drinks hit me at once and I was suddenly too drunk for my own good. To make things better, while I was walking to my seat, I did a huge four-foot zigzag when my muscle tone kicked in. Of course, right when this happened a group of police officers walked around the corner to see my drunken cripple waddle. One officer looks at me and said, "Whoa, are you okay, man? You look like you've had a few too many." It was indeed true, but I didn't want to get tossed from the game one period in. So, I replied with, "Yeah, officer, a few too many strokes, kind of makes it hard to walk sometimes." He responded with, "Yeah, I seen your arm, enjoy the game." "You too, officers," I said back as I went back to my seat feeling guilty I just used my disability to get out of trouble.

Every time I went to Toronto for a MADD victims conference, I brought my medical cannabis. However, they didn't catch it at security the first time even though they tore my mom's entire bag apart. Then when I went with my grandmother the next year, they missed it again but tore my grandmother's bag apart as well. We all found it funny how the one with the bag full of drugs went through just fine, but the ones with a deadly pair of nail clippers or a small bottle of shampoo not in a plastic bag was viciously torn apart like it was full of contraband. Because I never got caught or stopped or even asked, for years, I didn't know you had to declare your medical cannabis when taking a flight.

So, when I decided to go to Thunder Bay, Ontario by myself for a Survive and Thrive canoe expedition with twelve other amazing cancer survivors, I had not only brought my dried cannabis, but I brought marijuana gummies, suckers, drink mixes, and chocolate bars for the discrete medicating. I literally had a non-transparent, black bag full of nothing, but marijuana products and I went through airport security with it. My bag gets scanned, and I hear someone shout "rescan" before they rescan it and call for a manager. The manager comes and scans my bag for a third time before she came over to me with the bag. She reaches into my backpack and pulls out the non-transparent, black, plastic bag that's full of the marijuana products and asked me, "What's in this bag?" I responded with, "Oh, it's just all my weed." I grabbed the black bag, flipped it upside down, and dumped out the mountain of cannabis products all over the stainless-steel counter. The lady's jaw almost hit the floor and she immediately said, "I'm going to have to call the RCMP." Cool as a cucumber I said to her, "No worries, I know you're just doing your job, I'll be right here," while I stood on the other side of the big stainless-steel counter.

About two or three minutes go by and I still have all my marijuana sitting on the table while everyone taking flights is walking by as they pass through security. I saw the police officer coming up on the other side of the big counter and I pretend like I don't see him coming. The officer got closer to me and as soon as we made eye contact, just on the other side of the security counter from each other, I said, "Well it's time for me to go," and I started walking away. The officer flew around the counter and grabbed my right arm saying, "Where do you think you're going?" I simply, calmly replied, "I was just going to the washroom before my flight, sir." He then said, "You and I need to have a little chat first," as he takes me back to Weed Mountain still sitting on the security table and asked, "What is all of this?" My reply, "It's all labelled, as you can see, it's a variety of marijuana products. Probably a couple thousand milligrams of THC between the suckers, drink mixes, chocolate bars, and gummies, then my actual dried cannabis is in all these containers," as I hand him one. I was then *finally* asked if I had a medical marijuana licence. I took out my wallet and showed it to the officer who went to the manager and got my flight information as I sat there packing up my cannabis products. The officer came back with my medical licence, passport, plane ticket, and handed it to me saying, "Have a good flight." "Thanks, officer," I replied as I walked away to my gate. I saw a few people in the terminal that walked by me and Weed Mountain in security and they were looking at me as I walked to my gate like, "How the heck did he get through security?" This was also several years before Canada legalized cannabis.

Pain

Tragedy in this world is inevitable and the pain it brings can make it incredibly hard to want to live some days, and while you just think about how friendly death sounds in your head you are entirely drained with no energy, no focus, and no will or want to go do anything, even with your closest friends. Pain will have you wish that it was you who was killed just so you didn't have to deal with the reality you're stuck in. However, it's not just the physical pain that can cripple and break a person. The mental pain was, is, and always will be more than half the battle. The mental pain can be enough to make it physically hard to breathe, mentally unable to think or concentrate and bring you into a dark hole so deep that at some point, you'll truly believe that hole is where you belong, and you eventually call it home. But that's the negative mentality that one must shed in order to persevere. So, fuck that dark hole. You, I, and everyone else in the world doesn't deserve to live a life in a dark hole. **Life is meant to be bright, amazing, and beautiful, so make it just that.**

Before my last stroke, I thought I knew what pain was, but really, I didn't have a damn clue how painful life can be, and I know I still don't. For the first time in my life, I found the ability to distinguish the difference between physical pain, mental pain, as well as short-term and long-term pain.

My headaches can feel like a knife in the brain, it feels like I'm wide awake for an invasive brain operation and I can feel the sharp scalpel slicing through sections of my brain matter. If you live in the Calgary, Alberta area, you will have to deal with lots of chinooks (a warm gust of wind that comes from the Pacific Ocean through the mountains) several times a year or even several times a week. When this happens, it creates a huge barometric pressure change that will cause massive headaches to my mom, grandmother, myself, or anyone who suffers from migraines like us. When it comes through, you will see a straight line of clouds in the westward sky and the temperature will drastically increase as well. In the winter, it will be minus-fifty-degrees Celsius then a chinook will come through and it will suddenly be plus-five or plus-ten degrees. The drastic switch from winter to spring in a matter of hours is incredibly painful. Even for those who don't constantly suffer from migraines will come to Calgary, experience a chinook, and spend all day wondering why it feels as though a small bomb went off in their head. Some days, this pressure in the head is so bad you can literally feel every single heartbeat in your brain or your face, it's terrible.

Chinooks are not only terrible for migraines, but also for nerve pain. Every chinook literally feels as if I've been hit by a truck or fell off a tall building onto my left side. My fingers and hand will hurt so bad it feels as if they were blended off. They can hurt so bad I can't even feel them. This pain goes from my left hand into the forearm, up into the elbow, and through the upper arm into the shoulder before it goes into the left side of my chest and the left side of my back in my shoulder blade. It can feel as though I broke every inch of bone on my chest, back, and sometimes my face. The pain is excruciating, distracting, and incredibly debilitating all at once. On the really bad days, from time to time, this immense nerve pain even lingers into the left side of my face and feels like I just fought an MMA fighter.

Sometimes my shoulder will dislocate and pop out of place when I'm putting on a shirt, longboarding, or just going about my business. When it does go "POP," the pop is a very deep pop that sends this feeling from my shoulder into my stomach and gives it a little tickle. This stomach tickle isn't like a "hehe" kind of tickle. It's a very nauseating you're about to empty your stomach contents kind of tickle. If I don't puke on the spot, I dry heave, or at minimum, feel my stomach start to curl into knots. Even when I roll over onto my left side in bed it's enough to pop the humorous head out of the socket and the pain of the shoulder popping out wakes me up every time. It doesn't help that I roll like an alligator when I sleep either, I've had nights where it will pop out and wake me up to a dozen times.

Now when it comes to physical pain there is nothing that will ever be able to top the "phantom pain" I had experienced at the Foothills Hospital. The feeling of your hand being crushed so badly you can't feel it and have the pain hovering six inches in front of your face. Or to feel it in the corner of the room by the door was the single most physically painful and disturbing experience of my life to this day. I don't think there is much that will be able to top that.

Imagine being in a serious relationship or marriage with someone. This person was your everything, your heart and soul, and your true better half. Now imagine waking up one day and that massive inferno called love burning inside you, was just gone. It's been extinguished and you have no profound connection to that person any longer. But mentally you knew who they were, you knew what you've been through, but the raw emotion that bonded you together was extinct. The emptiness and loneliness I was left in, was unbearable to say the least. To this day, I still try to wrap my head around it, but just thinking about it breaks my brain and makes me feel sick. It was a mental pain like no other.

Now what if you spent years creating a plan to get your life on track. You finally find your life's greatest ambition and choose to pursue it almost getting close enough to see it through, only to have it all ripped away faster than you can think about your soggy ass. Having your life ripped away from you in mere seconds is not something anyone wants to experience. However, we are not even close to being in control of our reality no matter how much we believe we are. Every single one of us runs the risk of having our lives crumble beyond recognition on a daily basis. There is no way of entirely avoiding this because we cannot control another's mind or decision making. The only thing we can do is adapt to the change that is upon us and focus on a better tomorrow.

When it comes to recovering from the physical and mental pain, I find keeping physically busy doing things like walking, running, biking, swimming, or working out helps tremendously. The same applies to the mental healing. You need to keep your mind busy and active. For me, I found reading, playing poker, listening to music, doing speeches, and writing were all great mental distractions that helped get me by. The secret to my recovery was finding a balance between the two that worked best. I had to alternate between improving both my mental and physical health. I'd spend one day working on my mental healing and then the next, I'd spend on my physical healing and spend weeks in this routine of alternating back and forth. However, it's sometimes difficult to manage a social life in between all of it.

I have come to realize there are several forms of pain. As many ways as there are to be physically hurt, there are just as many ways to feel mentally and emotionally hurt. There is also the pain that comes and goes and there's the pain that seems to last forever. I find the short-term pain equals or very closely mimics physical pain. There are a tremendous number of ways to hurt yourself, just ask any guy; we do dumb shit, a lot. That's why women tend to live longer than us, however I consider physical pain to be more of a short-term pain, although it also can be long-term pain as well. For example, back in the 'longboarding with no shirt in Fish Creek Provincial Park days' when we're at the edge of the city and cheese-grate our body on pavement, it really sucks. You might have to spend a week or two sleeping sitting up just so you can heal. But two weeks is nothing, two weeks is a quick recovery. Breaking bones, also sucks but again an eight to twelve week heal is nothing. Stepping on a nail really sucks. But you can work through it and only takes a few days to heal if you avoid infection.

I consider the majority of physical pain to be short term. Even when I flew off a cliff and hit a tree on a mountain bike and ended up with internal bleeding, that only took a few weeks to recover from. However, serious physical injuries can also be in the long-term pain arena, and one hell of an arduous opponent. This may include but is not limited to cancer, stroke, and nearly every chronic mental/physical illness.

Long term pain I find closely resembles or mimics mental pain the most, however, again, serious injuries or illnesses belong here as well. For me, losing a loved one is one of the biggest and hardest forms of mental pain that I have had to experience. This pain lingers longer than any others. However, battling cancer is not only incredibly painful physically, but also absolutely debilitating mentally as well. A large number of cancer stories I've heard, take a long time of pain and suffering before treatments work, or death. There are also just as many stories where the cancer is found then the person passes within weeks or months. However, those few weeks or months are going to feel like years and decades of suffering. Then if the person sadly loses their life, that pain is felt by the loved ones that individual had in their life and leaves that pain to last for the rest of theirs.

Maybe it's not a death, maybe it's a heartbreaking, gut-wrenching divorce, or realization you have of someone. Either way, losing people you love is never easy no matter how you slice it. Even when it is necessary to cut off those individuals from your life, the fact that you're better off without them doesn't make things any easier. Eventually, time will show you that you were right (or wrong) but it's still a mentally difficult, heart-breaking process to put yourself through.

Family and Friends

Your family and friends are going to be your biggest support through hard times, I know without a doubt they have been for me. Spending time with friends, family, and loved ones is especially important because they know you more than anyone else. They're the best at making you smile, laugh, and feel good, which I believe to be one of the most important tools you need in order to successfully recover from a physical or mental illness.

That being said, your family and friends also know how to make you mad, frustrate you, and piss you off more than anyone else. They can and will push your buttons. They'll do it very easily, testing your patience more than ever. Sometimes you will just want to reach over and slap them upside the face over and over. But that's what friends and family are for, they test you, push you, and build you. In the end, it will not only make you a stronger person, but it will also reinforce your connection with that individual.

Your blood family is not your only family. For example, I have a huge longboarding family across Canada, I also have a huge MADD family across Canada, a cancer and stroke family across the globe, as well as a huge biker family in and around Calgary. All of these friends and families have had a huge impact on my recovery. Depending on the day, my mood, and what the situation is, I might reach out to people in every one of these families or just one or maybe none at all and go to my blood family. I feel confident there will come a time in your life when you'll see who is really there for you, who will fight for you, who is willing to help carry the weight of your cross, but most of all, why they are there for you.

For example, when I had my last stroke, it really brought the true people closer and pushed the fake friends and family away. It really showed me who cared enough for me to stay and fight by my side. That was a hard realization to see because some of the people I loved most, I ended up losing. That can leave you not even trying to rebuild those relationships, because if people are going to walk out of your life when you need them most, is there any point of opening the door and letting them back in? The reality is, when the going gets tough and tragedy strikes, you need them the most and if you let them back in, they will probably end up walking away again. They likely see having you around as a convenience or benefit to them but when that benefit or convenience is gone, well so are they.

These kinds of people are toxic, and I find they will only wear you out, bring you down, and be a catastrophic hindrance in your life and especially in your recovery. I think you are much better to cut the toxic people out of your life while continuing to progress forward. Life is too short to have anyone (family included) hold you back and or use you. Family should be there to ensure you live the best, longest, healthiest, and happiest life you will ever have. Not be a hindrance to your future and a negative effect on your success.

The ones that stick around and fight by your side, the ones that put up with your crappy attitude on your bad days, the ones that make you laugh and smile, the ones that support you in everything you do are the ones you want to keep by your side, hold onto, and fight for. They are the kinds of people that will help you out of your shell. They will help you fight through things like cancer or stroke, and they will help you see your dreams become a success. These are the kinds of friends and family you need to keep close to. Hold onto those relationships for the rest of your life, and most of all be grateful for the time you have with them because you might not have them tomorrow in this crazy, dangerous, and unpredictable world we live in.

The Little Things

It wasn't until my third stroke, that I realized how much the little things in life matter. It's not until you're unable to do these little things that you realize how much they truly matter and help get you through everyday life. For me losing the dexterity of being able to do small two handed tasks can bring an astronomical amount of frustration, which in turn brings on negative emotions, and that can really help me drive my days right into the ground. It took me a while to be able to zip up my coat or hoodie with one hand, sometimes I can do it within seconds and others it takes me up to five minutes. After my last stroke I gave up on dressing nice for a few reasons. First of all, I feel more comfortable in baggy loose clothing. I feel like baggy loose clothing hides my disabled stroke side better. Not to mention I am the biggest klutz in the world and if I was going to run the risk of ruining a shirt it's going to be the twenty dollar t shirt and not the hundred dollar dress shirt. But most of all putting on a button up shirt with 1 hand is a very meticulous and frustrating process. It can take me fifteen minutes to button up one button in the morning. Even with a button hook it can take me twice as long to get it on and off. The frustrations are enough to make me want to punch a (metaphorical) baby. The only two ways there are to get around this frustration is to force yourself to do it again and again until you strengthen the neuro pathways in your brain enough that it becomes easier and think of very different creative ways to go about the same task. I've not only had to become incredibly dexterous with my right hand, but even more so with my mind.

It's not just the little things in self-care and presentation that are important, but also the little things in every single daily activity. For example, trying to butter toast with one hand is very annoying. When you can't hold the toast with one hand and butter it with the other, the toast just slides around the plate. I now have to put my hip up against the counter and put the toast up to my hip on the plate then butter the toast towards my hip, so my hip is there to keep it from falling off the plate or counter. Then the same with the other piece. Again, it takes twice the amount of time to get the same job done. Not just buttering toast, but when you try to cut anything at all, like a lemon for example, you may be able to cut it in half on a cutting board once or twice but when you try to cut the smaller halves into halves without being able to hold it, you butcher the lemon, your hand, or both. Then by the end of it you have a juiceless squished piece of bloody lemon with more juices on the cutting board than in the actual lemon slice.

Getting snacks from the convenience store when you only have the one hand to use, can make it hard to grab more than one or two drinks or snacks at a time. I have to grab some items, then bring it to the counter and tell them I'll be back, then go get another handful and come back. Sometimes I hold up the line annoying everyone for the inconvenience at the "convenience store."

Post stroke, I now absolutely hate cooking with a passion. It's a mix of when I cooked lefty (my left hand) without realizing it and being reminded of the smell of my burning flesh whenever I think of cooking. As well as the pain, it is only having one arm and hand to cook with. For example, when you're making pasta and you need to stir the sauce and stir the noodles, you go back and forth, back and forth, back and forth, that's just for the pasta, now add your veggies, protein, and anything else you want. Now suddenly you have too much to prep, cook, and clean with one arm syndrome. When I do force myself to cook, I usually end up burning something and ruining it all anyway, so I now avoid cooking as much as I can which has made my diet terrible. I now pretty much live off of easy, quick things like cereal, toast, fruit, and light snacks.

Pretty much everyone knows how to tie their shoes. I know how, I just physically can't do it which is very frustrating because I have to keep my shoes loose enough to slip or force on. But when I have my shoes loose and my muscle tone kicks in, my shoe just falls off. I've had my shoe fall off as I'm walking down or upstairs in a busy train station. Or just when I'm walking down the street in the rain. It really sucks when its winter and I'm walking in snow and my shoe falls off. Not being able to feel it fall off until my foot is in snow really sucks because I then have to start back tracking through the snow to find my shoe that's usually then filled with snow.

When I do notice my shoe is untied in public I have to stop and ask a random stranger if they could please take a minute to tie my shoe for me. The normal response a twenty-five- or twenty-six-year-old gets when they ask someone to tie their shoe is usually judgemental remarks like people laughing and saying, "What, you can't tie a shoe?" It's not only embarrassing but it's also incredibly frustrating. I just have to say, "No, I can't tie my shoe," then follow up with, "I've had three strokes and my left hand is paralyzed." I recently started challenging people with an on the spot "Harrison challenge" when I'm in that situation by saying. "I'll give you a hundred dollars right now if you can tie my shoe tight enough with one hand." I then lie and say, "It will be the easiest hundred bucks you've ever made." To this day, not a single person has completed the on-the-spot challenge and claimed the hundred bucks from me. But it usually gets them to think about life a little differently and I tell them to try the "Harrison challenge" and see how long they can go through their day without using their non-dominate arm and hand.

I use a pocketknife to open almost everything I buy, but when you have the knife in your only good hand, it's tricky to open the packages because you can't hold them still. Sometimes I just stab away at it and end up breaking or damaging my purchase because I impatiently, and savagely stab, cut, and tear it open to get it. Having a small knife gets me through most of the things I can't open, as well works as a second hand in lots of situations. For example, most manufacturers use a stupid amount of plastic packaging for their products, so getting to them can be a challenge with one hand. Therefore, having a knife tremendously helps in my day-to-day life.

As much as the little things can bring you down and be a hindrance in your everyday life, it is also the little things you will come to appreciate and use to get you through the day. Since I have a huge hate for cooking and suck at it, I am always so happy and thankful when people cook me dinner or even help me cook dinner. I usually put off eating as long as I can. Sometimes unintentionally as my pain, broken brain, and medical marijuana are good at distracting me from feeling hungry. So, it's not unusual for me not to eat anything until supper or bedtime when my stomach starts making all kinds of gurgling noises that sound like a humpback whale's mating call. Once that happens, I know I have to cook something to eat but won't go cook because I hate it, I'm in a lot of pain and so sore I don't want to move, or I just don't feel I can stomach anything at the time. A lot of the time, even when I'm hungry after just a few bites I'll start to get sick to my stomach and stop eating. Then there are times I'll feel hungry no matter how much I eat. I either have an unquenchable appetite, or none at all, it's really confusing. Especially when I haven't eaten in days and eat only to feel worse than I did before.

I have noticed that setting goals (big or small) and getting them done on a daily basis is a nice little thing that will give you a sense of victory and good feels throughout the day. When I noticed that, I began to make "to-do" lists for everything. From food prep to many small goals that will lead to the success of a much bigger goal. I would make a to-do list, then get everything on it done, then make another, get everything done, and keep repeating the process until I got to where I needed or wanted to go.

Trying to hang up a coat when you have one arm is a bigger pain than you'd think, especially if you have no buttons and a zipper. When I go into a place or establishment where they hang your coat for you it's very nice. Also, when you have two arms full of stuff in one arm and hand, it's always a pleasure to have kind people open and hold doors for you. Even setting up the coffee machine before you go to bed so when someone goes to make it, they just need to press the button and turn it on before they can go about their morning routine is a nice little treat. Those are some of the little things that I've come to appreciate more as time goes on and as more time passes, I see, find, and experience more of these little things to get me by. I think it's imperative to be kind and do small acts of kindness like holding doors for people, because that small act of kindness can go a long way, just look at the tsunami that meeting Josh in the middle of the woods in Ontario caused.

Post-stroke Effects

I've had to deal with some of the most bizarre and unusual things when I came out of my coma. I not only lost the feeling and movement on the left side of my body, I had also lost my complete sense of balance. It wasn't only because I couldn't feel how my body was positioned when I was standing, but I would randomly lose all sense of direction out of nowhere. This was amplified when I was in the shower. The sensation of water running over my head confuses my brain and I lose all sense of direction when my head gets wet. It's like going from sober to the aftermath of drinking two forty-ounce bottles by yourself within a second.

Not only does water cause this, but even the wind can. On windy days or if I'm on the back of my uncle's motorcycle going for a rip, it happens. If I wear a half helmet, once the wind gets rushing over my head too fast, I lose my sense of direction, just like in the shower. The scariest part is, it happens as fast as flicking a switch, and let me tell you, when you're on the back of a motorbike ripping down a highway and all of a sudden you lose all sense of your balance, it can go from exhilarating fun and relaxing to absolutely terrifying real fast. If I wasn't on a Goldwing with my own lazy boy seat on the back, I would have easily fallen off going highway speeds.

My loss of kinesthetic awareness on the left side of my body causes all kinds of confusion and embarrassment. Because I can only feel the right side of my body, I only feel half as wide as I really am. Therefore, I'm constantly running into corners, poles, door frames, people and objects that are on my left side. To make things better, I still have a small blind spot in the lower left quadrant of my vision.

Nothing makes me feel like more of an idiot than reminiscing about when my buddy picked me up from the hospital and brought me home on a day pass so I could grab a few personal effects and escape the hospital for a bit. He picked me up and I was giving this new marijuana strain a try as we headed over to my mom's house. We got there, he parked out front, and then I grabbed the door handle on the passenger side of the car and opened it. I put my right leg out of the car and went to get out. But I just couldn't. I tried to get out of the car again, but my body was just not working. The last time this happened I woke up half paralyzed, so I started to freak out a bit with panic, worry, and anxiety.

I was starting to think, 'Oh my God, am I having another stroke,' as panic overcame me like a worried mother who can't find her child. I started to go over the stroke protocol, "FAST" (Face, Arms, Speech, Time) as I was going over that I realized I was not having another stroke and now I was just incredibly confused on why I couldn't get out of the car. I tried again, and again, and it was like I was glued to the seat. As I'm incredibly confused trying to figure out why I'm not able to move from my seat I looked down, and my seatbelt was still on. With the clip being on my left side, and not being able to feel my left side, I couldn't feel the strap holding me down. I unclipped it, got out, grabbed my stuff, and hung out for a bit before we left. One of the side effects from cannabis can be short term memory loss. So I blame that, the lack of feeling, and a dash of my own stupidity. I felt like such an idiot and can't help but shake my head and laugh every time I think about it.

I was walking in a store with a friend one day and as I came walking left around this big freezer bin, I didn't see the pile of milk crates that were stacked just around the corner in my blind spot and as I was minding my business talking to my friend, I tripped over the crates and flipped right onto my face. I couldn't do anything but burst out laughing and feel incredibly stupid at the same time. I peeled myself off the floor, dusted myself and my ego off, and we went back to shopping for groceries.

With the lack of feeling, sensation, and control of my left side, it causes all sorts of problems for me. Besides running into things, it seems to have a mind of its own at times. While on the train one day after watching a hockey game at my friend's house I was on my way home when my left arm fell off my lap in between me and the gentleman to my left. I didn't even notice or feel it fall at all. I only saw the guy look down at my arm after it fell to realize it had fallen. I went to bend my arm up and move it back onto my lap. Only with being incredibly rusty with it and being at the gym all morning training to finish my trek, my arm wasn't co-operating. When I went to lift my arm, it just did this chicken wing thing, and I nearly pushed the man on my left off of the train bench onto the ground. I could do nothing but break out laughing like an idiot, profusely apologize, and grab my arm to move it back while being super embarrassed.

There was no more embarrassing time than when I was on the train heading home and I gave up my seat to a lady with kids and a big belly with another on the way. The train moved one stop and it went from being relatively empty to being packed like the trains in China, there was no room for anyone. Just after the train filled up, we got on the move to the next station. While the train was creeping through the downtown core, I sneezed and when I sneezed my left arm flew out like it always does when I sneeze or get surprised, only this time it flew out and hit the bum of another passenger, of course it was a woman that was likely old enough to be my grandmother.

The woman turned around, looked me in the eyes, and then looked me up and down, totally checking me out. This woman then gives me an 'I'll take you around the block once or twice' kind of smiles just as I sneezed again. This time I caught lefty as it flew towards her buttocks, but it was too late by then and the embarrassment was done. As soon as she turned around and smiled at me, I felt my face go as red as a tomato. Luckily the second time my arm went flying at her, she saw and caught on that hitting her was a total accident. I profusely apologized for it, and all was fine, except my tomato-coloured face.

Sometimes these incidents are not so much embarrassing as downright frustrating to the point I want to throat-punch strangers. Again, on the train one day travelling north from the south end of Calgary, I got downtown to City Hall station and the train filled up. The booth I was in by myself was now fully occupied. Just after the train filled up, Limpy (my left leg) went into uncontrollable spasms. It wasn't my usual bouncing leg spasms it was a full-on tug of war between my quad muscles and my hamstrings. My quads were flexing and trying to kick my leg straight forward while my hamstrings and glutes were flexing trying to bring it back. As I was sitting there trying to fight the spasms, the guy now sitting in front of me just kicks my left leg, hard.

I looked down to see that my leg made its way to his side where my foot now lightly rested on his foot. Since I couldn't physically feel where my leg and foot was or feel that it was even touching him, I had no idea it was there. So, he just kicked my hypersensitive, paralyzed leg hard. It took everything in me not to punch him in the face on the spot, I know the old me wouldn't have even thought twice about it however between the combination of longboarding across Canada and my last stroke I was an entirely different person. I figured if I have nothing nice to say or do to him, I better just keep to myself and I did for once in my life. But my patience and emotions were sure put to the test.

It's not always on the train that I have these issues. Every single one of these issues can arise at any given time, in any location. I was at home having a pee one day, then I went to wash my hands, as I was washing my hand my muscle tone kicked in and pushed me to the right so naturally, I went to step my right leg out to catch my balance. Only problem with that was, the toilet was directly to my right. I was pushed to the right and went to catch my balance, but my leg wasn't able to move to the side and I toppled over the toilet into the wall taking out the toilet paper holder with my back in the process. Then to make matters worse, I was now stuck between the damn toilet and the wall. It took me at least five solid minutes of cussing, cursing, shimmying, flopping, and shaking to get un-stuck between the wall and toilet. It's the stupid things like this that make you late for appointments and buses which really aggravates the daily frustration and puts your patience to the test. For example, what if I was late for a date, what am I going to say? "Sorry I'm late, sweetheart, I was just stuck between my wall and the toilet." That's got to be the hottest pick-up line I ever did hear.

I've started to use the stalls in public restrooms because of my uncontrollable muscle tone. There have been a few times where I'm at the urinals trying to pee. For some reason after my stroke, it takes me like five minutes to get a pee going sometimes, even by myself, for whatever reason. I don't know if it's from my stroke or the catheters. But I'll be standing there and three people will come and go beside me and I'm still standing there. Then sometimes my muscle tone will kick in while I'm standing there and I'll accidently bump into the guy beside me who's just trying to pee in peace like I'm insinuating a sword fight and it creates a really uncomfortably awkward situation for me. So now I use the stalls and bounce off the walls like a crazy in the nut house instead of people.

At any given time, I can have the smallest of things put me on my ass. I was walking to the bus stop one afternoon. It happened to be an incredibly windy day and as I was walking down the main drag minding my business a big gust of wind caught me off guard. When this gust of wind hit me, it kicked up a white plastic coffee cup lid and threw it right in my face. Between the wind and the plastic lid hitting me, I went to do a back step to catch my balance only for my muscle tone to kick in and trip me as I stepped backwards. So really, I got hit in the face with a tiny piece of plastic garbage, and it knocked me flat on my ass.

I also have times where my body just doesn't want to work or cooperate with me, or completely fails to function at all. I was on my way to give a guest lecture at Lakehead University, October 2, 2018. While my friend (the professor) and I were walking up the stairs into the building, my left leg gave out like it did in Unit 112 when I tried to walk across the room to my bed unsupervised. Mid-stride, as we walked up the stairs with my laptop in my right hand, my leg gave out and I started to head for the ground almost tossing my computer down the stairs in the process. Luckily at the very last second, I caught myself and recovered, but my friend and I couldn't help but laugh at how closely the lecture was replaced with another trip to the hospital instead.

During that same lecture, I was in the middle of talking about something and Limpy went into spasms and started to shake my body. Luckily it was only a mild spasm that I was able to stop by putting weight on my left leg. But sometimes it goes wild, like it did when my therapist was balancing her whole body on my knee bobbing up and down. It just violently shakes and shakes without cause or any warning, which is another major cause of my running into poles, signs, walls, and tripping over milk crates.

One of my biggest problems post-stroke, is the effect it has had on my sleep, appetite, and body temperature regulation. The part of my brain that's had these brain aneurysms controls my sleep, appetite, body temperature, and some moods. My sleep has been drastically affected because I have an incredibly hard time getting to sleep, hard time staying asleep, and nine years later I have yet to feel rested when I wake up from a sleep. The four heavily-sedating medications I take from morning to bed time don't help the tiredness, drowsiness, and exhaustion at all. I am now tired every moment of every day. That alone can break a person down. Especially in the post-stroke life where walking across your living room can be utterly exhausting. You have one of two options. You can either fight through the drowsiness, set a plan of action, get your goals accomplished, and focus on getting things finished, or you can go back to bed to sleep your entire life away, do nothing, and get nothing done, ever. Seeing as we don't have a whole lot of time on this planet, sleeping your life away will get you nowhere. It will help you with nothing and will be absolutely sure you achieve nothing but a temporary moment of peace. But whenever you wake up again, you're still tired. I find I better stay out of the bed as long as I can. Going to bed and sleeping life away I think has a direct correlation to drugs, it momentarily provides you with that temporary escape, just for you to come back to reality and be exactly where you were beforehand. I just see it as a waist of precious time, so pain or no pain I make myself get out of bed and on with my day no matter how hard it may be.

My appetite is also very out of control because I hardly have any hunger sensation. For some reason, I don't feel hunger like I did before. I'll go a full day or two without eating and I won't even realize it. My hunger signal is no longer a hungry feeling in my stomach, although I do sometimes get that every now and then. Mostly, I realize I need to eat when I have a nasty headache, feel weak and drained with no energy, or I hear my stomach rumbling. I won't feel the rumble of my stomach, but I'll hear it and that's my cue to think, 'When was the last time I ate?' Sometimes that's the moment I realize it's been two days since I've eaten and I'll force myself to eat, occasionally making myself feel worse than before. On the rare occasion I'll wake up hungry and ready to eat, however when I go to eat, I'll take one or two bites of something and either feel sick or full and I'll stop eating. Then there are times I'll be hungry no matter how much food I eat. I could be hungry enough to eat a whole pizza by myself, do it, and still be hungry. Usually when I do manage to eat breakfast, I'm hungry again in an hour or two, then an hour or two after that. Or I'll just not eat all day and have breakfast at five or six in the evening. It's absolutely terrible not only for my body, but even more so for my mind.

Even more obliterated than my sleep and appetite is my body temperature regulation. I'll be cold for days, weeks, or months on end at times. I'll hide under a mountain of blankets, wear double socks, or winter coats over hoodies and shirts and it will do nothing for me. If I did put on tons of layers when I'm cold, I'll go from too cold to too hot in half a second and when I get a hot flash, I'll start to sweat profusely and it's really disgusting. Looking back, before I even had my strokes, I could tell that there was something wrong with that part of my brain because at the most random times throughout my early teens, I would get these uncontrollable hot flashes and I'd start to get incredibly sweaty for no reason at all. If I forgot to put on deodorant that day, I then became horrendously smelly which was embarrassing to say the least.

I'm very weird in the sense that I like to sleep in a slightly chilled room with the ability to warm up if needed. For example, at my mom's, I had a heated blanket under my bed sheets to act like a heated bed (awesome life hack by the way, especially in winter). Then I usually have my window open (slightly in the winter, and wide open in the summer). I'd also have a fan blowing air at my bed, and a heater in my room. All of this is so I can control my temperature in my bed. For example, the window open and the fan are to cool me down if I get too hot. If I get too cold the electric blanket and heater are there to warm me up. Since I'm constantly waking up throughout the night every night anyway, I'll wake up cold and need to warm up then I'll wake up again, this time too hot. If I'm too hot, I'll move the covers off and let the fresh air cool me off. If I'm too cold, I'll turn on the heater or the blanket to warm up. It's a constant battle to keep myself at a comfortable temperature just to try and get an hour or two of sleep.

Sometimes, it's incredibly frustrating as I'll be cold for weeks on end in the winter, then I'll be too hot for weeks on end during the summer. It's a constant never-ending battle. Especially in Canada where we complain about the freezing cold all winter then complain about the blistering heat all summer, there's not enough time that's just in the middle at a decent, acceptable temperature, we just go from one extreme to the other like flicking a light switch on and off.

I do have a few issues arise with my muscles being paralyzed and going into spasms. For example, since being paralyzed the muscles in my left eye have changed so much that I now have a stigmatism in my left eye from it changing shape caused by the muscles tightening or loosening. When it comes to muscle spasms, I'll have muscles I didn't even know existed go into spasms and throw me off balance, shake my body, or do weird shit. This is down to the tiniest muscles ever. For some reason at night time when I'm trying to sleep, and only at night time when I'm trying to sleep, my left tear duct will go into spasms. I'll feel it start to shake, contract, twitch, and vibrate. When this happens it's not painful, just more so annoying because once it goes into spasms it will leak tears. I'm not a crier so when I first noticed it, I was weirded-out and very confused on what was happening and asked myself, "Am I crying right now?" But nope, I'll be the happiest, luckiest, most grateful lad in the world not even the slightest bit upset, and it will go into spasms and leak. Sometimes it's only for a couple of minutes, sometimes it's for a couple hours, and at times it's all night long.

I'll wake up at my usual two to five in the morning and it will be like a small waterfall coming out of my left eye. I'll wipe my face off but it's of no use; sometimes it's so bad it literally looks like someone dumped a cup of water on my pillow. It can be funny too because I'll be able to see my face in the wet pillowcase. You'll see where my eye is because it's half dry then half soaking wet. Then you can tell where the outline of my face is, because of where the water seeps around my face it shows off my cheek bones and jaw structure. Sometimes I have to just toss my pillow off the bed for the night because it's so wet, uncomfortable, and gross.

It's not all physical damage I've come to notice. Since my last stroke I have noticed a significant change in my impulse control, which is not uncommon after a TBI (Traumatic Brain Injury) it can be in both good and bad ways. It's gotten me into trouble eating garbage food a lot. It's really exploited the unhealthy lifestyle in me, and it drives me crazy because I know better. But I'm just like 'meh whatever, I need to eat something at least' and don't really care. I still have to relearn how to control it, which is a lot like learning to walk; it's much harder the second time. I could see it getting me into a huge amount of trouble if I couldn't differentiate between right and wrong. Luckily, I still can, and I still have a conscience, probably more of one than I've ever had. The impulses can be good in the sense that when I want to do something like achieve a goal, I just do it. As soon as it comes to me, I get to work on it. Doing things in the "now" helps me tremendously because the "then" for me has become too unknown, now more than ever. I could be incredibly sore then, I could be hardly able to function then, I could be busy then, I could be stuck between a toilet and a fucking wall then, or like all of you, I could be dead then. Therefore, to me, there is no more of a better time to do things, than NOW.

Things I Was Ungrateful For

I can't even begin to explain how ungrateful I was for so many things, like being able to shower, go to the bathroom, dress, or care for myself in my day-to-day life. I truly believe that we all take these day-to-day life activities for granted until the day comes where we cannot do them and need help just doing the most basic things, we've done a million and one times before.

I spent one-hundred-and-fifteen days doing what I loved most in this world, Longboarding across my stupendously beautiful country. I pounded the pavement with my foot three-to-seven-thousand times a day riding some of the biggest and gnarliest hills the country had to offer loving every second of it, and I took it all for granted. One of the things I loved most in the world I took for granted. So, if you truly love something or someone, cherish every moment you have with it or them because you never know, it may just be your last time with it. Now when I say your "last time" with it, you may be able to get it back (like me and longboarding) but you may not be able to experience or feel it like you did before. I used to feel a great connection with my longboard. I used to be able to feel where every single wheel on the ground was and the sensation of the forward momentum, or the angle of the pavement, but now I can't feel any of it. I can only slightly feel half the board I'm standing on, everything else is gone.

Of course, I loved to play video games, but I now can't play the majority of games with one hand. I now have a huge hatred for video games because it's just a reminder of what I can't do anymore. However, on the bright side of not being able to play video games anymore, I can now spend my time on much more productive, life-changing things such as a career, hobbies, or my passions. So not being able to game doesn't bother me much until I'm at a friend's and they want to game, and I can't. Only then do I realize how much I took it for granted. Video games are nothing but a waste of time and a worthless distraction to me now, so I no longer care for them and have no desire to play them or to even try and get into them again.

I loved dirt biking and riding on 4X4's, but now I can't ride manual machines, I took that for granted. I spent hundreds of hours in my teens riding dirt bikes, and ATVs in the mountains of British Columbia, but most of it was at the Lloyd's place out in Langdon. Jake and I would ride them until they got so hot, we had to take a break to let them cool down for a few hours. From morning to dusk we would rip around the land having such a blast. It's been over nine years since I've ridden any machine and honestly, they kind of scare me with my new sudden loss of senses. Not to mention I no longer have a working left hand for the clutch, nor can I grip the handle with my left hand to help me in any way if I needed to shift my weight. So, putting me on any motorized ATV, motorcycle, or even a trike is now a very bad idea. I was riding a trike for the first time at Crystal Phillips Branch Out Bike Tour in the beautiful Panorama, British Columbia area. While I was riding on the road, it angled slightly towards the ditch which led to a ten- or twenty-foot drop into the river below and that slight angle of the road pulled me right towards the edge so I naturally would lean left so I wouldn't go right. But I was on a trike, and you can't lean on them like a normal bike as they ride the road, and I almost took a ride off the road into the river a few times. It was like when the pathway slightly tilted at the Royal Board Shop Wednesday evening cruise. I even took my sense of balance for granted and didn't even have the slightest clue until it was all taken from me. I guess that saying "you never really know what you have until it's gone" is a very true and harsh reality. I can't stress enough how important it is to be grateful and appreciate everything you have and can do in your life, because life has a horrific way of making you realize what you've taken for granted. From your ability to care for yourself all the way to the loved ones and family you have. "Appreciate them to the fullest extent and then beyond, because you never really know what you have, until it's gone." ("You never Know," Immortal Technique)

I took being able to care for and love my family and friends for granted. When your friends or family get sick or come down with an illness it is of upmost importance to care for them and nurture them back to health. Since my stroke I'm not the one that is easily able to jump up and go get icepacks, or drugs, or help them at all, but I still try my best. Mostly I am the needy one that needs help all the time and when you are physically unable to care for yourself there is no being able to help others, which leaves you feeling incredibly useless and helpless. I am just super happy I was back on my feet and walking again when my mom got her knee replaced so I was able to help nurse the nurse when she needed the help.

I even regretfully took the love I felt for my girlfriend for granted. Love is such a wonderful experience to have, and I am so grateful and blessed I got to feel, know, and experience what true love really was before I died. However, it took waking up half-paralyzed with no more feeling of love to realize that I had not only taken my entire relationship for granted, but I took that whole emotion of love for granted as well. I was incredibly disappointed, upset, and ashamed of myself for not being more grateful and appreciative of something so blatantly obvious.

I even took being able to stand or do the dishes for granted. The last thing me, or any teenage kid wants to do is simple household chores. I was never a fan of when mom came home and told me to do the dishes or clean up the messes my friends and I made. Then I'd have to stand there for a whole five minutes and go back and forth with the dishes. Not the most exciting thing in the world. However, shortly after I was home from the hospital my mom asked me to do the dishes and while I was doing them, I had flashbacks to therapy in Unit 112 moving a plastic ring from one location to another two feet away. I then realized I took being able to stand and move back and forth for granted. For the first time in my life, I was genuinely grateful to be able to do the dishes.

I was always good at working with my hands. Shop and welding classes were my best class's because I was so good at working with them. That was taken and I didn't realize how ungrateful I was for being good with my hands. I no longer have the ability to even tie my own shoes, button up my shirts, tie a tie, and it wasn't until my debilitating stroke, did I realize how ungrateful I was for this.

I was (and still am) a pretty active guy, I spent a lot of my teen's longboarding, biking, walking, and adventuring in Fish Creek. Strutting around exploring, climbing ridges, small cliffs, and trees. But it wasn't until now that I realized how ungrateful for all of that fun outdoorsy adventurous stuff I was. Adventuring is my number one go to when I am bored, sad, depressed, or just not feeling right. Now when you can't even walk there is no going to adventure unless it's the hospital in a wheelchair, but let me tell you, you can only roll through the same units, hallways, tunnels, and buildings so many times before you get super bored. Wheelchair adventuring was not my forte and was one of the biggest motivators for me to get out of my wheelchair and back to my feet. Only this time, I was going to be sure I was thankful and, even more so, grateful for every step I took.

When you have an event occur that makes you realize how ungrateful you were for everything in your life, it is a very eye-opening experience. I also found it can be very scary, because once you realize everything you took for granted, your mind draws a blank on everything else you've taken for granted. For example, I can almost guarantee all of us who have drinkable, running water and electricity, take it for granted. I guarantee your mind will draw a blank when you go to turn on the light and the lights don't come on or go to get a drink of water and no clean, drinkable water comes from the tap. It's not going to be until we are thirsty and in the dark that we will finally realize how much we took those things for granted. I can't stress enough how grateful you should be for everyone, everything, and every blessing we have in our lives before the universe makes you pay dearly for not. Because the universe sure has some sick ways of showing you your lack of appreciation for everything in your world.

The Power of the Mind

This blurb (chapter) in my book is also dedicated to my crazy old man. Dad thank you for opening my mind to the unlimited potential of the world and giving me access to one of the biggest keys of success in life. The plankton scale is the smallest unit of measurement we know at ten to the minus thirty-three.

The laws we know such as gravity do not exist here. Here there is a completely different set of laws that take place that are highly unusual. The way the world works at this small scale is very complex and astonishing. The study of this world is called quantum physics.

Looking into quantum physics I found that you can have anything or accomplish anything in this world by just thinking about it, envisioning it, and asking for it over and over and over, meanwhile setting goals that get you closer. You might not think you'll get it, but quickly giving up will never get you anything, you won't get what you want for days, weeks, months, years, or possibly even decades. But as long as you continue to ask for it, focus on it, envision it, and work towards it, it will come. No matter what it is you must be patient, optimistic, and hardworking.

When I was about thirteen or fourteen, my father showed me the movie "The Secret" and began to open my mind to the power of the law of attraction. When I saw the story of a woman that beat her breast cancer diagnosis by just thinking about it and willing it away, I was so flabbergast that I thought it was complete bull crap. There's no way someone could just think away one of the world's deadliest diseases. Being the arrogant, young teen, I brushed it off as rubbish and continued on with life.

Then about a year or two later, I had my first stroke and lost half my peripheral vision. Shortly after my stroke I was out in Langdon with the Lloyd family and while I tried to fall asleep on the couch in the basement, I suddenly remembered this woman's story and how she beat cancer. I thought about her story before I thought, 'Well, I have nothing to lose and everything to gain by trying.' So just like the woman explained in her story as I fell asleep, I went into a meditation of thinking to myself, 'Thank you for my vision, thank you for my eyesight, thank you for my ability to see again.' I repeated this again and again until I eventually fell asleep. Next thing I noticed it was morning time, I opened my eyes and stretched then immediately noticed there was a pinhole-sized spot in my blind spot that was now able to see. 'No way it works that easily.' I thought to myself. From that moment on, just like the lady battling cancer I thought to myself, 'thank you for my healing, thank you for my vision, thank you for my eyesight.' All day every day I was saying this to myself, and it wasn't long before I went from being half blind to only having a small blind spot in my lower left quadrant.

From that experience forth, I began to go into that meditation and just ask the universe for everything I want. Now you must be very careful what you ask for because the universe has really messed-up, sick ways of giving it to you. I feel positive that I can guarantee you'll get what you want in a way that you never would have imagined, guessed, or expected. It will leave you saying, "What the..." while shaking your head a few times over.

As an example, I spent years of my life on the wrong path trying to find the right one. I simply asked the universe for help changing me and my life for the better. Next thing I know I'm longboarding across the country and waking up half paralyzed. I never would have thought that these events would be what changed me and shaped me. It completely broke me, tore me apart, and literally crippled me. Now my life's biggest hardship, is also its biggest blessing because I got exactly what I asked for in the form of a seven-thousand-kilometre trek and a half-paralyzed body. I've used the same meditation technique for every situation I find myself in, for example I got caught in one of those situations where I spent a year and a half on probation where I was told I would never be anything, anyone, or achieve anything. So, I kept telling myself over and over in my head, "I can and will change my life for the better." I said this to myself over and over every night till I fell asleep. Then one day, I saw that Tupac quote that I really liked. It said, "If you can't find something to live for, you best find something to die for". Little did I know how drastically that quote would change my life for the better. If you want something, just keep asking for it and expect it to come in the weirdest way or in a way you never would have imagined. If there's one thing I've learned from it all, it would be to never underestimate the power of your mind and positive thinking, your thoughts can and will literally manifest your destiny.

The best personal example of being able to use my mind to ninja things away was about a year after my third stroke. After that stroke, I had so much brain damage that I was constantly having seizures. When I was having a seizure, I could tell only because it felt like someone was pushing me. If you've ever done salvia, lots of people experience an unseen force pushing them or pulling them to the ground. The feeling was just like an unknown force was pushing me to the right or left, but really, I was having a seizure and would be back in the hospital. I was at my friend's apartment one day when I got that sudden feeling of being pushed. As soon as I felt it start to come on, I screamed for my buddy. After screaming once or twice I thought to myself, 'This is really going to ruin my day.' That's when I thought to myself, 'No. This is not going to happen.' As soon as I thought 'no' the feeling of the seizure coming on just left and I didn't have another one until about five years later when I was on antibiotics for Pneumonia and having a few drinks with a friend while I played with a new toy and made some medications.

It was about 2AM when my right arm suddenly felt like I put it in a wall socket and a nice jolt of electricity went up my arm from finger to shoulder. I then flopped flat on the right side of my face cutting my right eye in an almost perfect X- shape. Now bleeding all over the kitchen floor and flopping from a seizure my friend quickly called an ambulance to come pick me up before calling my mother to let her know what happened. At the time, I didn't know that antibiotics and alcohol both reduce the effectiveness of seizure medications. Therefore, the combination of mixing them put me on my ass harder and faster than the personal bubble hash my roommate was stuck finishing for me.

Learning to Walk, Bike, and Longboard

When I was finally getting on my feet and walking regularly in therapy, it wasn't pretty. I needed four therapists and a shopping cart to assist me. I had one of my therapists watching my left knee, so I didn't snap it backwards, hyperextending it. I had another working on my core and gate position keeping me upright, standing tall with my shoulders over my hips, hips over my knees, and knees over my feet. I had another working on getting me to squeeze my shoulder blades together and engage my back. Then I had one poor therapist whose sole job was to hold up my pants as I was wearing baggy clothing and I lost a few inches during the five-thousand kilometres of longboarding, I also had no belt to put on.

The muscle spasms in my left leg were going uncontrollably and with my left leg just pushing across Canada for one-hundred-and-fifteen days it was still incredibly strong. My spasms started to go and my leg was bouncing like crazy so my therapist put her hand on my knee and pushed down to try and stop it, even with all her might forcing my leg down to try and stop it, it kept bouncing. As she stood at the end of my leg bent at a ninety-degree-angle as I sat in a chair, she then put her whole-body weight on my leg and was balancing on her hands on my knee. With her hands between her legs like she's in the middle of leapfrogging over someone she pushed her weight down till her feet left the ground hoping it would stop, but nope. She was still just bouncing up and down like it was a carnival ride. It was actually kind of comical to see. Since that didn't work, we just had to wait it out and let my leg do its thing for a good five or ten minutes.

Learning to walk the second time is much more difficult, although I can't really recall learning as a baby. However, post stroke, relearning to walk meant I had to relearn how to move every muscle individually. Once I was able to move the muscles needed to walk, I had to learn how to move them in sequence. This process is incredibly draining both physically and more so mentally. It was like I not only lost my physical ability to move and walk, but I also lost my subconscious mind that controls my ability to move and walk as well. When you walk, you just walk, there is no thinking about it your brain takes over and just moves the muscles like it does when you breathe. But for myself and every other stroke patient out there we actually have to stop and think okay use your quad muscles to lift and move your leg, then you have to think about engaging your glutes, hamstring, back, abs, and chest, all the while making sure you lift your toes when stepping, keeping your core muscles engaged, head up, as well as keeping your shoulders over hips, hips over knees, knees over feet, then still having to adjust accordingly when other muscles suddenly kick in from spasms.

When you add all of these things together it becomes incredibly physically and mentally exhausting. All it takes is one minor mistake while thinking about all of those things to cause problems and it will make me trip up. For me, it's lifting my toes and foot up. I usually forget to or can't from the muscle tone and I end up tripping over my own foot looking like I'm a super drunk guy, when I'm completely sober. It can be kind of embarrassing, but as the years went by my subconscious mind slowly began to get back into the rhythm of things. However sometimes on my bad days, my brain and body seem to not want to get along together. I can think of lifting my foot all I want, but if it's tired, in tone, or doesn't want to work, it has the mentality of a cat going, "Screw you, I won't do what you tell me," as it does the exact opposite of what I want. It will flop around and trip me up causing embarrassment, pain, and a stupid amount of frustration. On my bad days, I'm super slow because of how long it takes me to process every single movement. Between fighting the muscle tone, loss of balance, and physical control issues, it can take me a long time to go a very short distance.

I'll be walking just fine then mid-stride I'll have a muscle I didn't even know existed kick in without me knowing or even thinking about it. But I'll feel the muscle rub against my bone deep in my leg or I'll feel it stretch until it tears, causing extreme agony. When this happens, I really have to be lightning fast with my reflexes because I'll be going straight one second, then the tone will kick in and it's like someone just pushes me right or left out of nowhere, which is another reason why I'm constantly running into things. This usually happens first thing in the morning, I'll get up, get out of bed, start walking to the bathroom, then my muscle tone will kick in and suddenly I'm pushed into my wall or door frame or do a four-foot zigzag across the room. I'm just glad it usually happens at home in the morning and not out in public, although it does on the odd occasion.

Longboarding however is a bit different. When I get on my longboard, it's the same thing and I have to think of moving every muscle individually but in a different sequence. However, with my loss of balance it's a bit trickier. I'm also incredibly slower with my reaction time. It takes me two to five times longer to react to things. Like if someone decided to cut me off, I don't have the same control or reaction time to avoid them nor do I have the ability to stop. Also, if I hit something and or someone, I don't have the reaction time or control on my left to brace for the impact. I learned this at the Royal Board Shop Clinic one Wednesday afternoon when I was trying to cut around some pylons. I made it left around the first pylon, right around the second one, but as I went to cut left around the third one, the pathway was slanted and pulled me out further than I was expecting, and I hit the pylon with my front right wheel.

The board came to a dead stop on the spot, but my body kept going. With the momentum I had, I flew forward off my board and raised my right arm to brace for impact. My right knee and right hand hit the ground first. My left side did absolutely nothing but freeze still. The next thing to hit the ground, was my face. On the video (of the accident) you can clearly hear the plastic click of the front of my helmet hitting the cement as the front of my face smashed against the ground with the whole weight of my body behind it. My face smashed into the ground so hard it blew out the front Styrofoam part of my helmet. My nose exploded and started pouring blood nonstop for a good ten to fifteen minutes as I lay in the grass trying to recover. I bled and bled until there was an actual thick puddle of blood in the grass. I also busted open the bottom of my chin. The people around immediately sprang into action and began giving me medical attention. There was some debate if I needed to get my chin stitched closed or not. We were not entirely sure so a fellow rider and longboarding inspiration cleaned me up as much as he could before he rushed me back to Royal where my taxi was waiting to take me home. I got home and checked in with my ER nurse mother. After she cleaned me up some more, I then hobbled over to the hospital completely covered in blood from my nose bleed, split-open chin, and road rash still bleeding. I got a few stitches in emerge before I made my way back home for a much-needed rest. That's when I first realized all my senses and perception were so far gone that I shouldn't be on anything that moves.

I made the awful assumption of thinking I could still ride a bike and control it easier as it had a break, so I'd be able to actually stop or slow down on hills. So, I went out and bought myself a bike and it sat for a few weeks. Then on a beautiful day I went to go for my first post-stroke bike ride, by myself (what could possibly go wrong?). I took out my bike and put my left, paralyzed foot (I still can't feel) on the pedal. With my foot on the pedal, I then kicked off and started peddling away. I made it maybe one or two houses down the street when I suddenly found myself flying over the handlebars and into the middle of the road. I had no idea how or why it happened, so being the stubborn dipshit that I am, I got back on my bike and started to pedal away again.

Another fifty feet went by, and I was again on the ground after going over the handlebars. Now I was mad, sore, bleeding, and wondering what was going on. But I wasn't about to give up that easy, so I got back up hoping nobody saw that. I got back on my bike and started to pedal away for the third time. This time, I was looking down at my left leg to see what was going on. Then out of nowhere, as I was mid-pedal my left foot flew off the pedal and kicked the front tire of my bike sideways and I again go flying over the handlebars and eat the pavement. I realized I needed to buy a foot strap, so I have my foot secure. I did the walk of shame back home with my bike and put it back for a later date. Once I went to a bike shop and got some foot straps and new pedals with big teeth for extra grip, I got my little brother to put the pedals and left foot strap on for me. After they were on, I went for another bike ride. This one was going pretty well, and I rode around my community, over to the new, paved pathway that eventually ended at the end of the community beside ours.

I did have a few issues arise. As I was coming up a really small hill, I realized I couldn't get lots of torque into the pedals with only one arm to pull on the handle as I pushed down into the pedals. I got maybe halfway up the hill and stopped with the intention of getting off and walking up the rest of the hill. I grabbed the break lever, pulled it in, and held it till I came to a complete stop. Then I naturally leaned over to the left side to put my foot down, but I still had it strapped into the pedal. So, I just rode halfway up the hill, went to get off, but just fell over onto my paralyzed side instead. I couldn't help but think 'well that was dumb.' I had to take out my foot before I leaned over to the left, but it's harder than it sounds when you can't feel it at all or move it properly to take it out. I got up off the ground, walked to the top of the hill, then I got back on the bike and rode it to the end of the pathway before I turned around to head back home. On my way home, I got to the (only) busy intersection I had to cross. So, I went to get off my bike. I stopped, jiggled my whole leg, and pulled to get my foot out, then extended my leg to the ground. Again, I naturally leaned to my left thinking my foot was pulled out and put down as I stopped, but it wasn't. It was still strapped in, and I fell over, again. Of course, to the left side of the sidewalk was a foot drop into a pool of mud and water that I fell into.

Just as an extra needle, it had to be in front of the eight lanes of stopped traffic that was at the red light waiting. I climbed out of the mud hole now bloody, wet, sore, and completely covered in water and mud. Now I'm pissed off as I walk across the street. At the other side of the street was the bottom of a slight tiny incline that I had to go up so I could get back. I got back on the bike, put my foot in the strap, and kicked with my right leg until I got enough speed to coast to get my right foot up in time for the pedal, but I didn't put my left foot in the strap well enough. Once I got enough momentum to get my right foot up, I got maybe two full rotations with the pedals before I was again flying over the handlebars and on the right side of the sidewalk in some grass. I realized biking was much harder than longboarding and I started to think, 'maybe trekking downhill across British Columbia on a bike when I can't even go on a leisurely bike ride without injuries was the dumbest thing anyone could possibly do.' Yet I've never wanted to do something more in my life.

I got up again and walked to the top of the hill pushing the bike now bloody, wet, pissed off, muddy, and covered in grass stains, again questioning if I should attempt a twelve-hundred-kilometre trek across a province when I can't even go a single kilometre without ending up bashed, bloody, bruised, and dirty. After that fall, I got back on the bike and miraculously made it home without dying. But as soon as I got home, I rode over the lawn towards the side gate, leaned to my left, and fell over again onto the grass. The dogs heard me crash out front and started to go crazy inside the house as I got back up struggling to get my foot out of the strap for five minutes because I couldn't rotate my ankle. I then proceeded to put the bike back at the side of the house hoping none of my neighbours saw my sick biking skills, as I had enough embarrassment over the last few hours. Muddy, bloody, dirty, and sore I showered and cleaned myself up before I started to think, and plan to finish the trek across British Columbia. I figured I would walk the uphill, skate the flat, and bike down the crazy downhills. That seemed entirely possible, how hard could it be? I was walking, biking, and longboarding again. Sure, it wasn't pretty, but I was still doing it.

It was a good idea to me in theory, but I first had to learn how to stop without falling over and getting hurt or causing an accident on the highways. I was planning to leave in April of 2016 and spend as long as I could to go as far as I could. Everyday starting January 1, 2016, I was at the gym training which was a horrible mistake. For one, training on a stationary bike, stair stepper, treadmill, leg press, or any gym equipment isn't even close to training for a twelve-hundred-kilometre outdoor trip. In the gym you are just that, in the gym, with a roof over your head not exposed to all the natural elements of Mother Nature as you endlessly climb the empire state building on the stair stepper. I also spent all that time on a stationary bike not working on balance which I had next to none of and really needed to work on. Some days in the gym I would be walking like I'm loaded with a blood stream of liquor when I'm completely sober running into people and equipment. So, I'd be getting funny looks from people every once in a while. Then other times I'd be there walking around like nothings ever happened to me. As I recovered, I had my longboard stashed in my mom's car, when she was at work I'd go to the gym, then grab her keys, and go skate in the underground parking lot that was the size of a few city blocks.

Day after day, I'd spend hours in the parkade skating around the entire empty section that nobody ever parked in until someone called security on me. Then security would kick me out and I'd go back to the gym for a bit before I'd go back to longboarding in the underground parkade. I got to spend days in the underground parking lot learning to longboard again. After months of me coming back to skate after getting kicked out by security, police, and bylaw officers I think they had enough of it so they told me I could go skate in the tunnel there. The tunnel was short, flat, perfectly smooth and not fun so I stayed in the empty section of the parkade. Then they decided to change the parking on the campus and moved all the hospital staff into my self-designated longboarding section. That wasn't going to stop me so I kept on skating, but I now had the hospital staff that didn't know me, calling security on me much more frequently.

With more and more run-ins with police, peace officers, and security they began to ask me why I refused to leave and why I was always down there. I told them my mother worked there and her car was there with my belongings in it, and I came down here because it was much safer than the streets above us. Once they heard why I was down there, they stopped coming down to kick me out and instead they would come down to check on me and make sure I was okay and still progressing forward. I thought bringing my bike down there would be good for me as well, so I threw that in my mom's car and pulled it out instead of riding the stationary bike at the gym. I was biking the underground city blocks for a few hours when the peace officers rolled up on me to say hello and check on how I was doing. I pulled the break and stopped then went to put my foot down, but it was still strapped in. So, they rolled up to me and I stopped to say hello, only to fall over on my left side in front of them both. They asked me if I was okay, and I told them it happens to me a lot which was why I was always down there and not in the busy city streets. I think they then realized both me and the public would be safer with me there hidden underground.

Every day as I trained underground and at the gym (keeping the body healthy and active), I would go home to work on my public speaking skills, speeches, and presentation (keeping my mind healthy and active) between juggling that and the day-to-day life of outpatient therapy, doctors' appointments, personal appointments, and home therapy I began to plan out some of the logistical aspects of the trip. I got up one morning in one of those "there's no better time than right now, before you die" moods. I then showered, got dressed and walked to the store, got a map of British Columbia, and walked back home. I then spent all morning and into the afternoon planning the route. what way would be the safest way, I listed emails and numbers of media contacts for the major cities I would stop at, I got locations of campgrounds where I could stay, did my daily kilometre distances I needed to hit, and listed some of the items I still needed to make it safely. Once I had a rough draft of my plan, I decided to take a break and go to the gym for a few hours. I walked over to the gym and trained for hours and did a nice sixty-kilometre distance on a hard resistance then some squats, arm exercises, and then climbed stairs till I couldn't stand before I went back home ready to shower and go to bed at 4 p.m. I walked in the front door and immediately notice our dog Jake run away to cower in the corner, I then see little pieces of paper everywhere. It went from the front door, around the main floor, all over both couches, in the bathroom, beyond the basement stairs into the kitchen, and halfway up the staircase to the second floor, with a bit spread in the den and the bedrooms upstairs. I picked up a piece of the paper to see a bit of my writing on the back of it. I immediately looked at the table where I left my map to see all of the work I did was no longer there. I go upstairs to see Jake sitting there with the classic, "I'm just a cute-ass innocent dog, how can you be mad at me?" puppy dog eyes and smile. If you've owned a dog, I'm sure you know that look all too well.

After a much-needed nap, I was back up and off to the store for another map. Once I got back, I stayed up late working out the details of the trip, again. Of course, I wouldn't know if it was even physically achievable for me to do until I got on the road. After talking to some gnarly BC longboarding family who pushed across the province for the Ronald McDonald foundation a few years back I was given the flattest, safest way across the province and changed routes. Since I was seriously lacking in the independence department, I couldn't trek across the province alone, so I started looking for a support driver and volunteer for the trip. I began asking friends and family for help, hoping I didn't get another Mr. Driver. I found a volunteer and my grandparents stepped up and gave me their minivan to use so I didn't have to rent a vehicle. I set a date to leave all the while continuously going to the gym to train and going to Toastmasters both improving my physical and mental health. This routine went on for months from winter into the spring.

As it got closer to April, I was getting increasingly excited for the trek. But that evaporated when my volunteer driver backed out of the trip. So, I went looking for another, and found one. Only they bailed a few weeks later too. Therefore, I had to find yet another driver. However, only a week before the trek, they bailed on me as well. But the same day that the last volunteer bailed on me my little brother's dad stepped up. He was up for the monumental task of keeping me alive for five weeks as I attempt to hobble, kick, petal, and roll my way to the West Coast. Now really scrambling, I had to set up a new plan and leave date. Upon doing so, I realized by pushing the leave date back one more time by the week I needed, I would finish my nearly seven-thousand-kilometre-long trek across Canada, on the third-year anniversary of my third paralyzing stroke, to the exact day. It was a freaky weird coincidence that I saw as a sign from the universe that it was meant to be. I had been saving for months and set up a "go-fund-me" page to raise the necessary funds in order to get the food, shelter, equipment, water, and gas I would need along the way. The leave date was set, it went from April to August 2, 2016.

The Finish

August 2, 2016 quickly approached and my little brother's dad, Jason (Jay Jay), came over and under the supervision of his dog, Zoey, we packed up the minivan with the mountain of equipment I had been stockpiling over the months. After we packed up everything we jumped in and headed to Lake Louise. As we drove down the highway my nerves started to explode on my paralyzed side causing lots of fiery pain. I've noticed when my mental nerves start to get going the actual nerves on my paralyzed side start to fire and get incredibly sore as the overwhelming mental emotion brings on physical nerve pain for some odd reason.

After about an hour and a half we got to the village where my dad and I stopped to wait for his co-worker to come pick us up. I got out of the van thinking back to that day for a second, and I was off again. I went up and back over the bridge before I took a left going down to the westbound lane of the Trans-Canada. On the highway, I had a nice big shoulder to ride on and with Jay and Zoey in the van behind me making sure my wobbly, sketchy ass was at least protected by traffic coming from behind me, I felt pretty safe. It was only maybe thirty or forty-five minutes later my left leg started to go into spasms but I kept on trucking along on a mission as I felt muscles tightening and shaking that were trying to forcibly rotate and bow my ankle, however it was securely locked into my leg brace. An hour or two later I finally came to a long turn in the road that had a rest area on the right side of it with the "Welcome to British Columbia" sign so I pulled into the small area to take a picture. Jay and Zoey pulled in behind me as I sticker slapped the BC sign. Then I got Jay to take a picture of me and the sign as I put up an L with my right hand to symbolize "Love and Live Life" after that we got back on the road. I turned right out of the parking lot heading down the highway and as I rode on the shoulder some guy in a bright yellow convertible Mustang with the top down flew by me honking at me to get my attention, just so he can give me the middle finger out the open top of his car. I couldn't help but think, 'You damn loser, if you only knew what I went through to be here doing what I was doing.' I passed him off as another arrogant asshole judging a book by the cover and I continued on the move. But now I was in an incredibly salty mood and started to hate on every yellow-coloured wall magnet (Mustang). I took a second and looked at the ink on my right arm to remind myself that not every Mustang owner is like him. However, my blood momentarily turned as salty as the water in the Dead Sea.

With the anger of wanting to Hulk-smash yellow mustangs, I continued down the highway and after another hour, I made a right turn at the base of a mountain when it suddenly got incredibly windy, and I began to lose my balance. The lightly-covered sun was being rapidly covered by thick, dark clouds and it started to storm. With the wind and the rain both causing me to lose balance I was hardly able to get back into the van without falling over. Once I did, I hid out for five or ten minutes till the worst of the storm went by. Once Mother Nature calmed down, I got back on the road and continued to trek on. After about ten or fifteen minutes, I came around another right turn that went straight for a bit before turning left into the forest a few kilometres ahead. As I got to the straight part of the highway that was sandwiched at the base of mountains on both sides of me, I noticed what looked like yellow crime-scene tape on the right side of the ditch. As I came up to the tape, I could see that in the bottom of the ten-foot, bolder-filled ditch was a big white semi-truck and its load sitting sideways, almost completely upside down in the ditch. I signalled Jay to stop, and he quickly pulled up and got out. The yellow tape everywhere was caution tape that someone had already put up around everything.

Just to be sure, Jay looked in the windows of the cab calling out to see if anyone was inside needing assistance. After he took a walk around the truck and trailer to check for injured people we got back on the road. My curiosity really wanted to open the back to see what was in the truck. But the terrain of the ditch was a bit too much for me and knowing the load in the back had been majorly shifted I decided not to get crushed by its payload. After a few more hours on the road, we got to the area where I needed to be to get to Golden the next day.

Until then, I hadn't physically trekked that far (outdoors) since my last stroke, and I was exhausted with my leg now shaking like crazy. Realizing I shouldn't have trained in a gym or underground parkade and done it all outside like I did the first time in 2012 and 2013 we drove around to find a place to camp out for the night. We started to look for side roads off the main highway to find a secluded spot on crown land that we could camp on. We turned right off the highway, then made a left onto a random dirt road that started to go up the side of a mountain. The dirt road then took a right corner and as we came up to it on our right, there was an opening in the trees. In the middle of the opening was a huge pile of dead, cut-down trees. A pile that was much bigger than the van. JJ parked the van just off the side of the dirt road by the pile of wet wood and started to set up camp. I then realized I messed up big time with the assumption I would be okay to use a foot pump to blow up my air mattress after trekking all day. It took me a solid forty-five plus minutes struggling, utterly exhausted while shaking from spasms to pump up my air mattress. While I'm taking hours setting up my tent and bed, Jay managed to get some wood to burn and started a fire to cook us some supper. We camped out there in the middle of nowhere with a blue tarp strung off the van and a few dead trees to keep us and the fire dry. The next day we got up, packed up our things, and got back on the highway through the beautiful rock- and forest-covered mountains.

After all morning on the highway in the hot sun through the beautiful, forest-covered mountains we finally got to Golden where I contacted the Golden Star paper to see if they would be interested in a quick interview. Jessica and I set up a time and Jay drove me to the office for the interview. While I was talking to the kind woman, she brought up the event going on a few blocks over and suggested we walk over there to take a picture at the bridge for her article. So, after the interview Jessica and I walked over as Jay and Zoey drove over and parked the van before Jay put Zoey on a leash and walked down the path that led up to a little bridge where Jessica took a picture of me. As I was there, a few random local kids waved at me, so I waved back and went over to have a chat.

The first thing the young girl said was, "You're not from around here, are you?" I replied with, "Nope, how do you know that?" She told me, "You don't look like it." I then proceeded to tell them all why I was there, why I was geared up in a mix of longboarding and medical equipment, and what I was up to for the rest of the summer. The group of young girls and boy were intrigued and I got the usual interrogation of questions I always got. After a quick chat with them, I walked over to Jay and Zoey before we walked down the pathway to a decent look out spot where we could see the band play on stage. We hung out up there for a bit as everyone came up to Zoey to get their fix of puppy love. After we watched the band from afar for a bit, we walked down closer to the stage. On the stage's right side, they had tables and a little bar area we went to sit at but the dog wasn't allowed in the closed off section so we moved a table to the gates where Jay tied her up on the other side of them. We had a beer, watched the bands play, and had a bite to eat before we went over to our motel for the night.

We drove over to the "Selkirk Inn" where Jay Jay's friend paid for our room for the night. We arrived, parked the van, and got the keys to our room. Then while we were walking down the hallway, I saw something shiny that caught my eye, so as I walked down the hall, I looked to see what it was. It was a dime. I stopped and picked it up thinking about Uncle Tony and all the weird random places my mom's family has been finding dimes since his passing before going to our room. As soon as we got into the room my head hit the pillow and I crashed hard.

The next day, it was the same routine, we were on highway 95 heading south to Parsons. There, they had the smallest white sign that read "Parsons Unincorporated" on the right side of the road coming out of the bushes. Back on the road, I started to realize something I had never thought about before, and that was being able to operate the GoPro as I was on the road. If my attention was even distracted for a second, I would start to lose control and go into the ditch or onto the road a bit. My ability to multitask (including operating my iPod) while I was moving on the road was completely gone. It was actually depressing. However, the views were amazing. I was in a beautiful valley of Rocky Mountains and lush, green forest in every direction. On the right side of the road, the CP (Canadian Pacific) Railway tracks paralleled the highway. Then a kilometre or two beyond the tracks, huge mountain formations rose high into the atmosphere. To the left of the mountains were rolling hills for as far as you could see. The hills went on and on covered with more trees than you could comprehend counting. Once we got to our destination, we set up camp in a very beautiful spot.

Our spot rested on the edge of a small lake with the rolling, tree-covered hills behind it. I walked around and collected some small, dead brush to start a fire with. I then threw out my pop-up tent, made my bed, rolled a cannabis cigarette, and walked through the two or three trees that stood between us and the lake and sat by the edge of the water to have my smoke. As I watched the sunset over the mountains and rolling hills, I couldn't help but think about how grateful, lucky, and incredibly blessed I was and had an incredible moment of gratitude. Again and again throughout this entire cross-country trip I couldn't help but think, feel, and know like I'm the luckiest person alive. Not because I've dodged a roughly twenty-five percent chance of living four times, but because I am from such a stupendous, beautiful, peaceful, and clean country. I sat there basking in a moment of euphoria while I finished my smoke.

After spending another hour hating life pumping up my mattress, Jay cooked supper and we hung out for the night relaxing by the fire with the dog. After a while I went to bed and in the middle of the night, I was suddenly woken up to the sounds of howling wolves that came from right behind my tent where I knew the lake was. They were probably on the other side of the lake, but they sounded uncomfortably close as their echoes shot across the small body of water to where we were. I just hoped that they didn't make their way around the lake to our campsite and went back to sleep.

The next morning, I got up, walked over to the calm mirror like lake, and took a picture of the beautiful scenery. Jay came over and took a picture of me, so for the picture's sake, I gave him the middle finger. We had breakfast, I pounded down another protein shake, packed up our stuff, and got back on the highway towards Spillimacheen. The mountains on my left still stood tall reaching for the sky. On the right, the mountains were covered in a thick blanket of trees that tried going up the uninhabitable mountain sides. The weather turned out to be beautiful with nothing but clear, blue skies and sun, it made for another peaceful and beautiful riding day. After a few hours on the road, we came up to a sign on the right side of the road that said Spillimacheen was 14 km away, Radium Hot Springs was 53 km away, and Cranbrook was 198 km away. Jay took a picture of me and the sign while I had a sip of water before we got back on the road to Spillimacheen.

Once we got there, we began driving around looking for another place to camp. We ended up going way off road and took the minivan halfway up a mountain until we found an open area to camp. Jay parked the van on a patch of small rocks which made a clearing in the forest and as I got out of the van, I looked down to where I was putting my foot and I saw a dime just sitting there. We were literally halfway up a mountain in the middle of the thick, dense Canadian forest. The odds a dime would just be there waiting for me really freaked me out. I couldn't help but think, 'What are the odds?' as I picked it up and threw it in the cup holder with the other one wondering if it was a message from Uncle Tony saying he's watching over and sending me his love. I wondered if he was up there watching me finish my journey that started just after his murder. I couldn't understand why, but I would find out soon enough.

The next morning, I was still thinking about my late Uncle Tony as we had breakfast and packed up. We got back on the road, and I was maybe on the road for thirty minutes when my left leg went into spasms and started to uncontrollably flex causing an extreme amount of discomfort. I signalled Jay to pull over so I could get in the van to roll a joint. The dog decided to jump out and she hung out with me on the side of the highway as I had my smoke. We then got back on the road heading to Radium Hot Springs.

Once we got to Radium, we drove over to Canal Flats to stay at Craig and Whinny's place. They are good friends of Jays and have known him for many years. They had a secondary, small house behind theirs they called "the man cave" which was built by an old Calgary Flames player back in the day. There we hung out, chatted, and had a few beers before heading to bed.

The next day, we got up and drove back to the hot springs and I began to trek from there. Only today the head wind was so strong I was being blown all over the road and I couldn't hold a straight line with my dizziness, nor could I get very far without needing a break. We were still in a valley of mountains and trees, so it was definitely a striking and tranquil place to be. I was quite content with everything except the endless wind that had me being a huge danger to myself and everyone on the road as I was wobbling like a guy who just drank an entire bottle of whisky by himself. Even Jay Jay started to have some worries about me on the completely straight road. From the hot springs we continued to Invermere and once we got there, we drove back to Canal Flats for another night in the man cave.

The next day the same routine continued on, we packed up the van, drove back to Invermere, and began to trek down to Fairmount Hot Springs. We decided to drive into the springs once we got there and have a dip in the warm sulfur water. On the way into the springs from the highway we were driving on the gravel road that had a cliff at least seventy-five feet down if not more. If you drove over the edge, you were almost certainly doomed as you fell and rolled into a wall of trees that might have stopped you or bounced you around like a pin ball in a machine as you continued to roll down bouncing off the unmoveable trees. Just looking over the edge was giving me anxiety.

After our nice, short dip in the warm water, we headed back to the van. On the way back, Jay and I walked past an old hippy van and laughed so hard when Jay saw a sticker on the back that reads "Life is like a bowl of soup, you only get blown if you're hot." After Jay and I had a good laugh at that, we got back in the van and went back to Canal Flats for another night. After we got back, we hung out with their friends Todd and Sherri whose house was just down the street. Todd's son Thomas has cerebral palsy and he chased me in his wheelchair for a good hour or two around the big open grass area. As everyone had a chance to catch up, Thomas chased me around the big lawn giggling and laughing away. After we hung out at Todd's for a bit we went back over to Craig and Whinny's house. I got a chance to do laundry and Whinny said she would give me a back massage (as she is a massage therapist) the next morning before we took off to try and help me with the back pain that I was having. That night in the rain we walked over to the liquor store before going to another one of their friends' houses to have some drinks there. After that we walked back and had a good time and a few more drinks in the man cave. Curt even put on my helmet and pretended to be me for a minute, so I snapped a quick picture as we had a good laugh. We all stayed up pretty late that night and morning having a fun time. The next day it was back over to the turn off we stopped at, at the hot springs and we began trekking into Canal Flats.

    It was another crazy windy day, and I was again a huge liability being pushed all over the shoulder and roadways. As I struggled to get down the highway a black Ford truck with three mountain bikes hanging over the tail gate drove by, and gave us the middle finger out the passenger window on the way by. Eventuallys I made it back to Canal Flats without going into the ditch or causing an accident, just apparently pissing people off. Once we got back, we stopped at "Back Country Jacks" for a well-deserved meal. The owner took our orders then came back and sparked up a conversation. We started chatting and she politely asked me about my leg brace, shoulder brace, and what it was all for. I told her my story and what we were doing for the rest of the summer, and she was amazed. Our orders came out and I devoured my delicious cheeseburger and fries. After our meal I asked the lady for the bill and she told me, "Don't worry about it," and said, "It was on the house." I was grateful to have a nice surprise like that as we were going to need that money very soon. Jay Jay took a picture of me, the amazing owner and her daughter outside by their sign so I could put it online later then we drove back to the man cave for our last night. The next morning, I got up early to finish laundry that I forgot in the van the previous day. Before we said goodbye to everyone, I gave Whinny, Craig, Thomas, and Todd a few of my custom t-shirts for their generous hospitality, and we got back on the road.

    Shortly after we left, I was on the bike coming down a small steep hill and I started to have some more terrible bike realizations. On top of the wind rushing over my head causing me to be dizzy and disoriented, I realized I couldn't stop in a short distance. The hill I was coming down had some big holes and got rough, so I grabbed the break. When I pulled in the break lever it threw all of my body weight into the right side of the handlebars and threw me right onto the road. Luckily for me there were no cars coming that could have hit me, however it freaked out JJ so he honked and shouted, "Be careful, buddy!" at me over our radios. I had to take it incredibly slow because I was going to either fall over from the speed or be unable to stop myself in time if I had to. I also had to pedal downhill due to the incredible headwind at the time. As I'm riding all over the side of the road like an incredibly disoriented drunk because of the wind, I started to notice a weird clicking noise coming from the bike just as the downhill went right back up. I got off the bike on the side of the road almost falling into the outbound lane on the highway, which gave Jay another mild heart attack. Then I walked the bike up to the top of the hill that took a long, slow right as it went up. At the top of the hill on the other side of the road was a small pull-over spot so I looked for traffic and quickly hobbled over there as Jay pulled in and asked why we're stopping. I told him about the noise the bike was making and said, "I don't really trust it ripping down hills, something is going on with it," so he got on to see if he could figure out why. Immediately he started to do wheelies aggressively riding it. I saw with every pedal the derailleur was catching so I screamed at him to stop but he didn't hear me, so I called out for him again, but he was too far away and just as I went to call out again the derailleur snapped dangling on the left side of the bike dragging on the ground. He pointed out the little problem and I said, "Well, I guess we have to go find a bike shop."

We threw the broken bike in the back, and I googled a bike shop before we drove into the nearest town. The shop didn't have the size of part we needed so Jay tried to see if they could give us a deal on a new one or do a swap or something like that. They told us the best they could do is order the part, but it would take a few weeks to get there, and that was time we didn't have. So, we started driving around to look for pawn shops and found one nearby to see if we could find another part or bike before we got to a gnarly pass in the mountains. The passes were too much for me as is. The shoulders were nearly non-existent and with all the twists and turns having people, animals, cars, and boulders coming out of nowhere combined with my sketchy ass was too much for me to even do, let alone do it safely. So we would throw me in the back of the van, track the kilometres, then I'd spend a day or a few days on a safer part of the highway to make up the kilometres.

We told the man at the pawn shop we were looking for a bike and he told us to go look at the ones out front on the rack. We stepped outside and started to look for one I could ride. I pointed out the one I liked to Jay who asked the kind man working if he could take it for a quick spin. Jay jumped on the bike and rode around the dirt parking lot before he came back with his approval saying, "It might actually be better for you B." I went back inside to pay for it and the guy tells us it's going to be, "one-hundred-and-fifty dollars." Jay was like, "Whoa man, can't you give us a better deal than that?" and started to negotiate. JJ said, "Drop it down to seventy-five and we'll give you a free t-shirt like this," as he points to the shirt I was wearing. The man was interested in Jay's proposition and gladly accepted. Jay ran out to the van and got the size of t-shirt he wanted while I paid for the bike. I gave the guy at the counter his money, in exchange he handed me a receipt just as Jay returned with the t-shirt. We then drove back down the highway and got back on the move in the windy bush.

Once we finished trekking for the day, we had to find another place to camp out for the night, and after aimlessly driving around for a while we found one, so Jay pulled over and we started to set up camp. Master Campfire Chef Jay cooked up some awesome food over the fire and we sat around it, ate supper, and relaxed after another long day. With full bellies, we hung around the fire chatting before heading to bed. But what Jay said to me, caught me completely off-guard. After watching me struggle doing the simplest of things, like getting down a hill, staying on the right side of the shoulder, and not dying for a while he told me how impressed, amazed, and inspired by me he was. Followed by an "I'm proud of you B." Again, I found myself full of more unexpected, good feels and thought back to before the trek was even an idea for a minute. I couldn't help but feel incredibly happy. I was happy that I decided to finally change paths, I was happy that I was finally finishing my trek, and most of all I was happy that I had unexpectedly gained the respect of my peers in the process. I thought back to the reasons why I wanted to embark on such a gnarly journey to begin with. It was to throw a huge wrench in the life cycle of wasted shit that was my life at the time, it was to do something good with my life before I died, it was pursuing one of my passions, and to give back to the world, but most of all I wanted to do it for every single person that never got the second, third, or fourth chance at life like I did. I then couldn't help but think of the kind of person I became after making such a change. I detested everything about the person I was just a few years prior, and it felt really good that I was finally someone I was comfortable being. Again, I was unexpectedly experiencing the kind of happiness money could never buy. It was the same inner peace and happiness I felt the whole way across the country, minus most of the prairies.

Never did I think, let alone expect, doing something for myself and own personal needs would earn me the respect from my peers as well. Respect, money, fame, all these things were the furthest from my mind when deciding if it was something worthy of doing. So, to have gained something so phenomenally good, something that I was completely not expecting at all, was a nice bonus that again reassured me this was the best decision of my life. At one point Jay said, "I couldn't do what you're doing man," which in turn got the usual, "Not with that attitude you can't," that I tell people when they tell me, "they can't."

In the morning we got up, packed up camp, I chugged another protein shake, and we headed off to trek to Fort Steele. Once we got to town, we filled the van with gas then stopped at Walmart to get some supplies like a motorized fan to blow up our beds. I also saw a great deal on a fold-up camping chair and grabbed it as I walked by without reading or inspecting it closely. After we gathered supplies, we still had to find a place to camp. After driving around for a bit, Jay took a right off of the main road just after a small bridge and we went onto a random dirt road that led down into a valley. We easily got down the dirt road that was now essentially just two tire tracks going into the middle of nowhere. To our left side was what I called "can-alley." Hundreds upon hundreds of very old, rusted soup cans littered the beautiful natural surroundings. Once we saw this, we pulled over and were astonished at the corroding mess we stumbled upon. Our best guess was the hundreds of rusted cans were left by the old-time miners that were there dozens of years before. The trail of rusted cans continued on as we drove down the tire-marked pathway for a while, but it abruptly ended as fast as it appeared.

After following the tire tracks for a short while, we got spit out to where the CP rail tracks were for the trains and made a left down a gravel road and came across "Railway Spike Mountain." A short distance down the gravel road was a pile of railway spikes bigger than the van, probably twice as big. There were thousands of them just sitting there rusting in a big pile along with the big plates they pounded the spikes into, securing the tracks to the wood for the huge trains. We got out and each grabbed a spike as a souvenir, took a picture of them all, then got back in the van and drove down the gravel road that again turned left and brought us to what looked like a dry riverbed. We drove back to where the road turned left the last time and parked the van up against the bushes and decided to set up our tents there. As we were taking things out of the van and setting up camp for the night, an older man with a big, long, white beard down to his waist came walking upon us.

He asked what we were doing before I asked if it was okay we set up there for the night. He didn't care the slightest bit. He was just doing rounds making sure the local riff raff and hoodlums weren't down there causing a big mess again. After the chat with the older man, I decided I would make a little fire pit and get a fire going so I went around gathering big rocks before I put them in a circle between the van and our tents. Over at Railway Spike Mountain, I remembered seeing the steel plates and I thought they would be good to use for the fire pit, so I got in the van and drove over there and put a half dozen of them throughout the van. They were heavier than I was expecting, and I sliced my right pinky finger open when I was picking one up. I drove back over to camp, pulled out the plates one by one trying not to touch the rusty covered plates with my bloody pinky finger. Then I lined the firepit with the plates and went to clean my finger. I put some Polysporin on it and wrapped it up before going around to gather some wood to light a fire. We sat around the fire with the dog for a few hours hanging out while a few of the huge trains went past us only a short distance away in the trees before we went to bed. At one point, I took out the cheap chair that I bought at Walmart, so I wasn't pulling my expensive, heavy and bulky wheelchair in and out of the van causing a mess and I realized why the chair was so cheap. It was a fold-out kid's chair. The thing was tiny. It had a part that popped up over your head to protect you from the elements I suppose but that was so small it hardly fit over my head, and I was crammed into this tiny, blue kids chair for the night, very unimpressed with myself.

Next thing I noticed I'm woken up by the ground shaking and I have no idea what's going on. All I know is the ground is shaking, I see a bright light coming at my tent, with an incredibly loud noise. I started freaking out and got out of my sleeping bag, ripped open my tent, then tripped over the lip of the tent, half-naked in my boxers, wondering what the commotion was. I fell onto the cold, hard rocks outside my tent then looked up to see the minivan and I looked behind my tent to see a big CP rail train on the tracks go by us. I've never felt like more of a dumb-ass in my life, okay maybe a few times, like losing fights to toilets and walls, but it was definitely up there in the top five "dumb-ass" moments of my life.

I had completely forgotten where we were and that I was sleeping by the railway. Still in my boxers I climbed back into my tent, but my commotion woke up Jay. He asked, "Everything okay B?" I kept the fact I was a huge dumb idiot who had a mild heart attack, half-naked to myself and said, "Yeah, I'm fine, just tripped over my tent," and went back to sleep. The next train came by a few hours later and woke me up, but that time I remembered where I was and that the tracks were right behind me, so I didn't stumble out of my tent half-naked for the rest of the night, just woke up every few hours for a few seconds as they went by.

The next day it was a short trek to Cranbrook. There, we were going to spend a few nights until we got further out of town. We ended up finding a nice little campsite to stay at. Once we got unpacked and settled in, we took the dog for a walk and a swim in the nearby river. We got there and Zoey ran right into the river for a swim. We found her a stick and Jay and I were throwing the stick far into the river for Zoey to swim out to and bring back. Each time she paddled through the fast-running water with ease and grace before grabbing the stick, turning around, and bringing it back.

As we were standing on the side of the river, we saw a small eagle that had a fish in one of its claws. There was another eagle that was much bigger than the one with the fish swooping down at the smaller one picking on it. After being bullied for a bit, the smaller bird dropped the fish and within a second the bigger eagle swooped down and caught the fish in the air before flying off to enjoy its free meal. Jay says, "Whoa, that's not something you see every day." There was a family that was also in the river that saw it and the two young boys screamed out, "WHOA, COOL!" It was quite the cool, live discovery-channel moment.

We spent two or three days at the camp site until I made it to Moyie Lake then we would pack up and move basecamp before moving on to Yahk. When we got near Yahk, I realized I needed to do laundry, so I googled "coin laundry" and it said there was a place ten minutes away. So, we loaded up the van and started to follow the GPS. About five minutes later, I realized we were in the middle of butt-fuck nowhere in some vineyards, so I looked at my phone to double check that we were going the right way. My GPS said we were close, and the place was just up ahead on the right. My phone then says, "You have arrived at your destination." I got out of the van, still in the middle of nowhere, and this "coin laundry facility" was a hand-pump well on the right side of the road sticking out of the ground. I thought to myself, 'Sick laundry machine. I wonder where I put the coins.' I got back in the van, and I told Jay what a stupid waste of time that was. I googled a coin-laundry facility again and the closest one to us, that wasn't this one, was about a half-hour to forty-five-minute drive north. I guess someone took the time to stop and register the hand-pump well as a business and put it on google. It was a great **modern-day troll**, but I was pretty pissed.

We drove all the way up north just so I could do laundry. We got to the *actual* coin laundry place, and I threw my clothes in the wash and we hung out there for an hour or two until I was done. Once I was finished, I went back outside to see Jay and Zoey in the van just hanging out as a lady pulled into the parking lot on the right side of them. The lady saw Zoey with her big, cute puppy smile, and immediately smiled back.

Still smiling, she came over to the passenger-side window and asked us if we wanted to have her dog food and toys that she had in her car. She then proceeded to tell us her dog had just passed away and she wanted to get rid of all the stuff. We gladly accepted the free food and toys and told the lady we were sorry for her loss and gave her our heartfelt condolences before getting back on the road. We then had to drive all the way back down to our campsite.

The second night we were there, I remember a group of three or four girls showed up and took the camping spot that was across from us. They had set up their tents and took off to go get some things. It wasn't until after the sun went down when they returned. They all sat in the car for a bit when they pulled in. After being trolled myself, I thought about trolling them and creeping over to their site and hiding behind one of their tents to scare them once they got out. I then thought about their loud screams waking people up and me getting my ass beat up by a group of girls so I decided against it but still think it would have been funny, even after I hobbled back with a much-deserved black eye and bloody nose.

From Yahk, it was supposed to be a short day to Creston, however I was all over the road in the wind on that part of the highway. So, we got in the van and drove through the death traps and clocked the kilometres. I was going to make them up once we found a safe enough road for me to do it on. We found a nice campsite and it had a nice, paved road for me to trek down on and make up the kilometres. I headed down the paved road till it turned to gravel then I kept on going on the bike until the road ended and I had to turn around. I headed back to the campsite then back down to the dead end going back and forth as much as I could. On my last run, I was coming back to the campsite on my bike with my leg and shoulder brace on, struggling now that my leg was shaking in spasms from the tiredness. As I'm wobbling all over the random, secluded dirt road in the middle of nowhere, I noticed a car was following just behind me.

The car then pulled out in front of me and drove off before he parked on the right side of the road. I figured he was on the phone or something and pulled over to chat. I came up to the car and as I past the man in the driver's seat, I heard him say, "Wow, amazing." After I went by him, he continued to follow me and followed me all the way back to camp. I took the left turn into our camping ground and pulled over to wait for Jay to see this stranger in his car pull up behind me. He then got out and came over to talk to me just as Jay pulled in behind the stranger's car. The man starts asking me what I'm doing in the middle of the forest with all my braces and gear on trekking back and forth, up and down the road. Once I told him my story he was blown away. At one point he said he came to the forest "to do something stupid." What that was, we can only speculate. However, it seemed like he was having a hard time and was about ready to give up on life. But he ran into the one guy who has fallen plenty in life, but still gets back up no matter what. I don't think he could have randomly run into a better person at that time. Just talking to him for five short minutes, he was uplifted, inspired, and filled with the strength he needed at that moment in his life.

After he heard my story, he reached into his pocket and pulls out a few hundred dollars and said, "Here, this is for you, in case anything happens," and handed Jay the money. I asked him if he had Facebook to keep in touch, but he didn't have it. He told us his name was Pete and wished me the best of luck on my trek before he got back in his car and drove off out of the park. It was a totally random and strange situation, he seemed like he was having a tough time in his life at the moment and came to the woods to perhaps end it all, but after hearing my story, his demeanour quickly changed on whatever he was there to do, and he left the woods with a new perspective on life. We threw the dirty and dusty bike in the back of the van and drove through the camp to our site where the weirdness of strange things continued.

While I was looking for some dead wood around our site, that backed onto a small river, I looked over to the river to see a watermelon-headed, princess-guy wearing a purple scarf. Yeah, you read that right. This guy had a cut-in-half, hollowed-out watermelon with rectangular eye holes to see out of. On top of the watermelon was a princess tiara. Then around his neck was a dark-purple, fuzzy scarf. He was also wearing shorts and a muscle shirt. I couldn't help but think to myself, 'Are you high?' 'Is this really happening?' Like my friends and I did when the old, naked lady walked into my apartment. I looked, then looked away before looking back before looking away and back again. I probably did a quadruple take before deciding to have fun with it. So, I started to cat-call the watermelon-headed princess. "OWWW OWWW!" I called out to see his watermelon head turn and look at me. Once he was looking at me, I added, "Heeeey, do you like to party?" Right after I did that, his buddies to my right at the camp beside us burst out laughing. After a good laugh wondering how close to Shambhala I was, I went back to gathering wood for a fire and started our usual night routine.

We found out later it was watermelon-headed princess's bachelor party, and his buddies were dressing him up and torturing him for the night. Between Pete and the watermelon-headed princess guy, we had an interesting end to our day of travels. Jay cooked up another tasty meal, we sat around the fire, and had supper before we played a drinking game with a left-over beer or two and relaxed for the night.

The next day, we were up and heading to Nelson. Halfway there, we drove to my auntie's relative's house for the night. No one was there so we just camped outside in the front of the big yard. The next morning, I had a much-needed shower, ate breakfast, drank my protein shake, and we got back on the road.

From there, we drove back to the highway and began going west. That day we reached a very beautiful location called Christina Lake. It was a great place to stop for a lunch break. Jay parked the van and pulled out the camping grill. I looked over the barrier of the little rest stop. On the left, the right, and the end of the lake, the huge tree-covered hills held the beautiful body of water steady in its place. The hills and the lake went on for a kilometre or two, then the land on the left side of the lake came out of the ground raising the thousands of trees and ending the lake on the left. Down the right side of the valley a bit further, the hills on the right continued for as far as you could see with waves of green coming up and down. I found it kind of cool that you could tell not only in BC, but all across Canada, that the earth's crust, something we know as hard ground, wasn't always like that. You could tell at one point in our history the crust was soft, malleable, and rippled exactly like water before it solidified. With a nice sunny day and beautiful scenery, it was a great relaxing lunch break.

After our nice lunch break, we got back on the road to Osoyoos and once we got halfway there, we found a place to camp for the night. We went up a dirt road that led up into the hills until the road split left and right. In between the split was a big opening so we pulled over to the right and set up camp in the opening. I remembered seeing a group of big rocks and some wood just back around the corner, so I got the keys from Jay, drove down to the corner, put it in park, and started to load the right side of the van with the big rocks and wood. Most of the rocks were too big for my one arm so I grabbed the ones I could and a bunch of wood and drove it up the hill, over to camp. Jay was telling me to park it in front of him so I pulled up to him and when I went to put my foot on the break, I accidently hit the gas. The van lunged forward really fast for a foot or two before I hit the break to stop, right before running him down. I got out of the van and he said, "Whoa man, what are you doing?" I told him, "Sorry, I just hit the gas instead of the break by mistake." So, he gave me some quick driving tips as we set up camp for the night. I set up a small firepit with the rocks, lit a fire, and relaxed before bed. The next morning, I had my usual protein shake breakfast and got back on the road to Osoyoos.

Coming into Osoyoos was incredibly beautiful. There was a big switchback into the valley that was distractingly beautiful. In the bottom of the valley, you could see the entire city and beyond that, were rolling hills that went on forever. With the town surrounded by trees and hills I couldn't help but wonder what they would do in the event of a forest fire. The few-kilometres-long switchback hill was too much for me to do safely so I got in the van, and we drove down the hill without causing an accident. About halfway down I realized it was a good thing I didn't trek down it as I probably couldn't even have walked it without causing bodily harm to myself or spilling into the road causing a crash. In the distance there was a colossal, light-brown cliff face that rose one or two hundred feet in the air that was then topped with the trees of the forest. It was a cool and very beautiful sight of the valley.

Once in town, we went to the local store, grabbed some supplies, and filled the van with gas. As we left the store we drove around the mall and behind the shopping complex was a parking lot full of ducks. There were two bigger parent ducks and about a dozen baby ducks that took up the whole parking area which forced everyone to drive around them and park somewhere else. Instead of gathering in a group they all decided to hang out sporadically taking up as much room as they could. Zoey wanted to jump out of the window and play with them. However, I don't think any of the ducks would have felt the same, so she stayed on my lap with her tail aggressively wagging as she cried to get out, so I held her back from jumping out of the window.

We still had no idea where we were going to stay so we drove around town until we found a dirt road that led to the middle of nowhere and followed that until we found a big enough place to park the van and set up camp for the night. We pulled over on the right side of the road and set up our tents on the other side of the van. After we set up camp, I made a protein shake, then decided to go for a walk while I drank it. As I was walking down the dirt road with Zoey drinking my shake I looked down and found another dime, just sitting on the isolated dirt road in the middle of nowhere. I picked up the dime thinking about Tony while wondering, 'How many more weird places am I going to find dimes?' and continued on.

Just off the right side of the dirt road, I saw a small lake that sat behind a short row of two or three trees. I sat there with Zoey and slowly drank my shake for about ten minutes while soaking up the incredibly peaceful view of the calm, mirror-like lake that reflected the bright blue sky above and green trees all around it. Once I finished my drink, I walked down the road a bit more and past a single cow on my left who was standing there eating grass. I began to wonder whose cow that was and hoped I didn't stumble upon the wrong person's land and get shot at.

My left leg started to go into spasms again and I was hardly able to physically move so I decided I would head back to camp and rest my body. I did a five-step turn around with my left leg uncontrollably shaking like a jackhammer and struggled to come around the first left corner where the cow was. As I slowly hobbled around the corner on my shaking leg, I noticed the one cow had multiplied into about twelve. Zoey immediately took off running to check them out, I tried calling her back, but she didn't listen, and I couldn't help but worry she would get kicked or stepped on by one of the massive creatures. She ran up to one of the cows and the cow just looked at her as she slowly tried to inch her way closer to the cow. But when the cow moved, it scared her, and she abruptly jumped back before bolting down the road. I continued to walk down the road calling the dog and she slowly came back over to me just as a small, red car was speeding down the road. I hobbled out to the middle of the lane and stopped the car to tell them about the traffic jam of cows around the coming blind corner and told them to watch out. They thanked me as they drove off much slower than before.

I got back to camp where Master Campfire Chef Jay had started to cook supper, I threw the dime I found in the cup holder with the others, and we relaxed for the night. The next morning, we were up and heading north to Oliver. The campsite we ended up finding was five dollars a person and allowed dogs but there was a fire ban now in effect. We drove around the site until we found a place to set up camp and parked the van. The place was incredibly dry, dusty, and crazy windy. As we tried to set up our tents we got blasted with dust and the wind would catch them and throw them across the campsite. We had to place the tents down, fill them with big rocks, and hammer multiple spikes through the rings into the ground to hold them in place. After we finally got through the problematic task of setting up camp, I decided to go for a walk to see what was around.

I walked to the complete opposite side of the grounds and came across another beautiful view of the valley. Huge rolling hills went on for as far as I could see, completely covered with a thick blanket of forest. From there, I walked right to see how far the grounds went, sadly it quickly came to a dead end with a big fence around the perimeter. I began to make my way back to our site but, as I was walking between two sites, there were a group of guys at the site on my right who called me over. They were a bunch of young French guys working for the summer to pick apples and make some money. They were all incredibly drunk and offered me a shot of vodka as they poured themselves another round of shots. I sat down and they told me why they were there, and what they were doing. I then told them my story and, like almost every person across the country, they said, "HOLY FUCK!" I then asked if they wanted to play a drinking game if I got a few drinks and they said they were interested. I asked them where a liquor store was, and they told me it was right at the bottom of the hill that led to the camp site.

I walked back to camp and asked Jay if he could give me a quick drive to the store and we left. As soon as we got to the bottom of the hill it spit you out onto the main drag into town, so we slowly started to drive down the street until we got to the liquor store, but it was closed. I went to look at my phone to see if there was another nearby and realized I had left my phone on the bench with the group of drunk strangers. Just as I realized I left my phone behind and I'd be lucky if it was still there, the owner of the store came out and told me there was another liquor store down the road. So, we drove over to the other store and got a few beers for the drinking game and the end of our long days.

We drove back through town after we filled up the belly of the van with gas again and took off back up the hill. I was tempted to bomb down it on my board, but with the rough, rocky road and the intersection at the bottom I couldn't stop for, I decided not to. As soon as we got back to camp, I hobbled over to the site where I left my phone to see nobody was around. Thankfully, when I walked over to the table, I saw my phone was still sitting there at the end of the table where I had left it. Wondering where the drunk guys went, I headed back to camp to find a cute little kitty decided to come hang out and say hi.

The orange stray cat with stripes in its fur I quickly named Tigger as he just looked like a Tigger kind of cat. He was obviously hungry and started to eat the dog food that Jay had put out, thinking he might be thirsty too, I took out a bottle of water and poured some for our new, furry friend. He hung out, ate some dog food, drank water, and got a bunch of loving till he decided to jump in the van and go explore the inside. He climbed onto the driver's seat and popped his head out of the window. Zoey was interested in saying hello and jumped onto the door scaring the poor cat. With Zoey so interested we tried to see if Tigger and Zoey could be friends as Zoey has a little kitten back home that she plays and cuddles with all the time. However, Zoey was way too excited, and it freaked the cat out, so he ran onto the table and hid from the dog. Tigger wasn't having any of it and eventually ran off into the night. After Tigger ran off, Zoey, Jay, and I sat around and had some supper.

Just as we were getting things ready for dinner, a young French woman came up to us and asked if we could help set up her tent. The wind was still going strong, so it was hard for two people to set one up, let alone one. I got some big rocks as Jay got the hammer and some spikes, and we helped her set up her tent as she told us her story. She was having troubles with the family back home in Quebec and decided to get out for the summer, so she came to BC to work like many of the young kids from all over the country do in the summertime. I asked how she got there, and she said she hitch-hiked the whole way and then began telling us about those horror stories we all hear about when a creepy guy picks up a young, cute, hitch-hiking female. She told us how she almost threw herself out of a moving car just to get away from someone that had picked her up. What she had to say was very disturbing to say the least and I was both heartbroken and disgusted that she had to go through what she had to just to get there. After we had a good chat and shared stories, we took a picture before she headed off to bed just as I heard the sounds of fun off in the distance.

I walked down the campsite in the other direction from where I went before and came across a big group of people hanging out on benches. I went over to say hello and saw the same four or five French guys I saw earlier, now struggling to stand. They had met another group of young French workers who were camping out there as well. I went to ask if they still wanted to play a drinking game, but they were all so drunk they could hardly stand, so they definitely wouldn't have been able to handle a drinking game. They were even struggling to speak French to each other, so English wasn't happening anymore, I knew that much. I figured it would have been really ugly if I encouraged them to keep going so, I told them all to have a good night only to get five or six people trying to talk to me in mumbled French. I went back to camp where Tigger had made his way back and was on the benches waiting for me. I gave the little guy some more water and put out a sprinkle of dog food in case he was hungry, then got ready for bed. When I went to my tent the cat wanted to come in, so I let him and left a small opening in the door for when he decided to leave, but he didn't. He just sat on my chest purring as I pet him, and we drifted off to sleep. When I woke up, he was still there sleeping on my chest. I really wanted to keep him but knew that we couldn't.

Once I got up for the day, I went to the outhouse to go pee and when I walked in, I instantly wanted to vomit. There was human excrement all over everything and I struggled to contain my gagging as I peed in the hole of the piece of plywood. I went back to camp to have a chat with Jay and with the dryness, the dust, a fire ban, and unusable restrooms, we decided to pack up and find another place. One of my friends told me he was in the province staying at his grandparents' house in the Kelowna area. After he had a chat with them, he made a plan to put us up for a few nights and we drove up there.

I had a few days of catching up to do, so my buddy got on his board and spent one of his days trekking with me down the highway. But this is where I started to get incredibly uncomfortable and started to struggle more than ever. Over the few days we were there, the heat went from plus twenty-seven (my maximum post-stroke comfort level) to plus thirty-two on the second day, then up to plus thirty-seven, and on the fourth day it hit forty-two degrees Celsius. With my medications and paralysis making me hypersensitive to the sun I had to be covered head to toe. I had a long-sleeve shirt on covering my arms and some athletic pants, so I only had my hands, neck, and face exposed to the blistering sun. With my inability to regulate my body temperature, I started to get uncomfortably hot. I was stuck in a state of constantly wanting to pass out while doing six-foot zigzags back and forth on the bike struggling to keep going. With it being so hot, the sweat that came off of me was absolutely disgusting. I literally had a water fall of sweat dripping out of the front of my helmet, down my nose, then off my face. I felt and probably looked like I just crawled out of a lake; it was nasty. I struggled to differentiate what was harder to deal with, between the heat and the physically getting from A to B. To make things even better, I broke my leg brace which was a huge issue. After the relentless pounding, pressure and force I had exceeded its ability to hold and broke the medical-grade bracket on one of the sides. What's the worst that can happen when a medical necessity in order to properly function is suddenly broken and you're way too stubborn to stop?

Around the Summerland area was when it went from thirty-seven, to forty-two degrees and I couldn't breathe, it was absolutely dreadful. I wasn't having a very good time physically either. Intoxicated by the heat with a broken leg brace I was on the bike riding a path that rode along the water on a lake and I told Jay to go meet me at the end, so he took off just as I started to have crazy muscle spasms in my left leg again. I tried everything I could to get it to calm down, but nothing worked so I figured I would just continue to bike on and let my leg do its thing which was another stupid, fathead, stubborn decision to do. I'm minding my own business (well trying to) coming down the nice, paved pathway with the road on my left and the lake on my right. Then all of a sudden, I'm flying over the handlebars, and I hit the pavement on the right side of the paved path. I looked to my right and there was a five- or six-foot drop lined with big rocks that led into the lake. I was maybe a foot away from the drop, I looked down and couldn't help but think how lucky I was to not fall down the boulder-covered seawall into the water below.

After I said a little prayer on the edge of the lake wall, I looked up to see a guy walking my way who had to of seen the whole over-the-handlebar technique of dis-mounting myself from the bike. I looked up at him and he looked at me, then kept on walking by like nothing even happened, even though I'm there in front of him on the ground literally tangled into the frame of the bike on the edge of the embankment. I pulled my leg out of the frame, flopped over like a fish, too sore to move, and called Jay on the radio who quickly came back to peel me off the pavement and got me on the pathway moving again. I got to the end of the pathway and road wondering if I should switch to my board but was bummed to remember I needed my leg brace in working order for that, so I turned around to go back to the other end of the lake. I saw a chance to get off the pathway and onto the road as I was coming up to a busy pedestrian area, so I took it and started to ride on the right side of the road safely away from everybody. As I'm on the side of the road now coming up to houses, Jay pulls up on my left side to see how I'm doing. So, I stop to tell him. Instead, I did my usual stop, put the foot down as I lean, only to just fall over because my foot was still strapped in.

My head smashed against the right side of the van so hard it gave it a nice character dent and aggressively jerked my head to the right which gave me some whip lash. Right after I fell into the van making a loud bang with my head, I looked to my right to see an older woman out front of her house, gardening. I was really tempted to call out screaming in agony, then tell the lady I was just hit by this maniac, and I need medical attention, so she needs to call the police. But I decided to spare Jay's freedom for another day or two as he had proven to be the perfect man for the job of keeping me safe, alive, and fed in the isolated back woods. After that, I was hardly able to physically move with my body now in shock, so we decided to end it there for the day and we went back to Kelowna. The entire way back my neck was so sore from being suddenly dispositioned by the van door. My right forearm and elbow throbbed from when I fell the first time trying to brace for the impact of my over-the-handlebars X-Games manoeuvres, my left calf was in a constant state of spasms and continuously bounced my leg the entire drive back to Kelowna. We got back and I was hardly able to make it from the van to the front deck with my left leg going so crazy on me. I had to use the van, the garage door, and the walls of the garage just to physically get me from the van to the deck out front. Once I finally did make it up to the deck, I sat in front of the fan that rotated one-hundred-and-eighty-degrees as it sprayed a fine mist and finally cooled off. As I cleaned myself up, Jay and Shay's grandpa took my leg brace to the garage in an attempt to repair it.

Shay's grandfather was kind enough to order us pizza and we all had a nice chow down with a beer in their beautiful, cold, air-conditioned home that was about twenty degrees cooler than it was outside. I started to contact other friends in the area about places we could go set up camp once we got on the move again and one of my friends told me about a cool place. I also ran out of my medical stockpile of cannabis and needed more, now more than ever, with my body aching, throbbing, bleeding, and shaking like crazy. Luckily, we were in BC and there was no shortage of places to get legal medical cannabis. I looked up the closest place and Jay and I headed for the shop. Jay wanted to see what a legal store was like, so he came into the store with me. He explained how his entire generation was forced to go to shady, unreliable dealers and was very intrigued to see what a legally run storefront was like.

We walked into the store and the lady immediately checks us both out. I said to the lady, "Hello, I'd like to purchase some Sativa cannabis please." She ignorantly responds with, "You can't just come in here and buy weed." About ready to start a storm of curse words I reached for my wallet and said, "Actually, I'm a federally licenced patient so it's your job to do just that, if you have an issue, you can call your manager right now and we can sort it out." She then said, "Oh, well he can't come in the back," as she points to Jay. I told her not to worry he's just my ride. So, Jay waits in the main area as she takes me back to the purchasing area following federal government procedures and I purchase my small amount of cannabis before we left.

As we got in the van leaving the dispensary, Jay told me about the big container of marijuana he was left alone with in the front room, and I just laughed. I jokingly told him he should have just taken it and ran out on principle for them being so judgemental, arrogant, and apparently stupid. But, with how unprofessional they were, I was kind of serious. I told Jay we were not going to come back to that dispensary ever again and there was another place in Vancouver I was already registered with, so I only got a little amount to hopefully get me through to Vancouver as I aim to support the businesses that treat me well.

From there, we got on the road and drove south so I could take the highway west to Vancouver. As we were driving, my left leg went into spasms again and started to get incredibly sore, so I got Jay to pull over. Jay pulled off the highway and onto a side road and we started to drive into a lightly wooded area down a dirt road. Jay then saw another dirt road that had just 4X4 tire marks and went downhill so he turned right and took a few seconds to figure out how he was going to position the tires on the side ruts so he doesn't bottom out the minivan on the way down the four 4X4 trail.

He slowly began to head down the steep dirt road and somehow made it down the hill onto the riverbed without a single scratch or bump to the van. I rolled my smoke, got out with the dog, and Zoey had a quick run around and went pee as I had my smoke. Just after I finished my joint, I came walking around the bushes to see a lady, her daughter, and their dog going for a walk so we stopped to have a chat. I told them my story and they were astounded. I then asked if they could wait a second while I grabbed them a card and I walked around the bushes where the van was to grab one. When the woman came around the corner and saw the van down there, she was blown away and literally shouted, "YOU GOT YOUR VAN DOWN THAT HILL? I DIDN'T EVEN TAKE MY 4X4 DOWN THAT HILL!" I gave the lady and her daughter a card to find me on Facebook and follow my trip and we had a short chat before we got back in the van with the dog.

We pulled up to the bottom of the hill in the van and I hoped Jay wasn't going to drive it over the right edge of the cliff or bottom it out. Jay looked at the hill for a minute then he put the van in first gear, stepped on the gas, and we started to make our way back up. It started off easy then made a right turn around a tree before going at a much steeper incline to the top. To our left, there was a hill that went almost straight up. To our right was the opposite and there was a steep hill down with a wall of trees and bushes. The very top of the hill was the steepest part and was very loose dry dirt, so the traction wasn't very good, and the tires started to kick up lots of dust as they spun trying to grip the ground. At the top of the steep road were mountains covered in trees and cliff faces just on the other side of the highway.

We turned left to go back to the main highway and headed towards Princeton. On the way there, I remembered the lady we met in the riverbed had told me about some old train tunnels to go check out when we got to Princeton. We found a place where you could rent fully furnished cabins for the night and decided to stay there. After being on the road for a few days, just the shower alone was worth the cost. Once we checked in, we headed over to the Kettle Valley Rail Trail to check out the train tunnels. As I was walking around having a smoke, I checked out what was around the cabins and I came across a young man and I asked him, "Hey buddy, do you know if there is a dispensary in town?" He told me, "No, sorry man there's none here." Once I got back to the cabin finishing my last smoke, I connected to the Wi-Fi and Google told me there was a dispensary in town only a few kilometres away. We got back in the van, got some cannabis from a very questionable dispensary that tried to pass off the same strain as the five different kinds I wanted to try, and then headed to Kettle Valley. We arrived at the parking lot, I got out with the dog, and we started walking down the trail on the gravel path. I took a moment and looked right at the massive wall of light-brown rock. What wasn't light-brown rock was covered with green moss that had grown over the years. After a few high-hazard warning signs about the tunnels, we came to the opening of the first one.

After more warning signs we began to enter the tunnel and I dropped Zoey's leash so she could stop and smell all the walls and rocks as we walked through. As we got deeper into the tunnel, we lost all the bright sunlight, and it went completely black. I suddenly got so disoriented I lost my balance and fell like a tree that was just chopped. It was like going from sober to being so drunk I couldn't even stand in a matter of a few steps. After hearing me splat against the rocky ground and curse once or twice Jay called out, "Are you okay B?" I told him I was fine as I took out my phone and used the flashlight to get a sense of where things (like the ground) were. I was literally warned it's dark and to use a flashlight by a few of the hazard signs. But of course, I was too stubborn to listen to it, so it was no one's fault but my own dumb ass. After the first tunnel, we came into an opening that was maybe one-hundred feet until we entered another tunnel in a cliff face.

After the short tunnel, there was another opening where massive stone blocks stood on each side of the pathways to keep people from falling or venturing off the trail. On the right side of the opening was a huge cliff face that went straight up. Most of it was brown rock with a smooth, flat surface and where it was more jagged, moss managed to grow. On the very top of the rock face, you could see there were trees and small bushes that extended towards the bright blue sky.

I walked to the concrete blocks on the other side where Jay and Zoey were and looked over the edge of the manmade barrier. It dropped down ten or twenty feet, then there was a small creek. On the other side of the creek was another rock wall that stood vertically. This one was more jagged and rough, so it managed to be comfortable enough for a few small trees and lots of moss to grow. The creek at the bottom of the cliff was small; but where it pooled, it was a very light-green colour. The creek ran through the canyon of rock that stood a hundred feet tall on both sides.

As we entered the mouth of another tunnel, I looked up and saw the huge cliff face was all broken, jagged, and completely covered in green moss. On both sides of the huge rock faces, the tops were lined with trees and bushes all along the edges. It was like a huge crack in the earth's crust that they made tunnels through; it was really cool. It reminded me of a miniature version of the canyon I saw with Favourite and her family in Ontario before we parted ways just outside Thunder Bay. It wasn't nearly as big or epic but still neat, especially since you could go for a walk through the monstrous sheet of rock.

The next tunnel was very short, and we could see right through it with another entrance to a tunnel shortly beyond that one. With the hot sun beating down on us as we exited one tunnel and entered the next, we continued our walk. We came out of the tunnel, and I looked to my left to see one lonely tree that grew off the cliff before it dropped down into the creek filled with lots of rocks and medium sized boulders. On the other side of the creek was the huge rock wall that was completely covered in dark-green moss and was able to hold a few small trees. Looking down the creek you could see it took a long slight right before a hard left and disappeared behind the rock face.

After we came out of that short tunnel, we came across a tiny bridge that had massive wooden boards down the sides keeping people from falling off of the edges. To the right, was another cliff face not quite as big as the others but it was covered in dark-brown moss and a few dozen trees. We then entered the second of the bigger tunnels of rock. At the end of that one, the pathway ended, and we turned around to go back to the van. As we walked back through one of the longer, dark, cold tunnels I made a short video of my possible last words and said, "It's dark, I'm heading into a tunnel, and Jay Jay is a pervert, there is no telling what's going to happen." We continued walking, and when we came to another one of the longer tunnels, Jay stopped with the dog for a minute so I thought I would continue down the tunnel and hide along the wall in the dark and try to scare him.

I stood tall against the hard, cold rock on the right wall of the tunnel and waited. I heard someone coming and thought it was Jay, so I slowly pulled myself off the wall and quietly crept close to the person. As I got closer, I started to make out their facial features and I suddenly realized it was a lady with long dark hair by herself. It was definitely not Jay so I crept back into the darkness of the wall from which I came, and this woman passed me without knowing I was just a foot or two away from her ready to scream. As I crept back onto the wall, I couldn't help but think, 'I should have scared her anyway,' and how funny it would have been. Which was then followed by how funny it would have been when I got beat up by a woman in a tunnel in British Columbia. When Jay did come through, I pulled myself off the rock wall and tried to scare him, but he didn't even flinch, I did however scare the crap out of the dog. After our adventure, we went back to our cabin for the evening, I had a shower, Jay made dinner, and we relaxed for the night.

At one point, we went outside so I could have a smoke. I then realized all my stuff was still locked in the glove box of the van and asked Jay to get the keys for me. He saw the window to the van was still open and went to open the locked door from the inside. As soon as I saw him reach for the inside I said, "No don't!" but it was too late. The alarm on the van started blaring and going off at two in the morning. Jay ran inside to get the keys as the car horn screamed. He came out, turned the alarm off, and then said, "Sorry," to anyone that was woken up. I got my Indica cannabis, rolled a smoke, smoked it, and then went to bed.

From Princeton, we made our way southwest heading towards Hope. We spent a couple days heading that way on the Crowsnest Highway and once we got near, we had to find a place to stay. One of my friends told me while we were in the Kelowna area about a beautiful lake to go camp at. I looked it up, and we headed that way following the GPS. Only I forgot she told me the main way that you can get there is with a 4X4, or you have to go around the long way.

Following the GPS, we started to head up a mountain on a dirt road. We got halfway up the mountain when the terrain turned into big boulders that protruded out from the ground by a few inches. Jay was going slowly over them making sure the van was always high centred and not rubbing the undercarriage or scratching the van. At one point, the trail made a long, slow left turn, then went almost straight up before it took a right at the top. With us almost being there we decided to try and make it all the way up. The minivan had been a beast of a machine thus far, so what was one more hill?

Jay stopped the van, put it in first gear, and we began the vertical climb in the minivan on the side of this mountain trying to get to Jones Lake. We got about halfway up the incline before it got even steeper. With the van in first gear Jay is giving the gas to the point where the front tires were spinning as they lost traction and the front end of the van was sliding back and forth, left and right on the trail trying to pull us up the hill. Just as this was happening, a guy came around the top of the hill going back down in his raised black 4X4 jeep and when he saw us in the light-brown, soccer-mom minivan trying to make it up this colossal vertical hill, with the front end sliding and tires spinning he just shakes his head and palms his hand into his forehead like, "What the fuck are you idiots doing?" It probably made sense to him once he saw the red and white Alberta tags, as it was "red and white plague" season. Which is what people from BC say when half of Alberta goes to BC for the summer. We realized we weren't going to make it up to the lake that way, so Jay reversed the van down the main trail backwards until we spotted another side trail. This trail wasn't such a crazy incline, and the van easily made it up to the top into the bush.

I made a protein shake and we began to set up camp for the night. With the fire ban now lifted, I gathered some wood and started a small fire in the dugout pit that was already there in the ground. Jay started to cook supper and had the radio in the van playing as I sat around the fire drinking my protein shake. After my shake, I got up and looked for some more wood before it got too dark. As I was walking around the far end of our camping spot getting into the woods by myself, I started to hear this weird noise I had never heard in person before. I thought I may have just imagined it, so I stopped and listened, when I heard it again. This time it was a very recognizable sound, the sounds of a bear grunting. I waited and heard it again then again, and it sounded like it was getting closer. Way too close for comfort especially since the sun had set so we only had a light glow in the western sky for light to see, and Jay was in the process of cooking chicken over the fire for supper.

I hobbled over to the van as quickly as I could and turned off the radio. Jay said, "Hey man," as I interrupt his tunes. I told him to be quiet and listen for a second. Then again, the sound of the bear grunting was heard. Jay cooked and we ate as fast as we possibly could keeping our flashlights out checking the surrounding area, just completely paranoid. I went back to the van to try and find the bear spray I bought just in case the bear stumbled upon us. With the dog there we had a little bit of protection, but Zoey was no match for a huge bear. At best she could notify us if one was coming too close. I was honestly surprised she wasn't already barking or freaking out.

After tearing the van apart, I couldn't find the bear spray and the paranoia really hit me. As we sat by the fire, we could hear the bear just off in the bush walking back and forth making grunting noises. I don't think my flashlight was turned off or turned away from the depths of the bushes where the noise was coming from. The noise of the bear roamed closer and closer for around an hour or so before it slowly faded away.

After hanging out for a bit around the fire I headed to bed. With ears wide open listening for the sounds of the bear, sleep that night wasn't too great. Next thing I notice it's morning and I'm woken up to the sounds of a girl screaming, "FUCK HER RIGHT IN THE PUSSY!" which was this online video that went viral and was going on for months now. I laughed because I knew what it was from, but I don't think Jay did, he just got to wake up to it. He woke up to that and asks if I heard the woman just down the hill on the road to our left screaming. I told him I did, and he said something about people being wild and going hard at nine in the morning on like a Tuesday.

I gave Jay the background story of the viral video and he had a laugh as we packed up camp. We got back on the road and after a few hours, I needed to stop and have a break, so I crossed the street to a rest stop on the oncoming side. Right when I stopped, I looked down and there on the pavement on the side of the highway, in the middle of nowhere, was another dime. I couldn't help but think, 'What the hell? What are the odds I would stop right here out of all the places to stop at, and there would be a dime?' Another coincidence or a sign from the spirits, I had no idea at first, but it was really starting to freak me out. With the frequency of these dimes and being in the most random, unpopulated, isolated places. I wondered, 'Was it Tony watching me finishing my trek from above? Was he letting me know he was there watching?' These dimes were having me think of all the good times we had growing up together and that it would all be okay. We would be reunited as a family again eventually.

Wondering if Uncle Tony was watching over me, I had a marijuana cigarette as I took a break on the side of the road. Zoey decided to jump out to join me and go for a pee. While I had a puff on the side of the highway, I looked at my phone and thankfully I had some cellphone service, so I looked up the alternate way to Jones Lake that wasn't a 4X4 off road trail and took some screen shots for later. I also took a quick look at Facebook and saw posts about the coward that killed Tony and how he was released on parole after serving eighteen months of his seventy-two-month sentence. My mind exploded with so much unmeasurable anger I couldn't think or see straight. I was so enraged I had to have another joint just to calm my nerves. But one thing was now abundantly clear to me. Finding these dimes was no coincidence, it was a clear message from Tony up above. He was watching me finish my trek and he was making sure that I knew it. It was enough of a tug on my emotions I cried out a few tears as I continued through the forest on the road.

After I was done trekking for the day, we drove back over to Jones Lake which was easy to get to the alternate way. Once we got to the lake, we began to drive clockwise around it looking for a place to camp. However, it was really busy and the only spot available was the area by a boat launch ramp on the other side of the lake. We parked the van, and I was horrified when I got out. There was about half a dozen black garbage bags full of trash some lazy cowards just left there. The place itself was incredibly peaceful and amazingly beautiful. The light-blue lake water sat at the base of completely tree-covered hills. Where the lake ended on the far end to our left, there were huge Rocky Mountains that came soaring out of the ground and reached into the sky. They still had lots of snow on them, even though it was the end of summer now. The huge Rocky Mountains then turned into big, tree-covered rolling hills that came our way touching the sides of the lake. Then to the right of the lake the tree-covered hills went on for as far as you could conceive, eventually getting lost to the distance. As I was enjoying the sights and setting up my tent I looked down and another dime was just sitting there on top of the dirt.

I bent down and picked it up while thinking, 'What is going on here? Why am I finding dimes in literally the most random areas of the country on mountains and roads.' It was really starting to freak me out and also got me thinking about my hero Tony again. Finding each dime brought on a lot of lingering negative emotions which in turn brings on nerve pain, so I decided to roll a smoke and go for a walk. But first, I pulled out my tent and got everything ready to be set up for when I got back. As I was getting my things out, another lady and her teenage son pulled in and started to set up their camp. When they saw the mountain of garbage left by the previous pigs, we hatched a plan to split the garbage between us and remove them from the area to dispose of them properly.

I sat in the van behind closed doors and rolled a smoke with the new Princeton cannabis. Since people were starting to come in and pitch tents in what seemed to be the only available spot, I decided to go walk down the road that went around the lake. I got to the road and my spasms kicked in again and I could hardly even move my leg. I put my smoke in my mouth really wishing I brought my vaporizer because it's discrete, doesn't smell as strong, and it's much easier on the lungs so doctors prefer it, and I've had a huge increase in my cannabis intake over the last few weeks to physically be able to get across the province. With a half-pound of dried cannabis and nearly an ounce of oil smoked in the last four weeks I could only imagine how black my lungs were getting. But mainly I like my vaporizer for the discreteness of it, I could just sit in my tent, and no one would know I was puffing anything unless they came into it.

I sparked my smoke and within a few puffs my leg calmed down enough I could slowly start to walk down the road on the right side. As I was walking, I looked down into the ditch and saw a Frisbee. Thinking the dog might have fun with It, I grabbed the hard red disk and kept on walking. Once I was finished half of my smoke I started to walk back just as this black truck came flying down the dirt road and passed me, kicking up a dust cloud that quickly enveloped me and I started to choke on the dust and cough harder than I was when I was smoking my cannabis.

I got back to the camp still dusting myself off and saw the black truck pulled onto the other side of the boat ramp. As I left for my walk there were two other cars that were just pulling in and now the only remaining place was just crowded with cars, trucks, and tents with a path only for the boat launch that not a single person used. We sat around and talked with the other people as we had a beer or two that they offered us before bed. As I was getting ready for bed I got in the van and started to roll a smoke as my leg was killing me from the day's ride. I was usually able to take off my ankle brace after the day on the road but today my ankle and leg were so weak that anytime I took a step, my ankle wouldn't be able to handle it, and it would roll which isn't pleasant even though I can hardly feel it as it happens. But after walking on a sideways ankle for a while it gets very sore and throbs like crazy which was currently happening.

As I was rolling my smoke, this one guy was obviously watching me. He was looking where I was putting my marijuana things and watching every movement I made. I rolled my smoke then locked my stuff in the glovebox and gave the keys back to Jay. My ankle and foot were in so much pain I couldn't bring myself to go for a walk, so I lit my smoke and threw the Frisbee for the dog just as another car pulled into the right side of the boat launch. Zoey went running after the flying disc, only when she brought it back, it was broken in half, so I tossed it to the garbage pile and had my bedtime Indica smoke before I crawled into my tent and went to sleep.

As I was just about asleep, I was woken up to the sound of someone at our van and I assumed it was Jay. However, Jay was in his tent in bed as well. Jay also heard the person and hit the lock button on the key-fob to be sure it was locked then heard someone say, "fuck" as they walked away. No idea who they were or what they wanted. My only assumption was that the one guy who was staring at me rolling my last smoke was possibly trying to find my medications. That or another drunk was going around car-hopping.

After the stranger walked away, I fell asleep, and I woke up to the sounds of the other campers getting packed up and leaving. I slowly got out of my sleeping bag and started to pack my things for another day on the road. Jay called out to me to see if I was alive and getting ready. Once I replied he said, "Oh good morning, Bee-anna, how did you sleep?" I told him, "It was good except for the guy at the car in the middle of the night."

Because the camp was so overcrowded and now had a fire ban on, we decided to find another place to stay. Just a day away from Mission, we drove around and tried to find a place to camp that was closer and eventually found a site that was much less busy and began to set up our tents and covered them in blue tarps as it was raining on and off that day.

The fire ban was finally lifted however everything was soaking wet. Jay pulled out the small green camper stove and began to cook the steaks he had marinating in some beer and spices. We took out the couple bags of garbage from Jones Lake and threw them out in the garbage bins at the new site before we had our dinner. After dinner, Jay and I played a simple drinking game with our few beers and a deck of cards. The game consisted of a few questions. The first question was guessing if the card was red or black, the second was higher or lower (than the number on the first card), and the third was in between or outside (the range of the previous two cards). Every time you got an answer wrong you had to take a sip of your drink. After that, we relaxed for the night. Now that we were getting into populated areas again, I finally had some cell service, so I started to contact a few local media outlets. I remember the night being very calming. With the sounds of a river maybe thirty feet from my tent I lay there and listened to the relaxing, tranquil sounds of the running water as I fell asleep.

The next morning, we got up and packed, I called the RCMP to let them know I would be on the side of the highway and asked if they had any requirements of me. But they gave me the same answer as the ones all across the province did. They all said, "As long as you're not obstructing or slowing down traffic in any way, you'll be okay." But I always called them when I could, just to be sure. After I got up and called the RCMP, I heard things hitting my tent and had no idea what it was. I then heard Jay screaming and swearing at someone. I got out of my tent and Jay was still cussing and cursing before he told me that the things hitting my tent all morning were from squirrels up in the tall trees dropping pinecones on us. I couldn't help but laugh as every now and then a random pinecone would fall from the sky on us as we tried to pack. The aim of the little critters was surprisingly accurate too, this definitely wasn't their first human pelting rodeo.

As I came out of the empty woods and into the densely populated area of the West Coast of Canada, I started to be a problem on the road. With my inability to safely walk, longboard, or even ride a bike I was becoming a danger, a liability, and starting to become problematic for the general public. So, once we got to Mission, we decided to get me and my zigzagging-wobbly ass off the highway and make up the kilometres from Mission to Vancouver in a safe place. Jay suggested we go to Stanley Park and ride there.

I started to contact friends in the Vancouver area looking for a place to crash for the next few nights as I made up my kilometres. I was told we should go crash at "the Stoop" skate house. They are awesome people that put up travelling skaters that come in and out of town for events or just passing through. I contacted them and they said we were more than welcome to come crash for a few nights. We drove over there and hung out on the back deck and chatted for hours as everyone asked me all kinds of questions about my trip across the country. At one point, someone pulled out the bearings from the last guy (that wasn't my father) who longboarded across the country. The same amazing man that snapped me out of an immense drug-like state with a gold metal when I was in ICU, Striker. As day moved into the night, everyone started to go to bed, and we debated whether to throw out our tents or crash on the couches on the back deck but that was easily determined when someone mentioned their dog might have fleas. Jay took Zoey to the van so fast and started to throw out the stuff we needed to get to bed. We popped out our tents and began to fill our air mattresses that both now had holes in them from the dog's claws. So, we would go to bed on a mattress and wake up on a half-filled or completely flat one. Jay's mattress had a huge hole in it, so he decided to just lay down the seats and sleep in the back of the van with the dog.

I made my bed and as I lay there listening to the sounds of police sirens and cars, I couldn't help but miss the peace and quiet of the nature we just spent the last five weeks in. It seemed to take forever to get to sleep that night. I wondered if it was because I wasn't out in nature and back in population or if it was because I was so close to finishing my trek and I was filled with anxiety that had not hit me yet.

Once I finally fell asleep, I was suddenly woken to the sounds of tires screeching followed by a loud crash and the sounds of debris scattering everywhere. I quickly got up and popped my head out of the tent to see a small glowing fire quickly drive off. I didn't see anything worthy of staying up and reporting and wondered if I should get out half naked and go investigate but I decided I would be of no actual use to anyone as I only saw a moving flaming object between the cracks of the white fence. After hearing people coming out of their houses all around me, I decided to mind my own business and go back to bed. That would be easier said than done as for the next few hours it was fire trucks, police, and people talking about the incident everywhere around me.

The next morning everyone was still talking about the three in the morning wakeup call. It turns out some drunk crashed his wall magnet into a parked car just beside the house, then tried to drive their flaming wreckage away but was stopped by police and arrested just a few blocks away. We sat around chatting about things and Jay was worried about Zoey possibly getting fleas and didn't even want to risk a vet bill and medications even though it was not entirely clear there were any, so I started to talk to some friends in the area to see if they could put us up for a night or two while I caught up on some kilometres.

My awesome French friend in Maple Ridge was more than happy to have us over for a couple nights so we headed over to Stanley Park for the day before we went to her house. We got to the park, and I started to skate along the seawall. Across the waterway, I could see a big, tree-covered hill that came out of the ground and was now halfway over-taken by houses. There was a huge bridge that came out of the tree lines on my left and stretched all the way over the water to where the houses on the hill were. As I was going around the sea wall again, I started to notice I was getting dirty looks from people, like everyone.

As I continued to ride it was like every person I rode past was giving me bad looks and someone said something to me so I pulled out my headphones and everyone was complaining to me about how I "shouldn't be riding my skateboard there." They were genuinely upset and agitated I was doing such a horrific thing in their presence. I brushed it off the first time and the second time. But as I came back to the statue of a mermaid on a rock, I almost collided with someone after my muscle tone threw me off balance and I jumped off my board to miss him. The guy was incredibly upset I had interrupted his run and started to give me a piece of his mind. He stopped complaining and all I could say was, "I'm leaving, sorry I almost hit you, have a great day," as I grabbed my board and hobbled off back to the van. It took me forever to walk back and when I saw a few other longboarders riding the trail, I wondered why I was getting grilled and they just floated on by people, so I put my board down and got back to pushing when an old man looked me in the eyes as I approached, then took a big step to his left and deliberately cut me off and I nearly collided with him. He too stops me to tell me I'm not allowed to skateboard there. I badly wanted to tell him, "Until I see a sign that permits me from doing so, I'm riding, and I just saw a few riders pass me on longboards, so where were you on that one, dip shit?"

Completely infuriated and fed up with people, I was turning more and more into an asshole by the minute while wishing I was back in the bush. I got back to the van and told Jay I was not welcome to ride my board there, so he suggested I bike as he knows there is even a bike rental place there. He pulls down the bike and I get my foot in the strap and he gives me a push to get going. No one was saying a thing, so I continued biking around until I ended up getting spat out into a parking lot after taking a wrong turn. I also started to notice people would deliberately cut me off and get in my way. Between having to dodge people and not knowing where I was going, I got lost and infuriated as this young Asian couple did the same thing the old man did. They looked me in the eye, then took a big step in my way. I was getting more and more salty by the minute so I went back to the van and asked Jay if he could come lead the way as he knew his way around the park and could ride ahead of me clearing people out of my way.

We went to the bike rental place, got Jay a bike, then began to bike around. I followed Jay and realized I was going the wrong way as we were in a different parking lot than I thought. I got my ways mixed up. We went around for a bit then we got to an area where you had to get off and walk for the kid's park and I was pretty much pushed into the poles by the impatient crowd of people and struggled to just get my foot out and I ended up falling over in front of at least thirty people taking someone's handle bars to my left ribs as I went down, which wasn't all too pleasant. I was more embarrassed than hurt but as soon as I got up off the ground, I felt the pain and walked my bike over to Jay who was waiting on the other side of the kid's park. Now I was getting impatient and more aggravated by the second, with so many people everywhere it was causing lots of problems for me.

With my left knee now throbbing and a sore left ribcage we continued. I got back on my bike and tried to get my foot into the strap only to realize it was now broken from my fall. Once I got my foot in, I tried to get going but the angle of my foot was bad, and my foot was catching on the arm of the pedal keeping me from a complete rotation. With my inability to move those fine motor muscles to rotate my foot, I had to have Jay come over and twist it for me. However, my fall really irritated my leg, and it was now going crazy, shaking with spasms. After we got going, we realized we forgot to pay for parking again after we went to the bike rental place and parked in a different parking lot when we returned. So, we turned around and headed back to pay for another few hours of parking.

I actually made it back without falling again and right when we got to the top of a small hill overlooking the parking lot, we saw the van and there beside it was parking authority with pen and paper in hand. Jay zoomed down there as fast as he could as I just kind of slowly coasted down the hill knowing what would happen if I got going too fast. Just as I pulled up, Jay was thanking the man as he decided to let us "out-of-towners go because they really target the locals that abuse their parking privileges." Just as the nice man walked away, I felt my phone ringing in my bag. I got off the bike feeling the ache in my knee as I placed it down and answered the call. It was a lady from

CBC radio calling me back asking if I was available to do an interview. I asked if we could do it in Stanley Park and she was more than happy with that. So, I biked around for a while as we waited for the young woman to arrive.

I got back to the parking lot using my best guess as to when she said she would arrive and just as I got to the van, she called me and told me she was at the parking lot. I rushed around trying to find her with no success wondering if I had made a mistake. I told her what I saw around me, and she realized I was in the other parking lot. She zoomed over and we walked around and talked for a bit before I got on my board and rode around which was rather hard with my shaking leg, left aching knee, and ribs hurting with every push and expansion of my breathing. I still wasn't fully recovered from my Summerland adventures as it takes me so much longer to recover from wipe outs post stroke. However, she just wanted some sounds as it was for the radio, so it wasn't too painful.

After the interview, we got back on the pathways and began biking. I thought Jay's presence would help but people were still looking me in the eye as I was coming then would step into my way and cut me off. I was wondering what was going on with people as I'm hardly able to manoeuvre around them in time and nearly crashed into every person. We came around a parking lot and down a hill that split two ways and there was a big traffic jam of people there. Jay hit his back break, locked his back tire, and skid to a quick stop. Me on the other hand…

I grabbed the back break, but I tried to stop too fast for my abilities, and it threw me into my right handle bar turning me left on the sidewalk and I ran into the back of Jay, who was there waiting for the traffic to clear. I saw him last second and threw my body limp to the right to try to avoid hitting him and hopefully hit the grass instead. But when I ran into Jay I was back at the X-Games for the disabled, flying through the air, over my handlebars, hoping I would make it to the grass. It was like one of those scenes you see in a movie when the person is flying in slow motion through the air and looking at the soft place they want to land. But then the slow-motion stops, the reality of that thing called gravity takes over, they stop moving forward, and just go straight down. SPLAT. I hit the cement hard flat on my chest and stomach a foot or two short from hitting the grass. I hit the pavement hard on my right and on my left arm that seemed to naturally curl up into my chest as I was airborne before hitting the ground and rolling into the grass, cussing and cursing. I remember a woman let out a blood curdling scream when this happened, "OH MY GOD! ARE YOU OKAY!?" She screamed bloody murder like I was just brutally shot or stabbed multiple times and in life threatening condition.

After I swallowed my pride, I told her, "I've been through worse, I'm sure I'll live." I got up and I looked at Jay and said, "Yeah, screw this place. I don't think this is the best place for me." I really hurt my left arm and my back when I belly-flopped onto the pavement with my arm between my body and the ground. Jay looked at me, in obvious pain, and asked if we should stop for the day. I told him, "yeah, we should definitely find me a better spot." So at the end to another day of the

X-Games for hobble-heads, we headed over to my friend's house for the night. Being so incredibly sore I had to remind myself **never give up and live life to the fullest no matter what life throws at** you.

But before we left, we had to make a traditional Stanley Park stop at the "big tree." We drove over to it and parked the van. There stood the shell of the "big tree." The sign there reads, "It was a monument to the original forest of the giant trees. It had survived extensive logging in the eighteen-hundreds. It had endured colossal windstorms that knocked down thousands of trees in the park. It had lost its top; however, the circumference is nearly fifty feet."

I walked into the preserved "hollow tree" with the dog and looked at the big, black steel bars cemented into the ground that held the shell in place. Jay took a quick picture of Zoey and I, before I went straight back to the van so we could get out of there and I could have some pain management which I desperately needed. As I hardly walked back to the van, I could feel my tone kick in and started to walk on my left tiptoes which bends my foot in half and really hurts. The pain in my left arm hurt really bad and after seeing the swelling I wondered if I should go get it looked at by a doctor or X-rayed. However, with growing up in hospitals and with an ER nurse my whole life I knew what to look for to tell if it was broken or if there were any problems, so I let the bicep tense up my arm into the fetal position it goes into when it's hurt and let it do its thing. Only when my left arm tenses up like it does, it pulls on my left shoulder blade which causes upper back pain and/or a shoulder dislocation as well.

Jay got in the van, and we headed over to Maple Ridge for the night. Since Stanley Park wasn't an adequate place for me, we decided to go to "Mile 0" where the other Terry Fox monument in Canada is located. As we left Vancouver, we drove through the nice and quiet scene in East Hastings. First, there was a guy wearing green shorts that sat at his knees, wearing no shirt and with no boxers or underwear on. His junk was probably hanging out of the front as his white ass was hanging out the back. He's like this, just walking down the street like it's a normal Saturday afternoon of showing off his bird. Next up, was a lady with her tube top down to her waist and her breasts out hanging down to her stomach. Then there was a guy sitting on cardboard boxes with a needle shooting something up his right arm and then on the corner of the street was a cop in full uniform just standing there watching for violence so he can keep the peace or do whatever he can to help people in need.

We continued to drive through what seemed to be the homeless capital of Canada and I remembered one of my friends telling me about this place and the methadone clinic that was giving out free needles and a place to shoot up. Which sounds messed up, but it drastically helped cut the spread of disease, helped clean up the dirty, used needles on the streets that were becoming an overwhelming issue for the city, and kept lots of individuals from dying from overdosing. From what I've heard, it was actually doing a good job at it. The uniformed officer was just there to stop violence and let the people do their thing and kept it all contained to the one area of the city. We continued down the street and stopped at a red light behind one other car who was pulled over talking to someone. As the light went green, we sat there stuck with people honking behind us. We sat there so long we all missed the green light and had to wait so the guys in front of us could do their hand-to-hand business.

We finally got moving and I began to notice there was a stream of water running down the side of the road, which was odd for being a dry, sunny, hot day with no rain or clouds in sight. We continued down the road a little farther and I looked to Jay and said, "Well this guy is making a mess," as I pointed to the stream of fluids that was pouring out the back of a big cube van from under the back door. We finally got to Celine's house and with the fire ban gone we had a small fire in the back yard as Zoey and her two dogs played. I was taking pictures of them playing when Celine's bigger dog Gibson got a little too pushy and Zoey snarled and snapped her jaws together at him to put him in his place. In one of the pictures I took, you could see the anger in Zoey's face as she's growling and showing her teeth. Then you can see the fear in Gibson's face with his eyes wide open, looking so scared. His facial expression screamed he knew he messed up. It was a great capture. That night, Jay folded the back seats down and I pumped up both our air mattresses and stacked them and slept in Celine's place as Jay crashed in the van for the night.

The next morning, we got to the ferry and headed over to Victoria. I thought about finishing my trek in Vancouver but I didn't want the massive landmass of America in the background, so I thought the west side of the island would be the best place to get nothing but water in the background. As we were on the ferry, I got a message back from the Heart and Stroke foundation. So, we made arrangements to stop in and say hello while we were there.

In Victoria, the Thunder Bird Motor Inn put us up for a night which was super awesome of them. That night my anxiety sucker-punched me and it was going so crazy I wasn't able to get to or stay asleep. I asked Jay if he could turn off the TV, as my head was in this endless loop of, 'Tomorrow you're finishing the trek you thought was over at one point,' and, 'Tomorrow is the third-year anniversary of your last stroke.' I couldn't help but think about the whole trek across the country from tattoo to where I currently lay and how gnarly, painful, and difficult the last few years of my life has been. It ended up being a pretty sleepless night for me as I was encased with so much thought and emotion.

The next morning, we were up and off to go meet the woman from the Heart and Stroke office in Victoria. Jay had put the bike on top of the van with the wheels in the air and as we pulled into the back of the parking lot, the bike hit the height sign that was dangling from two chains. "Whoops" Jay said. I also wasn't paying attention to the height of the van at the moment, and we both learned a quick lesson to pay more attention to that.

When we got out of the van, I looked at the bike which was still in one piece and didn't see any dents in the roof of the van so I grabbed my board and again struggled to skate around the building to the front doors and called them to let them know I was there. A short time later, Jay appeared from around the corner with Zoey and we waited for a brief moment before she came outside. We had a good talk about things and took a picture with the Heart and Stroke sign trying to avoid the massive dentist sign just above it. As Jay was trying to use my phone, Zoey came over and sat with us for the picture.

After our quick meeting we got back in the van and drove over to "Mile 0". When we got there, I got my board, stepped over the wire fence, and walked right through the field to go look at the Terry Fox monument. I took some pictures, checked it out, and took off on my board trying to avoid a trip to the ER. As I skated around, I came through a small tunnel of trees before I went down to the ridge area and looked around. The view of the ocean was beautiful, and I could have sat there on the ridge all day but I skated down the path before I came back and ran into Jay who was walking with the dog. He handed me the leash, I took it from him, and Zoey started to pull me around. Then she started going really fast and straight into a group of older people. One poor man didn't know where to go or what to do, with the dog and I quickly coming flying around the corner, so I turned off into the grass then waited before I gave Jay the leash back, saying, "Yeah, that was a stupid idea."

I started to push the other way, away from the older people and came around a slow left turn that had a few more elderly people walking towards me. One gentleman was on the pathway in his lane, and I was in mine coming up to him. To his left walking in the grass on my right side were two older women and as I came up to them on the path one lady looks at me then steps off the grass and directly into my way on the pathway. For a split second I thought, 'Ok. I'm just going to send you flying,' as I was so fed up with people at this point. Instead of taking out the old bag I just rode into the grass where she was walking before she cut me off. I looked at her and said, "Really lady, really?" And without saying anything they walked on. When Jay walked by them a short time later, they were still complaining about me and Jay said, "He's not going fast; he's had a massive stroke." Apparently, the lady just said, "Oh," and walked on. I remember thinking, 'I can't believe I missed longboarding and being treated like shit,' even with my leg brace and shoulder brace on, people only saw the longboard and treat you based on their perception of what long boarders are to them. I told Jay, "Screw this, let's go find a place that isn't filled with old people or people in general so I can skate in peace," and began skating back to the van. Once we got back to where we parked, I saw the big "no skateboarding" sign on the pathway that I missed rushing across the grass to the "Mile 0" sign and the Terry Fox statue. As soon as I saw the sign, I realized I was the asshole here and it all began to make sense.

We took off heading down the 14 highway, across the big, beautiful island but it wasn't long before my spasms kicked in and I could hardly walk again. We got to the Port Renfrew area where I saw a little rocky beach just off the west side of the highway. I used my board as a cane to get down the ditch that had big roots I used as stairs, but with my muscle tone kicking my foot straight down and violently shaking in the process, my foot was catching them, and I almost fell face first down the small embankment three or four times. If it wasn't for my board, I would have fallen for sure. Once I finally made it down to the small rocky beach all I could see was the water of the Pacific Ocean, it was perfect. Jay came down with the dog as I sat there reflecting on the last three and a half years and smoked my strawberry-flavoured victory blunt. Sadly, it wasn't even an enjoyable time for me. You'd think finishing the trek I'd feel ecstatic and proud or something. However, it was all so overwhelming I couldn't even stand to be there. The tsunami of overwhelming emotions, experiences, stories, and past hardships came vividly flashing threw my mind which caused my nerve pain to go absolutely crazy. It was like the left side of my body had spontaneously combusted. It hurt with such an intense burning sensation from the inside. I half expected to burst into flames on the spot as I chain puffed my blunt trying to ease the burning nerves. I finished my smoke but from my eye level down to my ankle, the left side of my body still burned. 'Well, this is pretty shit,' I thought to myself, wanting to immediately leave, not even able to enjoy the monumental moment in my life, at all.

As I stood there in full spasms and pain on the left side of my body, I gave Jay my phone to take a few pictures. I wanted to raise my left arm in the air facing the water. My left arm because at one point I couldn't even move the thing let alone lift it over my head and facing the ocean to symbolize facing the rest of the world beyond the water. I told Jay to stand behind me and take some pictures as I raised my left arm up in victory. Only every time I raised my arm higher than my shoulder, my shoulder would pop out of place and dislocate which would cause my arm to drop in agonizing pain and make me nauseous. I probably dislocated my shoulder three or four times if not more just to get the picture I wanted. Jay also took pictures of me dipping my board and Limpy (my left foot) into the water. I really avoided the wheels in the ocean this time as I didn't want to destroy my bearings like I did with the Atlantic dip at Middle Cove Beach years before.

As I sat there, trying to reflect on the cross-country trip and my third stroke for a brief moment my emotions ran wild, and I could no longer enjoy the moment. So, with my wobbly leg I started to walk back to the ditch just as Jay called me over to see the small star fish he found. I told him, "I really need to go and get more medications," as my blunt on the beach was all I had left, and it didn't do anything for my pain. Jay found some seashells and I collected three of them for me to give to important people in my life there and back home.

With populated areas not being a good place for me, Jay and I made a plan to take our time and take a few days in the bush to finish the last kilometres and we began to head back to Vancouver. After we caught the ferry back to the mainland, we stopped at a coin laundry place so I could wash my dirty clothes. After a quick stop at a legal provider of mine in the area we headed over to the Amsterdam Café for my Vancouver tradition where I rented a volcano and sat down to medicate. After a few bags I was feeling a bit better and started to function better as well, so I gave my love to the little kitty that was there before we went back to Maple Ridge again. As we left and went back around to the parking lot, I remembered I completely forgot to pay for parking and was expecting a ticket as I know they monitor that spot hard. My friend paid for a ticket in front of a parking enforcement guy and put it on his dash before we left, and the officer still gave him a ticket because it wasn't clearly visible when it slid down or something as he shut the door.

Luckily Jay remembered to throw some change in and paid for parking before I was even physically able to get out of the van, so I dodged a bullet there and we headed over to my friend's for one last night in Maple Ridge. But first we went to grab my laundry. I grabbed my clothes out of the one dryer as Jay grabbed my hoodies from the other, threw them in a plastic bag, set them down for me to grab, and we took off to Maple Ridge.

We arrived, the dogs said hello as we said hello to Celine and her son Sedrick. We were all in the back having a small fire hanging out for a while when Celine told me to bring my things inside for when I go to bed. She and her son went inside, and I began to fill the air mattresses from the left side of the van that Jay backed in. As I was trying to shimmy myself between the fence and the van trying not to rub the air mattress on anything, I heard the blast of a loud train horn that scared the pants off of me and my already sore lefty(left arm) jumped and punched the wooden fence on my left really hard. My right side did nothing but for some reason, post-third stroke, my left side jumps like crazy when I get scared or hear an unexpected loud noise.

As I was wondering why I just heard a loud train horn in the city on the street, Sedrick came out, looked at his phone, then asked, "Did you hear a train horn at all?" I replied, "Yeah, man, it scared the crap out of me and I punched the fence when I jumped." He had a laugh and said it was his buddy letting him know he's back in town. I told him, "Call him an asshole for scaring me," as I brought my stuff inside still laughing about what just happened. I set up my bed and went back outside for a bit longer. Jay, Celine, and I accompanied by Zoey and Gibson sat around and chatted for a couple hours relaxing before bed. I was getting cold so I went to put on one of my freshly cleaned hoodies and I couldn't find them anywhere. I then remembered Jay put them down for me in the laundromat and I never grabbed them as I thought Jay was going to. I suddenly realized my two one-hundred-dollar Ephin hoodies were in a laundromat in the heart of downtown Vancouver. I called the store and asked the person if they could see them, but they were long gone, and I was furious that I just lost a couple hundred bucks while knowing someone's going to be stoked on life to find them. Celine went inside and grabbed me a grey sweater to put on, so I at least had something to wear. A short while later, Jay decided to crawl in the van and sleep with the seats down again and the rest of us went to bed inside.

The next morning, I woke up and I was just on the floor as both mattresses completely deflated again. I went and brushed my teeth before creeping outside to see if Jay was up. He heard me coming and said, "Good morning, Bee-anna," like he always did. Knowing he was up, I popped the back hatch of the van and it was completely filled with cigarette smoke. I gave him some attitude about it as I knew I was going to get it by my grandparents once we got home in a couple days. After I got upset with Jay, I started to think about our route home and where some adequate places for me to catch up on kilometres would be. I thought the highway from Fort Steele and all the way up to Golden would be the best isolated location for me to safely push as there was hardly any traffic or population between the two places.

As I was pondering places to ride, Celine came out of her house just as I hear Jay get a phone call. Jay answers the phone saying, "Hello," then shouts, "WHAT!?" as he bursts into tears. Celine asked me what was wrong, and knowing the death of a loved one was the only thing that has ever done that to me, I told Celine, "I don't know. I think someone has passed away." Jay came over in an absolute mess and said, "B, we have to go right now my friend was just killed in a car accident and another is in the hospital fighting for her life in ICU." **There are some things in life we can't control** and the passing of a loved one is definitely one of those situations.

There was no arguing at all, as death seems to be the only thing the world will temporarily stop for. I told him, "I'm so sorry to hear about your friends, Jay Jay." He had spoken so highly of the wonderful couple the entire trip across British Columbia, and I was really looking forward to meeting them one day. I ran inside and rushed to gather my things and we tossed everything we brought into a big unorganized mess into the belly of the van, and we left within five minutes of that phone call. We left mid-morning probably around nine or ten and we got back to Calgary well before dinner, it should have taken several hours more. I'm surprised we didn't get pulled over as we were probably doing well over the speed limit with Jay in shock. However, I think we did get one ticket just as we got into the city of Calgary from a speed trap on the side of the road.

Like I said earlier, my journey will inevitably end with death. It just so happens it wasn't mine, yet. But it's only a matter of time until me, like all of you, will have to face it. It may be today, it may be tomorrow, or it may be in a few decades from now. All I know is I'll be living life to the fullest until my time on this beautiful planet runs out and I'll be giving it my all everyday no matter what life throws at me. The entire way home I sent Jay's surviving friend all the love, happiness, and healing vibes I could. I prayed for her to recover, which she did physically. However, the mental pain of losing a loved one is much more of a never-ending, arduous battle.

After Jay dropped me off, I walked into my room where I was quickly enveloped by the love of the Reston School kids get-well cards. I took a minute to walk around my room and read all of the uplifting messages while thinking, 'I can't believe it's all over.' It came to a very fast, abrupt, and tragic ending and I wished it could have ended on a better note but there are some things in life we can't control. That phone call would have ended the trip wherever we were, and by some mystery of the universe, it was on the very last day when we were planning on turning around. It struck me how it should have ended three years prior in September of 2013 while I fought for my life in the ICU.

Again, I couldn't help but think about how that it should have been me who died. Time after time after time and time again. But I made it, throughout it all. I began to think about how before I left Calgary with my dad, I wanted this trip to change me and my life forever and I couldn't get over how much more of a genuine, caring, and positive human I am now, compared to before. I got exactly what I wanted. I finally not only finished a monstrosity of a challenge without dying, I forever changed who I am and the way I view things with a better outlook on life. I am a better person, happier, and for once in my life I am the most grateful I've ever been. I have come to realize that no matter who you are or where you come from, tragedy in life is inevitable. However, I believe these tragedies are what shape you into the person you're going to become. But it's up to you to decide whether it's going to change you in a negative, or a positive way.

Now that I was finished my trek, I started to think about what's next for me. As soon as I walked into my room and saw the get-well cards still plastered all over my walls and re-read them, the newspaper articles, the signed deck from Ryan at Royal, and the signed longboarding posters I have. I realized that I now should have the credibility behind my name and story to start speaking. So, I began building onto one of my Toastmasters projects and re-enrolled with them. A month later I felt confident enough, so I contacted Lori at the Reston School and began to plan a date I could come give her and the school a very long overdue thank you.

My two current goals were to go do a speech for the kids in Manitoba and get to being stroke free. Lori talked to the school and booked a date for me to come down. I took the bus down to Manitoba almost getting the boot off the bus in Saskatchewan after the older, uneducated and misinformed bus driver tried to tell me my federal cannabis licence (valid anywhere in Canada) wasn't valid in Saskatchewan, and I needed to look into the laws. However, I finally got to Manitoba and Lori picked me up before we drove over to her house for a delicious taco casserole dinner. After dinner, I gave her a quick overview of my presentation and asked her about the one thing that I was unsure about, but she said it was fine. The next morning, we got up and headed over to the Reston School and I did my first public presentation.

My mental nerves were unreal as they all piled into the gymnasium, however, oddly, my nerve pain wasn't going crazy like I expected it to. I delivered my presentation before Lori and I had a quick talk with some of the students. Then I was suddenly signing kid's hoodies, backpacks, binders, notebooks, and a longboard. It was also funny to see some of the kids losing their minds trying the "Harrison Challenge." After my speech and the little autograph party, Lori and I walked around the school and I went to say hello to a few classrooms and teachers. I had a nice talk with a fellow student who had a stroke in his mother's uterus before he was even born which blew me away as I didn't even know that was possible at the time.

I was given a big poster signed by all the school kids who left me uplifting positive notes. It was a day or so later, I started to get messages from students who were at the speech and every one of them said how motivated, inspired, and moved by my speech they were. They told me how it impacted them in a variety of positive ways. I then started to realize every single person I told my story to was motivated, inspired, and impressed all at once. I realized I needed to do it more and began contacting charity's, hospitals, and other schools to deliver my hour-long presentation to anyone that could use some inspiring. It was something that I went from hating and avoiding school over, to absolutely loving and enjoying. I had finally found my mental escape. However, it was definitely odd going from the shy, quiet, strong type who rarely shared my story, to sharing it to the world.

After Lori and I left the school, we went back to her house and hung around while the rest of her family arrived. Once everyone was there, we got into the car and took a drive to a restaurant just on the other side of the Saskatchewan border where they treated me to another delicious dinner at a great steak house to celebrate before going back to their house for a quick nap. Then at around 2 a.m., Fred drove me to the bus station so I could get on the bus and go back home.

As luck would have it, both my current goals were accomplished within a few weeks of each other as I was booked in for a brain scan a short time later. On November 24th 2017, I was up at 5:30 a.m. for a brain imaging procedure called a cerebral angio. My ride showed up around 6:15 and I made my way over to my home-away-from-home, the Foothills Medical Centre (FMC). My medical appointment letter told me to go to the diagnostic imaging department on the main floor in the main building, but I got dropped off at the other building, the special services building (SSB) where I spent most of my hundred and five days in the hospital after my last stroke. I took a quick lap around the physio department to see if any of my old therapists were still there, sadly they weren't nor there a single person I recognized. I then took the elevator to the 5th floor where I was put in Unit 58 to see if any of my nurses were there. Every time I come to the hospital I try and see if I can say hello to any of the people who helped me get back on my feet. Luckily for me, one of my nurses was working and I got to have a quick chat before I gave her a hug and took off for my appointment. I went back down the elevator to the main floor then walked down the hall that connects two of the buildings together before going into the diagnostic imaging department.

I headed into the department and told the lady I was there for a CT angio. She told me I was in the wrong place and told me to go down to the other desk and check in, so I went there. Once there, the lady working told me I was in the wrong place and told me to go back to the desk I was just at, so I did. I then told the lady again, I'm there for a CT angio, and she, again, told me **now you** have to go back to the desk I was just at. Starting to get frustrated, I hobbled back over to the lady and told her I was there for a CT angio. She, again, told me I was in the wrong place as the CT machines are in another location. I then handed her my passport and told her my healthcare number I have come to remember.

She then figured out that I was there for a cerebral angio not a CT angio. I had gotten my words mixed up and caused the whole confusion myself. I finally got checked in and was waiting with another man and his wife in the waiting room. The wife started asking him questions about the procedure, but he didn't know the answers to them. I overheard the questions and told her all about what was about to happen from what I was told and what I could remember from my past experiences.

I was then called over to the changing room where I was told to change into the clothing provided on the bench. I got in and shut the door, then stripped down nude and grabbed the first thing I saw to put on. I put the robe on, then realized I couldn't tie it up at the back and my white butt was full-on hanging out with it open at the back. I then grabbed another house coat and put it on so it was open at the front to cover my exposed, hairy, paper-white butt. But again, I couldn't tie it up, and it was falling off every two seconds. I left my stuff and hobbled over to the desk to get the lady to tie it up for me. Finally tied up, not realizing I just put on two house coats and not the normal gown and housecoat I got on the hospital bed and waited for my porter to come push me to the procedure room.

Once there, I had to wiggle over from my bed onto the procedure table. To the left of the table were three or four massive forty- or fifty-inch flat-screen TVs directly beside the bed going down the left side of it. Above me was a machine that comes down from the roof connected to big tubes and wires, then it has a flat end on it that hovers just above your body. It almost looked like a small white side table that had the legs cut off before it was flipped upside down and attached to all the tubes and wires. I took a look at the label on it and it said, "Siemens made in Germany." I thought, 'Holy, that came a long way to get here,' and I was kind of intrigued by it and wondered how far the other machines I've been in had to travel to get here.

Finally, everyone came into the room washed up and ready for the procedure. The only person that was not ready was me. This was my first time being completely awake for this. The first three or four times I was put under or in a coma, so my nerves started to get the best of me and I was rubbing my hands and a bit shaky. The doctor came in, saw my anxious state, and asked me if I wanted something to take the edge off once the girls got my I.V in my arm. I told him I would, and he went off to grab something before I could tell him I didn't want any opiates. Of course, he came back with a low dose of fentanyl. I then told him I don't want opiates because they make me sick, so he went off and got me some Ativan instead.

He injected it into my I.V and I took some deep breaths trying to relax. I got a tiny bit of help and began to settle enough for them to start. They pulled up my housecoats and exposed the groin area where they gave me a quick shave on both the left and right sides of my groin. Then they put down sterile working pads around the site they are going in and after a quick wipe down with a first cold then burning hot sterilizing solution, I was then given a needle with freezing to the right of my groin area where they are going to puncture my Femoral artery. I got the needle, and they began to push the tube up my artery. At first it was okay, but then all of a sudden it was like the freezing wore off and I started to feel every millimetre of the tube being pushed up my artery. It felt like I was having a razor blade shoved up it and I began screaming in agonizing pain.

The doctor slowed down to see if it helped, but it did not. The feeling of a razor kept coming up in my right inner leg/groin area. The doctor then asked if I wanted the drugs I refused before. At this point, I would have smoked crack to alleviate the pain and I told him I would. So, he went off and returned with the small dose of drugs then put it into my I.V and **I'm** instantly overcome by this warm body high from head to toe, I felt pretty good, and he began to work again. The pain was now mild enough I could handle it. But then out of nowhere I felt sick and told them, "I'm about to puke." The ninja-like nurse grabbed a puke bucket and put it to my right as fast as I was able to turn my head, and I spewed right there. I'm sure it had a bit to do with the drugs and more to do with the fact I wasn't supposed to eat or drink after midnight the night before and I showed up with a coffee in my hand. After a quick puke, I was calm enough and felt well enough to continue the procedure.

The flat, white German-made device was put over my stomach area and then it made a funny sound that took a picture of my tummy. This image then showed up on the bottom left corner of the massive TV to my left beside my head. I looked at it and I could see the faint outline of my body, then I could see the tube he had in my body, in my body. It was super strange to be able to watch this small tube coming up my body on the TV as he was doing it.

I was really worried about the part where they come up the back of my neck and into the brain to inject the contrast dye because after having it done a few times I have lots of scar tissue in the back of my neck that is very painful at times. I was concerned and in enough pain that before the procedure I went to my doctor to tell him specifically not to go through my right side because of that. But I saw a resident who argued with me over what I felt or didn't feel on the procedure table so my hopes were not very high after that meeting as by the end, I was so frustrated that I wanted to hit the guy and I just left.

Then they immediately started working on my right side and I was really frustrated and mad that they were going up the right. Then, as I'm lying there watching this tube on the screen go up my artery, I see the tube start to cross over from the right side of my body to the left side. Now I'm watching this on live TV maybe six inches from my head. All the while also feeling this tube cross over from the right to left, inside my body. Watching it and feeling it happen at the same time was one of the most uncomfortable feelings I've ever experienced, and I nearly vomited again from the very unnatural feeling of this thing moving across my gut inside my body. It was like feeling and watching a tape worm make its way through your body at the same time; it wasn't pleasant. Once the tube was crossed over to my left, they continued to put it up towards my brain (turns out my argument with the resident didn't fall on deaf ears). Once the tube got up the back of my neck, I didn't even feel it, which was nice because feeling something crawl up the artery in the back of your neck into your brain is also way up there on the most uncomfortable feelings-you-will-ever-feel list. Finally, they got to the brain where they injected the "contrast dye" to get into all the very small vessels and make them more visible on the scans. Once they start injecting the dye, two very weird things happen. The first weird thing that happens is you get the taste of metal in your mouth. It literally tasted like someone put aluminum metal shavings in my mouth, it was weird. The second strange thing that happens is you feel like you peed yourself. My entire groin area suddenly got warm like I just peed.

After the dye is injected, they started taking pictures. They move the white flipped table looking scanner around to one side of my head then took a picture. Being awake for the first time having this done I got to feel it all, and it was incredibly unpleasant. When they take the picture, you can literally feel the inside of your brain heat up, and it's not just a little bit. They took the first image, and I felt my brain in the back part of my head heat up. It got hotter and hotter and hotter, then it got so hot I almost screamed out in agony but as fast as the pain came, it subsided. They moved the machine and again I felt the right side of my brain feel like it was an egg being fried in a pan. Then they moved it again, this time it felt like they cooked the left side of my brain. I then wondered, 'how much damage just happened to my brain,' because feeling your brain being cooked like a hot meal on the stove from the inside has to cause a considerable amount of damage you would think, especially with the insurmountable pain it brought.

They then took the tube out of my groin and put an angio clip in to close the open artery. When they do this, it feels like someone takes a small impact gun to your groin. It doesn't hurt at all; you just hear a funny clicking noise and feel the vibrations from the tool as they clamp the hole in the artery shut. After that, I was transferred back over to a bed and brought to the day surgery recovery room in McCaig tower on the 4th floor just behind the hospital. The worst part about having this procedure done (for me) is the four to eight hours of not being able to move or bend your leg afterwards. You have to lay down flat with your leg straight for four hours minimum. It's easier said than done, especially if you have lots of energy and always want and NEED to be moving, or you flop and roll and turn when you sleep like I do. Before my four hours were up, I got an unexpected visit from my neurosurgeon. At first, I heard him (through the fabric curtain walls) deliver some not-so-great news to another patient, then he came into my area to talk to me. This is where I got the best and most terrifying news of my life.

He came in and told me that the images came out great and it was another job well done. Then he told me that the AVM in my brain was gone and the odds of it coming back were nearly impossible. It was like the greatest stress, the stress of death, was suddenly taken off my shoulders after nine agonizing years living with the possibility of dying every day, which was incredibly relieving. However, I then started to think about the five plus years that stress had me driving my life into the ground and destroying any future I could have had, which was the terrifying part. Here I am now finally able to have a foreseeable future, but I was completely naked and unprepared for it. Now what am I to do? I was then told I could get up and go home but to take it easy for the next few weeks to let my groin properly heal. My nurse walked by, and I asked if she could help me to the washroom as I was still connected to the I.V pole. As I got off the bed, I nearly flashed her my junk, forgetting I'm still naked in a house coat. Finally, I got to the washroom and returned. She said she would be right back to take out my I.V for me so I sat and waited. After five minutes I saw her walk by, and she told me she will be right back. So, I waited for another ten minutes, and she came by to tell me she got a new patient and that she will send someone over when she can. Being me, I decided, 'Screw that, I'll take it out myself.' So, I started to peel off the tape that held the I.V down before I started picking at the bigger piece of clear tape that held the I.V needle in my hand.

Once I got most of it off, I was ready to pull it out, but then I realized I couldn't hold and put pressure on it to prevent the bleeding, so I sat and waited. My ride text me twenty minutes prior saying she was there so I said screw it, got up and I went to get a paper towel for the blood. I grabbed the I.V to pull it out and right when I went to pull it out a nurse came in. I gave her my hand and said, "Here you go. It's almost done." She asked, "What are you doing? Were you going to take that out yourself?" I said "Yup, my ride's been here for half an hour now, I have to go." She then took it out and taped a cotton ball on the puncture site. I changed, grabbed my stuff, and started heading for the exit. Right when I got to the door that left the unit, I was told I could not leave until a family member got me. I started arguing saying, "I can walk, I'm fine, I will be okay, and my ride's been waiting." However, because of the drugs they gave me, it was against policy to let me go by myself, so my favourite of my three sisters, Bella, had to come find me before I was able to go home.

I couldn't for the life of me stop thinking about why the stroke-free news was so incredibly terrifying. You'd think it would be the biggest stress relief ever, which it was, but it also wasn't. At a young age, I realized how painless having a stroke was. In my experiences, the only painful part about having a stroke, was surviving one. It happens before you can comprehend what is even happening and I considered myself incredibly lucky that I would be able to just die and go out like a light switch. I thought I'd have a fast and painless death. Now that I am no longer at risk, it's highly unlikely that my AVM will ever come back, let alone rupture again. Now all of a sudden, like almost all of you, I have to deal with the unknown mystery of how my passing will come. When it comes, I'll know, and if I'm lucky it will be fast and over with before I even know what is happening. But until that day comes, I'm never going to give up on what I love to do and I'm going to live life to the fullest no matter what life throws at me.

For almost half my life I had to deal with dropping dead without cause and my "fuck the world" and "I don't give a fuck" attitude was like a negative side effect from this stressful, sickening, mental entrapment. But now that it was gone, I was guaranteed a future and that didn't take stress off my shoulders, it brought on a ton of it and compounded it. I wondered why that was before I came to the realization it was because I had a conscience again. My negative, horrid "I don't give a shit" attitude had completely worn out my conscience. I didn't care about the world, about life, or about its inhabitants, and especially didn't care about myself, my health, my future, or what I did and who I did it too. I had a true Tupac "fuck 'em all" mentality for the world.

But that's all changed. I have a future now, so I now have to care. I must care about what I do, who I do it to, why I do it, and who might be affected by my actions. Well, I don't "have to," but I do. I went from not caring the slightest bit to now caring way too much about everything and everyone to the point where I'll go out of my way and move mountains for someone who needs it. I used to see people struggle and think, 'Yeah, well I got my own problems.' Now, I see people struggle and I think, 'How can I help them?' or 'How can I make things less of a burden for them?' It was like bouncing from one polar opposite to another. I went from not caring at all and having no conscience to having a conscience and caring a lot. But I've realized I would rather care too much and help others and make a positive difference, than not care at all, ignore others, and make a negative impact on people's lives. Because I finally realized when you do good things in life and to people, you attract good things and people into your life. I had a chuckle at how I used to be the son that would steal money from my mom's purse to being the son that would steal her purse and fill it with money without her saying anything or asking anything of me, and to know I've made that drastic of a change in my life was a beautiful moment to have.

I couldn't tell if it was my cross-country endeavour or the third massive stroke that had sealed the deal on changing me forever. Obviously, the paralyzing stroke changed me forever, but that was in the physical form with paralysis. I'm talking about the mental mentality change. I'm very certain that the trek across, the people , the stupendous beauty, and the awesomeness of my country had a profound overview effect that changed my outlook on life, forever. This is the life I dreamt of, this is the life I always wanted, and this is the life that I have always longed for. Now that life and that future I once thought I'd never have, has only just begun.

Hard Work

Before my last stroke I didn't have a clue as to what working hard was. However, there are definitely a few things about working hard and the rewards that come when you **work hard** that are worth noting. I spent the majority of my life not giving a damn about anything, so I never actually tried or gave things much effort. However, when you're given a cancer diagnosis or have a massive stroke, not putting in effort or working hard will inevitably lead to your death and or a much lower quality of life. When I came out of my coma half paralyzed, I could have easily played the stroke card and given up to spend my life in a wheelchair, and if you saw my physical and mental state after my third stroke, I don't think many people would have argued much with me about it. But being in a wheelchair can drastically reduce your quality of life. Or it likely would have for me. The freedom and independence taken, compounded with the lack of mobility that comes when you're stuck in one is incredibly frustrating which made me very irritable and I wasn't willing to spend the rest of my life like that if there was anything I could do about it. Also, this was my dream and if there was ever a time in one's life never to give up, I'd say that would be on your dreams and making a positive difference in your world.

This was the first time in my life where I was physically held back from achieving my dreams. I had been held back plenty by people like my probation officer who only tried to bring me down and my teachers who could never understand where all my anger and hate for the world came from, not knowing I could drop dead at any second without warning. But for the first time in my life, I saw firsthand how incredibly beautiful, positive, and wonderful the world and life could really be, and in my world the love, positivity, and good will always outweigh the hate, negativity, and bad that can be in one's life. I believe it all depends on what way you choose to look at your situation. When I came out of my coma, I was still entirely enamoured by all my explicit memories of the journey with my father across most of the country. However, my half-paralyzed state and the copious amounts of morphine being pumped into my veins definitely let in a tsunami of negativity at first. But thanks largely to cannabis and the Reston School in Manitoba I was redirected and got back to focusing on what was truly important—positivity, never giving up, and accomplishing my dreams.

When you reap the rewards of your astronomical amount of hard work, the rewarding feeling you get is absolutely unmatched by any amount of money. Plus, the unexpected benefits of improving both your physical and mental health in the process is also priceless, I'd say. Another huge benefit of your hard work will be seeing your quality of life improve and when you see your quality of life improve, whether it be physically, mentally, or financially, you feel successful which is pretty self-empowering on its own. So, when you're chasing your dreams and life's ambitions, remember that if you don't have to work hard for it, it's probably not worth it, but working hard to see your dreams through, most definitely is. Throughout my life, I have found that the temptations of quitting come when you're on the verge of a breakthrough, have almost achieved your next goal, or when you can see the finish line. I don't think most people realize how close they are to success when they finally make the decision to quit.

For example, on my eighteenth birthday, as I spent the night in jail, I was ready to give up on life. I was ready to just jump off a bridge or blindly step into traffic and the temptations of doing just that were so gut-wrenchingly real that I spent hour after and hour contemplating how to end it all. I was in the deepest, darkest pit of my life and there seemed to no longer be any light at the top of the hole—it was just hopelessness, anger, frustration, and a dark pit of negativity and I feel that hole is a very influential place to be to quit. You're detained, trapped, hungry, cold, and dealing with every negative emotion you could possibly think of. I understood that the system could physically detain me, but they could never mentally confine me. I was more ready to quit and say screw it all, but I still had the freedom of my mind and the life-manifesting powers that come with it, so instead of giving up I told myself over and over, "I can and will change my life for the better," and I began to focus on a better life. A year and a half later, I was out of jail, off probation, on the road, and improving my life.

Then after one-hundred-and-fifteen days on the road with my father we got to the doorstep of the last province on our journey and I fell, hard. We could literally see the tape that was the finish line (the mountains) and I was suddenly in a position where I couldn't even stand up. I'm still not sure what was more frustrating, being paralyzed, or being so close to finishing the biggest thing I've ever done with my life and being held back from doing so. I'm quite sure that if there ever was an excuse not to finish something—waking up half-paralyzed with zero independence would be a pretty reasonable one. But I was so close to the finish I just couldn't give up. I knew this journey was going to be a lot of hard work, but this kind of astronomically hard work was so far beyond my understanding and abilities to achieve at the time. It was unlike anything I had to face before, but I knew that I couldn't give up. My reasons for not giving up were more for others than it was for myself, so one therapy session, one day, one goal, and one step at a time I began the relentless hard work of finishing my goal.

Patience

Patience is a virtue. We live in a world where patience is being slowly and methodically robbed from us more and more one generation at a time. Drive through fast food, takeout and delivery, same-day mail order sites, and online shopping are just a few examples of the result of our laziness and lack of patience. However, when it comes to achieving life goals, accomplishing tasks, or trying to recover from a severe physical or mental-health issue, patience is an absolute MUST. If you don't have patience, I think one won't get to where one wants to go, recover, or get through much of what life throws at them in their world. Even surrounded with a copious amount of convenience, there are some things we cannot force and must be patient for. Off the top of my head, speaking from experience, I know love, trolling the masses, changing your life, recovering, and medical appointments are just a few of the things that cannot be forced, but patience sometimes can. I feel there will come a time in one's life where that patience is tested, flexed, distorted, and pushed beyond one's limits to withstand it. I think patience is one of those things that life will inevitably test you on. Personally, it's one of the most consistent forms of mental battles I have ever had to endure on a regular basis.

 Since my third stroke, I've been forced into being patient with everything. It takes two or three times as long to do the simplest of things from zipping up coats, untangling headphones, and walking to places. To getting ready for the day, making food, putting away laundry, or just making my bed. Because I was childless most of my life, I've never had my patience tested on a daily basis until being half paralyzed. For example, if I need to see a doctor, I book an appointment, and wait. If said doctor sends me for a brain scan, it can be up to a three-month wait for that. If my doctor is not around for a week or two, more waiting. I can't even tie a shoe, so I have to stand around and wait for someone to help me with that. Over thousands of hours of therapy and I still can't use my left hand, no choice but to continue to **be patient** with that. If you think you have patience, then I encourage you to try the "Harrison challenge" and see how far you can go throughout your day without using your non-dominate arm and hand. It will not only show you how much patience can suddenly be thrown one's way but will also help show you the many things in your life that you have come to take for granted. But use your best judgment and try it when you're not doing anything dangerous that may cause you or others injury or harm. Like, waving a loaded gun while hunting with your buddy is not the time to use only one arm, pretending you've had a stroke. Try it when you're doing things like folding and putting laundry away or putting a fresh fitted sheet on your bed, that's a fun one-handed task.

I can't stress it enough: We all need to be more patient with others, but more-so with ourselves. Unless they win the lottery, I don't see someone having their life do a complete three-sixty for the better in a day. Hell, it took me one-hundred-and-fifty-days on the road, one-hundred-and-five days in the hospital, and six years of consecutive resiliency, hard work, and patience to accomplish my successful life change. "Good things come to those who wait," is another very real and true saying, so BE PATIENT!

Hidden Message

please note this may ONLY APPLY TO a physical copy of the book and may not work in e-book formatting

I can only assume most of the individuals reading this saw the bolded words throughout the book and have been questioning why they're there. If you saw them and asked yourself, **are you stoned?** I'm here to say no you're not, well maybe you are...but the words are definitely there, and they are bolded. My entire life I've never really had an interest in books and reading because of how non-interactive they are. I wanted to do something a little different in my book, so I put together a hidden message within the book for all of you to take part in. It's at the end of my book because I made you all be patient with it. Grab a pen and paper and write down the word or words in the order of the list. Keep in mind its not exactly grammatically correct and you will need to put a comma, period, and capitalize a letter in it here and there.

1 Page 215, bold in 1st sentence-

2 Page 279, 2nd paragraph-

3 Page 120, 3rd paragraph-

4 Page 219, bold in 1st paragraph-

5 Page 40, 1st bold, second paragraph-

6 Page 44, 2nd paragraph-

7 Page 274, 1st sentence-

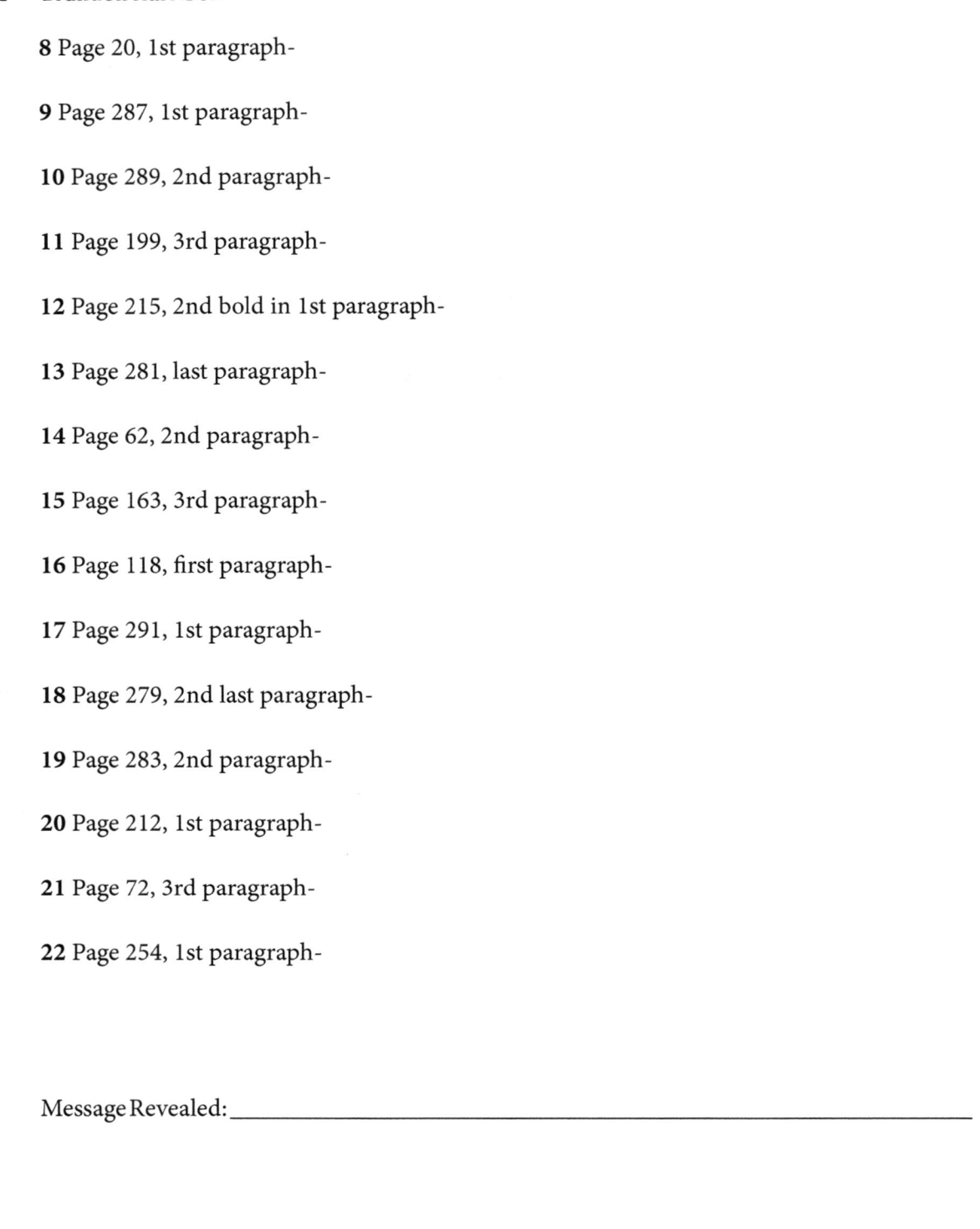

8 Page 20, 1st paragraph-

9 Page 287, 1st paragraph-

10 Page 289, 2nd paragraph-

11 Page 199, 3rd paragraph-

12 Page 215, 2nd bold in 1st paragraph-

13 Page 281, last paragraph-

14 Page 62, 2nd paragraph-

15 Page 163, 3rd paragraph-

16 Page 118, first paragraph-

17 Page 291, 1st paragraph-

18 Page 279, 2nd last paragraph-

19 Page 283, 2nd paragraph-

20 Page 212, 1st paragraph-

21 Page 72, 3rd paragraph-

22 Page 254, 1st paragraph-

Message Revealed: _____